# Dental Materials: Latest Advances and Prospects - Volume II

# Dental Materials: Latest Advances and Prospects - Volume II

Editor

**Vittorio Checchi**

MDPI

Basel • Beijing • Wuhan • Barcelona • Belgrade • Novi Sad • Cluj • Manchester

*Editor*
Vittorio Checchi
University of Modena and
Reggio Emilia
Modena
Italy

*Editorial Office*
MDPI
St. Alban-Anlage 66
4052 Basel, Switzerland

This is a reprint of articles from the Special Issue published online in the open access journal *Applied Sciences* (ISSN 2076-3417) (available at: https://www.mdpi.com/journal/applsci/special_issues/Advanced_Dental_Materials_II).

For citation purposes, cite each article independently as indicated on the article page online and as indicated below:

| Lastname, A.A.; Lastname, B.B. Article Title. *Journal Name* **Year**, *Volume Number*, Page Range. |
|---|

**ISBN 978-3-0365-9776-8 (Hbk)**
**ISBN 978-3-0365-9777-5 (PDF)**
**doi.org/10.3390/books978-3-0365-9777-5**

Cover image courtesy of Vittorio Checchi

# Contents

# About the Editor

**Vittorio Checchi**

Vittorio Checchi is an Associate Professor of Restorative Dentistry, University of Modena and Reggio Emilia, Italy. He is the Head of the Restorative Dentistry Department of the Dental and Maxillo-Facial Unit of the CHIMOMO Department at the University of Modena and Reggio Emilia (Italy). He graduated with honors in Dentistry at the University of Bologna (Italy) in 2006. He was an Adjunct Professor at the University of Bologna (Italy) from 2007 to 2009. He attended the Postdoctoral Externship Program at the Dental School of Columbia University in New York (USA) in 2009. He received his PhD in "Biomedical technologies applied to dental sciences" at the Second University of Naples (Italy) in 2010. He was Assistant Professor at the Dental School of the University of Trieste (Italy) from 2012 to 2017. He was Assistant Professor at the Dental School of the University of Modena and Reggio Emilia (Italy) from 2019 to 2022. He has been a lecturer in the Master of Aesthetic Restorative and Prosthetic Dentistry at the University of Bologna since 2016 and in the Master of Prosthesis and Implant-supported Prosthesis at the University of Modena and Reggio Emilia since 2022. He is the author of more than 100 scientific papers published in national and international journals, with an H-Index of 21.

*applied sciences*

MDPI

*Editorial*

# Special Issue on Dental Materials: Latest Advances and Prospects—Volume II

**Vittorio Checchi**

Department of Surgery, Medicine, Dentistry and Morphological Sciences, University of Modena & Reggio Emilia, 41125 Modena, Italy; vittorio.checchi@unimore.it; Tel.: +39-0594224763

Many fields of dentistry are firmly connected to innovative materials, and the highest clinical improvements frequently come with the development and creation of original and high-performing equipment, instruments, and biomaterials. Nowadays, the application of these dental materials leads to effective clinical dentistry, with many remarkable advancements. In recent times, many fields of dentistry have used these newly developed materials: implantology, prosthesis, restorative dentistry, orthodontics, and endodontics. However, this production often presents a lack of reliable scientific research, and, unfortunately, clinicians tend to make use of materials that are not necessarily better than the previous ones.

The aim of this Special Issue is to publish high-quality research articles, clinical studies, and review articles centered on the latest advances regarding dental materials.

A total of 15 papers (9 research papers and 6 review papers) are presented in Volume II of this successful Special Issue.

Hadzik et al. evaluated the long-term effectiveness of using the guided-bone-regeneration (GBR) procedure to correct small peri-implant bone dehiscence, using a xenogeneic deproteinized bovine bone mineral material and a xenogeneic native bilayer collagen membrane. The authors concluded that using xenogeneic bone and a xenogeneic collagen membrane in a GBR procedure could be used to correct small peri-implant bone dehiscence [1].

Fernandez Castellano et al. focused on maxillary sinus lift procedures performed on animal models, using a balloon elevation control system technique. The maxillary sinus lifts performed via this innovative device associated with the balloon technique are minimally invasive procedures. The elevations achieved sufficiently allowed the future placement of implants of varying lengths and diameters without any risk of perforating the membranes, even in the presence of extremally resorbed bone crests [2].

An Italian study group evaluated the influence of manual expertise on static computer-aided implantology (s-CAI) in terms of accuracy and operative timings. After the cone-beam CT scanning of eleven mandibular models, a full-arch rehabilitation was planned, and two different operators performed s-CAI. Finally, the distances between the virtual and actual implant positions were calculated. The mean value of the operative timings was statistically inferior to that of the expert operator, with an improved accuracy over time for both operators. The support from digital surgical guides did not eliminate the importance of manual expertise for the reliability and shortening of the surgical procedure, and it required a learning pathway over time [3].

Felice et al. hypothesized that virtual planned guided bone regeneration (GBR), with the aid of customized meshes, could optimize the treatment of extended alveolar defects by reducing the risk of dehiscence. The authors concluded that a careful evaluation of the soft tissues and knowledge of their final relationship with the implant and prosthesis can improve digital mesh/membrane manufacturing, with a suitable healing process occurring up to implant placement and loading, as well as favoring peri-implant tissue stability over time [4].

**Citation:** Checchi, V. Special Issue on Dental Materials: Latest Advances and Prospects—Volume II. *Appl. Sci.* **2023**, *13*, 10787. https://doi.org/10.3390/app131910787

Received: 13 September 2023
Accepted: 25 September 2023
Published: 28 September 2023

A systematic review by Desnica et al. evaluated current in vivo research on regenerating critical-sized mandibular defects and discussed methodologies for mandibular bone tissue engineering. Out of the 3650 articles initially retrieved, 88 studies were included in the review. Using scaffolds with bioactive molecules and/or progenitor cells enhanced success in mandibular bone engineering. Therefore, scaffold-based mandibular bone tissue engineering could be introduced into clinical practice due to its proven safety, convenience, and cost-effectiveness [5].

A narrative review by Selahi et al. aimed to review the literature on using autologous blood preparations, which can aid regenerative processes when applied to extraction sockets. The authors stated that, unfortunately, there is a lack of studies in the current literature comparing the amount of pro-inflammatory cytokines in a patient's peripheral blood to their levels after centrifugation in blood concentrates. Therefore, more studies are needed to clarify the correlation between pro-inflammatory cytokine levels and alveolar healing after extraction and assess the risk of treatment with blood concentrates in patients with systemic diseases causing chronic inflammation [6].

A retrospective study by Mummolo et al. aimed to evaluate a possible correlation between the characteristics of the mandibular ramus and lower third molar impaction by comparing a first group of subjects to an impacted lower third molar and a second group to normal eruption for an early prediction of this pathology. This comparison was made using linear and angular measurement, taken via digital panoramic radiographs. This manuscript showed that the angle of a lower third molar, in relation to mandibular pain, can be an index to predict tooth inclusion [7].

A narrative review performed by a Mexican study group summarized the characteristics of dental stem cell (DT-MSCs)-derived biomaterials and their classification according to their source, bioactivity, and different biological effects on the expansion and differentiation of DT-MSCs. Also, the advances in research into the interactions between these biomaterials and the molecular components involved (mechanosensors and mechanotransduction) in DT-MSCs during their proliferation and differentiation were analyzed. The authors concluded that these kinds of biomaterials can contribute to research into regenerative medicine and the development of autologous stem cell therapies [8].

Recently, digital dentistry began to play a crucial role in many dental disciplines, especially the orthodontic field.

Regarding digital dentistry, Shopova et al. aimed to demonstrate and compare the capabilities of two different digital approaches (intraoral scanning and digital examination of occlusion) in the final analysis of occlusion after orthodontic treatment. The authors found that there is a good collaboration between intraoral scanning and digital occlusion determination, since the digital occlusion imaging system provides comprehensive results and allows the analysis and treatment of occlusal dysfunctions. It can provide information on the first contact, strength of the contacts, contact distribution on each tooth, sequence of contacts, maximum bite force and maximum intercuspation, path of the lower jaw movement, and occlusion and disocclusion times, as well as record videos with the active sequences and distributions of the contacts [9].

Bucur et al. published a manuscript with the aim of determining the intensity of pain perception in patients undergoing fixed orthodontic treatment, analyzing the severity of pain during four routine procedures (placement of separating elastics, ring cementations, arch activations, and elastic tractions). Patients suffered differently from the intensity of perceived pain as they grow older; most of them showed moderate pain after following the studied orthodontic interventions and required analgesic medication. The least painful procedure was the elastic traction procedure, while the most painful period was the first 3–4 days after procedures [10].

The original article by Cameriere et al., conducted on a sample of 538 cephalograms derived from healthy-living children aged between 5 and 15 years old, proposed a statistical model to assess pubertal growth spurt using the ratio of the anterior height projection to the posterior (Vba) of the fourth cervical vertebra body (C4), as well as calculate the residual proportion of skeletal maturation and the time for the pubertal growth spurt to end for a given Vba. The validation process results showed that the proposed model did not produce any incorrect forecasts. Therefore, this proposed method could estimate the beginning and end of the pubertal growth spurt, together with the residual proportion of skeletal maturation for a given Vba [11].

An in vitro case study, Jakubowicz et al. discussed the multiscale analysis of the reproduction accuracy of jaw geometry obtained using selected orthodontic materials. An accuracy assessment of the model geometry mapping was performed using noncontact systems, including a fringe projection optical 3D scanner, computed tomography, and a focus-variation microscope. Measurements were taken in three modes for comparison, as were the silicone and polyether impression materials. Data analysis showed that deviations were the smallest in the case of silicone and the best fit occurred between the silicone impression and the plaster model. The conducted research confirmed the validity of the assumptions considering the use of multiscale analysis for geometric analysis [12].

To achieve proper esthetics is one of the main challenges associated with using modern dental materials, both in prosthesis and restorative dentistry.

Porojan et al. analyzed the finishing and thermocycling of five resin matrix CAD/CAM ceramic surfaces (a polymer-infiltrated ceramic and four types of nanoparticle-filled resins) to assess their consequences for optical properties. Surface microroughness and optical and hardness evaluations were achieved before and after artificial aging. The authors demonstrated that the optical characteristics of resin matrix ceramics were not significantly modified by thermocycling and thermocycling significantly decreased the microhardness, especially for glazed samples [13].

Unosson et al. described a material made of novel amorphous calcium magnesium fluoride phosphate (ACMFP) core-shell microparticles that may be applied in preventive dentistry for the prevention of caries and the treatment of dentin hypersensitivity. The remineralization and dentin tubule occlusion potential of these particles were evaluated in vitro using acid-etched dentin specimens, and treatment with the ACMFP particles resulted in complete tubule occlusion and dense mineralization layer formation. A cross-sectional evaluation of dentin specimens after treatment formed high aspect ratio fluorapatite crystals and poorly crystalline hydroxyapatite. Therefore, these studied particles provided a single source of readily available calcium, phosphate, and fluoride ions for the potential remineralization of carious lesions, as well as exposing dentin tubules to enable a reduction in hypersensitivity [14].

Finally, this Special Issue also involved research dealing with endodontic materials.

A systematic review by Ferreira et al. aimed to assess the effects of non-thermal plasma treatments on root canal sealers' adhesion to dentin. While there was no consensus about the effect of non-thermal plasma (NTP) on the AH Plus sealer's adhesion to radicular dentin, NTP seemed to positively influence the adhesion ability of BioRoot RCS and Endosequence BC. However, the authors recommended cautiously interpreting these findings due to the scarcity of studies on the topic [15].

Although submissions for this Special Issue have been closed, more in-depth research in the field is being collected for inclusion in a new Special Issue: Dental Materials: Latest Advances and Prospects—Volume III.

**Funding:** This research received no external funding.

**Acknowledgments:** I give thanks to all of the authors and peer reviewers for their valuable contributions to this Special Issue 'Dental Materials: Latest Advances and Prospects—Volume II'. I would also like to express my gratitude to all of the staff and people involved in this Special Issue.

**Conflicts of Interest:** The authors declare no conflict of interest.

## References

1. Hadzik, J.; Błaszczyszyn, A.; Gedrange, T.; Dominiak, M. Effect of the Lateral Bone Augmentation Procedure in Correcting Peri-Implant Bone Dehiscence Defects: A 7-Years Retrospective Study. *Appl. Sci.* **2023**, *13*, 2324. [CrossRef]

2. Fernández Castellano, E.R.; Marquez Sanchez, M.T.; Flores Fraile, J. Study of Elevation Forces and Resilience of the Schneiderian Membrane Using a New Balloon Device in Maxillary Sinus Elevations on Pig Head Cadavers. *Appl. Sci.* **2022**, *12*, 4406. [CrossRef]
3. Pellegrino, G.; Lizio, G.; D'Errico, F.; Ferri, A.; Mazzoni, A.; Del Bianco, F.; Stefanelli, L.V.; Felice, P. Relevance of the Operator's Experience in Conditioning the Static Computer-Assisted Implantology: A Comparative In Vitro Study with Three Different Evaluation Methods. *Appl. Sci.* **2022**, *12*, 9561. [CrossRef]
4. Felice, P.; Lizio, G.; Barausse, C.; Roccoli, L.; Bonifazi, L.; Pistilli, R.; Simion, M.; Pellegrino, G. Reverse Guided Bone Regeneration (R-GBR) Digital Workflow for Atrophic Jaws Rehabilitation. *Appl. Sci.* **2022**, *12*, 9947. [CrossRef]
5. Desnica, J.; Vujovic, S.; Stanisic, D.; Ognjanovic, I.; Jovicic, B.; Stevanovic, M.; Rosic, G. Preclinical Evaluation of Bioactive Scaffolds for the Treatment of Mandibular Critical-Sized Bone Defects: A Systematic Review. *Appl. Sci.* **2023**, *13*, 4668. [CrossRef]
6. Selahi, D.; Spiegel, M.; Hadzik, J.; Pitułaj, A.; Michalak, F.; Kubasiewicz-Ross, P.; Dominiak, M. The Appliance of A-PRF and CGF in the Treatment of Impacted Mandibular Third Molar Extraction Sockets—Narrative Review. *Appl. Sci.* **2023**, *13*, 165. [CrossRef]
7. Mummolo, S.; Gallusi, G.; Strappa, E.M.; Grilli, F.; Mattei, A.; Fiasca, F.; Bambini, F.; Memè, L. Prediction of Mandibular Third Molar Impaction Using Linear and Angular Measurements in Young Adult Orthopantomograms. *Appl. Sci.* **2023**, *13*, 4637. [CrossRef]
8. Aguilar-Ayala, F.J.; Aguilar-Pérez, F.J.; Nic-Can, G.I.; Rojas-Herrera, R.; Chuc-Gamboa, G.; Aguilar-Pérez, D.; Rodas-Junco, B.A. A Molecular View on Biomaterials and Dental Stem Cells Interactions: Literature Review. *Appl. Sci.* **2022**, *12*, 5815. [CrossRef]
9. Shopova, D.; Bakova, D.; Yordanova, S.; Yordanova, M.; Uzunov, T. Digital Occlusion Analysis after Orthodontic Treatment: Capabilities of the Intraoral Scanner and T-Scan Novus System. *Appl. Sci.* **2023**, *13*, 4335. [CrossRef]
10. Olteanu, C.D.; Bucur, S.-M.; Chibelean, M.; Bud, E.S.; Păcurar, M.; Feștilă, D.G. Pain Perception during Orthodontic Treatment with Fixed Appliances. *Appl. Sci.* **2022**, *12*, 6389. [CrossRef]
11. Cameriere, R.; Velandia Palacio, L.A.; Nakaš, E.; Galić, I.; Brkić, H.; Kalibović Govorko, D.; Jerković, D.; Jara, L.; Ferrante, L. The Fourth Cervical Vertebra Anterior and Posterior Body Height Projections (*Vba*) for the Assessment of Pubertal Growth Spurt. *Appl. Sci.* **2023**, *13*, 1819. [CrossRef]
12. Jakubowicz, M.; Gapiński, B.; Marciniak-Podsadna, L.; Mendak, M.; Mietliński, P.; Wieczorowski, M. Multiscale Evaluation of Jaw Geometry Reproduction Obtained Via the Use of Selected Orthodontic Materials in Dental Implants and Orthodontics—In Vitro Case Study. *Appl. Sci.* **2023**, *13*, 6932. [CrossRef]
13. Porojan, L.; Toma, F.R.; Uțu, I.-D.; Vasiliu, R.D. Optical Behavior and Surface Analysis of Dental Resin Matrix Ceramics Related to Thermocycling and Finishing. *Appl. Sci.* **2022**, *12*, 4346. [CrossRef]
14. Unosson, E.; Feldt, D.; Xia, W.; Engqvist, H. Amorphous Calcium Magnesium Fluoride Phosphate—Novel Material for Mineralization in Preventive Dentistry. *Appl. Sci.* **2023**, *13*, 6298. [CrossRef]
15. Ferreira, I.; Lopes, C.; Ferreira, A.; Vaz, F.; Pina-Vaz, I.; Martín-Biedma, B. Effect of Plasma Treatment on Root Canal Sealers' Adhesion to Intraradicular Dentin—A Systematic Review. *Appl. Sci.* **2023**, *13*, 8655. [CrossRef]

applied sciences

MDPI

Article

# Effect of the Lateral Bone Augmentation Procedure in Correcting Peri-Implant Bone Dehiscence Defects: A 7-Years Retrospective Study

**Jakub Hadzik [1,*], Artur Błaszczyszyn [1], Tomasz Gedrange [2] and Marzena Dominiak [1]**

1 Department of Dental Surgery, Faculty of Medicine and Dentistry, Medical University of Wrocław, 50-425 Wrocław, Poland
2 Department of Orthodontics, TU Dresden, 01069 Dresden, Germany
* Correspondence: jakub.hadzik@umw.edu.pl

**Abstract:** Guided bone regeneration (GBR) is a well-documented and widely-used dental surgical procedure for the treatment of various types of alveolar bone defects. The aim of the study was to evaluate the long-term effectiveness of the GBR procedure in correcting small peri-implant bone dehiscence using the xenogeneic deproteinized bovine bone mineral material and a xenogeneic native bilayer collagen membrane. The present study was designed as a retrospective study. Seventy-five bone-level tapered two-piece dental implants Conelog®, Camlog (Biotechnologies AG, Switzerland) were divided into two groups G1—no bone augmentation (no GBR)—44 implants and G2—bone augmentation (GBR)—31 implants. For both groups, the closed healing protocol with a primary wound closure was used. The incidence of peri-implantits was evaluated, the quantitative assessment of soft tissue thickness was performed using the ultrasound (USG) device, quantitative assessment of marginal bone loss (MBL) was done. The prevalence of peri-implantitis was 5.3%, with a three-fold increase in peri-implantitis comparing the groups without and with bone augmentation (G1 = 2.27%, G2 = 9.7%). The average keratinized gingiva thickness was 1.87 mm and did not differ significantly between groups. No statistically significant differences in MBL between G1 and G2 were found. When dividing patients by gender, no statistically significant differences were observed. When dividing patients by age groups, statistically significant differences were observed between the youngest and oldest groups of patients. Within the limitations of this study, it can be concluded that the use of xenogeneic bone and a xenogeneic collagen membrane in a GBR procedure can be recommended to correct small peri-implant bone dehiscence.

**Keywords:** guided bone regeneration; GBR; implant; soft tissue; marginal bone loss; bone graft

**Citation:** Hadzik, J.; Błaszczyszyn, A.; Gedrange, T.; Dominiak, M. Effect of the Lateral Bone Augmentation Procedure in Correcting Peri-Implant Bone Dehiscence Defects: A 7-Years Retrospective Study. *Appl. Sci.* **2023**, *13*, 2324. https://doi.org/10.3390/app13042324

Academic Editor: Antonio Di Bartolomeo

Received: 14 January 2023
Revised: 9 February 2023
Accepted: 9 February 2023
Published: 10 February 2023



## 1. Introduction

Dental implants are nowadays considered a highly predictable treatment option to replace missing teeth with a reported long-term (10–20 years) survival rate of 89.5% and 92.7% [1,2]. However, when bone dehiscence is present at the time of implant placement to place a dental implant, different bone regenerative techniques, such as guided bone regeneration (GBR), need to be used. GBR is a successful, well-documented and widely used dental surgical procedure used to treat various alveolar bone defects [3,4]. GBR requires the application of a resorbable or non-resorbable membrane to exclude non-osteogenic tissues from interfering with bone regeneration and can be used as a surgical procedure preceding implant treatment [5,6].

Currently, a broad spectrum of grafting materials of different origins, such as allografts, xenografts, and alloplastic materials, is available [7,8]. Similarly, materials of different origins are available in various forms ranging from blocks to bone chips, and this provides the dental surgeon and patient with many treatment options. The situation with membranes is no different; the choice between non-resorbable (including Polytetrafluoroethylene

PTFE; expanded polytetrafluoroethylene e-PTFE, high-density polytetrafluoroethylene d-PTFE; Titanium-Reintforced PTFE Membranes, Titanium Mesh and Cage membranes) and resorbable membranes of different types and origins is wide [9]. Depending on their origin, resorbable membranes used in GBR can be divided into natural polymers (collagen membranes) and synthetic polymers (aliphatic polyesters (e.g., poly (lactic acid) (PLA), poly (polyglycolic acid) (PGA), poly (ε-caprolactone) (PCL) [10,11].

Undoubtedly, the treatment options are wide, but most importantly, they require adaptation to a specific clinical situation. Since the beginning of dental implantology, implant placement in the aesthetic zone in such a way that implants imitate nature and, at the same time, maintain healthy tissues has been challenging. The perfect three-dimensional position of the implant is critical for proper prosthetic restoration, especially in the aesthetic area. When a proper prosthetic-driven implant positioning of the implant requires covering small fenestration or dehiscence caused by an exposed implant surface on its facial aspect, the GBR technique, in combination with xenogeneic bone and resorbable membranes, can be used [12]. In these situations, the GBR can be used simultaneously with implant placement since, according to Chiapasco and Zaniboni [13], guided bone regeneration procedures are a reliable means for treating dehiscences and fenestrations created during implant placement.

The first objective of the study was to evaluate the long-term effectiveness of the applied GBR procedure in correcting small peri-implant bone dehiscence using the xenogeneic deproteinized bovine bone mineral material and a xenogeneic native bilayer collagen membrane. A secondary objective was to evaluate factors that may influence marginal bone loss.

Hypotheses of this study were:

1. When the GBR procedure is used for implant dehiscence treatment, it does not influence the marginal bone loss around the implant in 7 years of observation;
2. There are no gender-related differences in marginal bone loss around implants;
3. There is no difference in marginal bone loss around implants between age groups.

## 2. Materials and Methods

### 2.1. Study Design

The present study was a retrospective study aimed at evaluating the long-term effectiveness of the applied GBR procedure in correcting small peri-implant bone dehiscence. The study was performed in Wroclaw Medical University Dental Clinical and Teaching facility. Among the group of patients who received Conelog®, Camlog (Biotechnologies AG, Switzerland) implants as part of a clinical trial conducted in 2012–2014, a group of patients was selected who received implants with lateral bone contour regeneration and placed with no bone regeneration. Medical records of a 7-year follow-up were analyzed. A bioethics approval for this follow-up study was granted by a local bioethics committee of Wrocław Medical University (registration number 861/2021). The study has been conducted in full compliance with the Declaration of Helsinki. All patients gave two written consents: the first was general consent to have dental implants placed, and the other consent involved participation in the clinical study. The original clinical study analyzed changes in soft tissue thickness; detailed data from the clinical study and 12 months of follow-up can be found in our study [14]. In a 5 years follow-up period, the soft tissue augmentation with CTG (connective tissue graft) 3 months prior to implant placement was found to be the most effective method in terms of the soft tissue thickness gain—1.035 mm (SD = 0.73 mm) over the entire follow-up period (5 years) [15].

The purpose of the present study was to evaluate previously unanalyzed medical data in terms of the influence on MBL. The influence of lateral GBR procedure, gender structure, and age structure was analyzed. The prevalence of peri-implantitis was also assessed.

### 2.2. Clinical Data, Groups of Patients, Surgery, Implant Loading

The medical records of 67 patients (27 male, 47 female) who had 75 bone-level tapered two-piece dental implants Conelog®, Camlog (Biotechnologies AG, Switzerland).

The 3.8 mm and 4.3 mm diameter implants of different lengths were used in the study. Implants were placed in the healed bone in the aesthetic area of both jaws were selected (no prior GBR allowed). Specific exclusion criteria for this group of patients were presented previously [16]; briefly: generally healthy adult patients were included, and patients with periodontal disease, noncontrolled metabolic diseases, and heavy smokers were excluded.

The implants were divided into 2 groups: G1—no bone augmentation (no GBR)—44 implants, and G2—bone augmentation (GBR)—31 implants, Figure 1. All of the patient records analyzed and included in the study contained full details of the procedure, including the depth of the implant placement and the GBR procedure used in case of dehiscence presence. Forty-four implants were inserted and completely embedded in the native bone, placed equicrestally. In 31 implants where the dehiscence (to the implant first thread) was present, the external lamina of the alveolar process was augmented during implantation with the deproteinized bovine bone mineral material (Bio-Oss®, Geistlich Pharma AG, Switzerland) and a native bilayer collagen membrane (Bio-Gide®, Geistlich Pharma AG, Switzerland) to cover the exposed implant surface on the facial aspect. For both groups, the closed healing protocol with a primary wound closure was used (Figure 1).

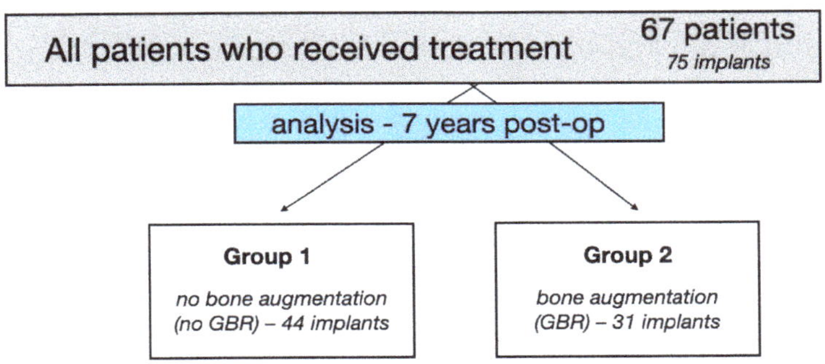


**Figure 1.** Allocation of patients, size of the groups. Guided bone regeneration (GBR) G1—no bone augmentation (no GBR)—44 implants, G2—guided bone augmentation (GBR)—31 implants.

Implant loading took place after 6 months. Conventional impressions were taken using the polyether (PE) impression compound Impregum Penta (3M, Maplewood, MN, USA). All implants were restored on a standard abutment provided by the implant manufacturer's Camlog (Biotechnologies AG, Switzerland) with metal-ceramic cemented single crowns with semipermanent cement (Implantlink®, Detax, Germany). A follow-up clinical appointment for all the patients included was conducted by the same investigator (AB).

### 2.3. Clinical Outcomes

Patient clinical evaluation included bleeding on gentle probing and biological complication such as peri-implantitis. Peri-implantitis, according to the 2017 World Workshop on the Classification of Periodontal and Peri-Implant Diseases and Conditions, involves bone levels $\geq$3 mm apical of the most coronal portion of the intra-osseous part of the implant together with bleeding on probing [17]. During the clinical examination, the thickness of keratinized tissue (TKT) in the surrounding implant site was examined using the Ultrasound (USG) device Pirop® (Echoson, Poland) as described previously in our study.

### 2.4. Marginal Bone Loss

Since all the implants in G1 were placed equicrestally, and in G2, the bone augmentation was performed to cover the first implant thread, the level of 0 was taken as the initial value for further measurements. The MBL was reported in mm and referred to millimeters of bone loss compared to the initial value.

The intraoral radiographs were done using a holder (Visualize HD®, Gendex®, USA). The radiological evaluation and X-ray measurements were done using the Gendex software

(Gendex®, USA). X-ray image was calibrated using build-in calibration Gendex VixWin Platinum (Gendex®, USA). The known diameter of the dental implants was used for the calibration. The same device and software were used in all cases.

### 2.5. Statistical Analysis

The statistical analysis was performed using the GraphPad Prism 9 software [GraphPad Software, Inc., USA]. The data obtained in the study were tested to check the normal distribution (Shapiro–Wilk and Kolmogorov–Smirnov tests). Depending on the criteria met (normal distribution), an appropriate test was selected for further analysis. A parametric and nonparametric statistical approach was applied depending on the data. An unpaired *t*-test was used for parametric, and a Mann–Whitney U test for non-parametric data. All data are means ± standard deviation (SD). $p < 0.05$ was considered statistically significant.

## 3. Results

### 3.1. Implant Survival Rate

All of the 75 placed implants remained integrated after 7 years. This resulted in a 100% implant survival rate.

### 3.2. Peri-Implantitis

A total number of 4 implants met the criteria for periimplantitis [17] (bone levels $\geq$ 3 mm apical of the most coronal portion of the intra-osseous part of the implant together with bleeding on probing). This corresponds to 5.3% of the total implants placed in the study.

Among the G1 group with no GBR, based on clinical and radiological examination, one patient (2.27%) was diagnosed with peri-implant disease. However, in the G2 group, where the xenogeneic bone substitute was used in the GBR procedure, three patients (9.7%) were diagnosed with peri-implantitis. This indicates a three-fold increase in peri-implantitis comparing the groups without and with bone augmentation.

When dividing patients into groups by gender, 11% of male patients were diagnosed with periimplantitis and only 2.1% of female patients.

When patients were analyzed by age groups, in the youngest group (25–40 years old), a 4.35% rate of peri-implantitis was found; in the middle group (41–60 years old), this rate was 2.94%, and in the oldest group (61–72 years old) 10.5% of patients were diagnosed with peri-implantitis.

It was decided to include the entire group of patients in further analysis; however, due to the severe peri-implantitis cases found that might affect the results, especially in some groups, the results are given separately (see results all figures) for the whole group (75 implants) and for the group excluding the peri-implantitis cases (71 implants).

### 3.3. Marginal Bone Loss

For G1 with no bone augmentation, a mean MBL = 0.63 was nominally lower than in G2, where a bone augmentation was performed, and the MBL was 0.98. However, no statistically significant differences were observed between these groups (Figure 2A, Table 1). In this case, all patients were included, including those diagnosed with peri-implantitis, and importantly, even after excluding cases of peri-implantitis, no significant differences were observed between the groups (Figure 2B).

**Table 1.** Marginal bone loss (MBL) for Group G1 and Group G2.

| | G1 | G2 | G1, Excluded Peri-Implantitis | G2, Excluded Peri-Implantitis |
|---|---|---|---|---|
| mean MBL (in mm) | 0.63 | 0.98 | 0.60 | 0.72 |
| SD | 0.6 | 1.0 | 0.57 | 0.65 |
| minimum | 0 | 0 | 0 | 0 |
| maximum | 2.12 | 3.97 | 2.17 | 2.60 |

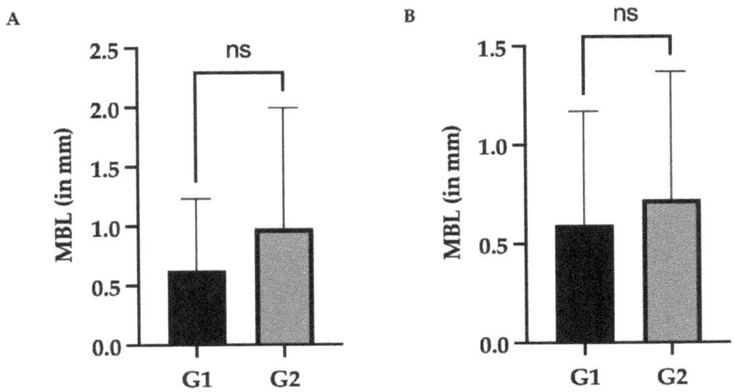


**Figure 2.** Marginal bone loss (MBL) in G1 (no bone augmentation) and G2 (bone augmentation) (**A**) all patients included in the study; (**B**) patients with peri-implantitis excluded. Error bars shown in this figure are means ± SD. The abbreviation non-significant (ns) is used for statistically nonsignificant, satistically significant at $p \leq 0.05$.

When dividing patients by gender, no statistically significant differences were observed between men and females (MBL = 0.85mm and MBL = 0.73mm, respectively). Similarly—after excluding patients with peri-implantitis, no statistically significant differences were noted (Figure 3, Table 2).

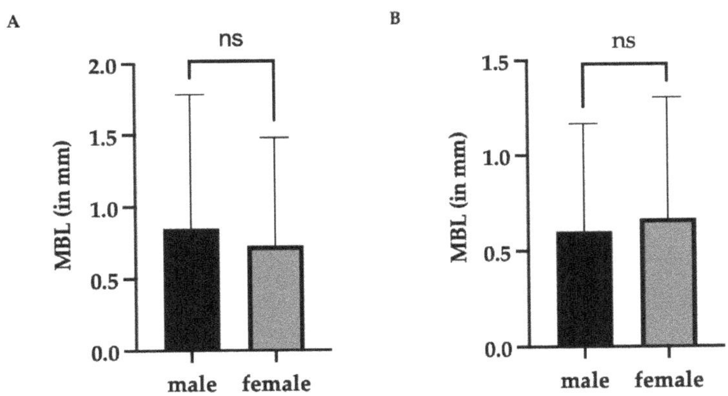


**Figure 3.** Marginal bone loss (MBL) for both gender groups. (**A**) all patients included in the study; (**B**) patients with peri-implantitis excluded. Error bars shown in this figure are means ± SD. The abbreviation ns is used for statistically nonsignificant, statistically significant at $p \leq 0.05$.

**Table 2.** Marginal bone loss (MBL) for both gender groups. Data are means ±SD.

| | Male | Female | Male Peri-Implantitis Excluded | Female Peri-Implantitis Excluded |
|---|---|---|---|---|
| mean MBL (in mm) | 0.85 | 0.73 | 0.60 | 0.67 |
| SD | 0.93 | 0.75 | 0.56 | 0.64 |
| minimum | 0 | 0 | 0 | 0 |
| maximum | 3.97 | 3.5 | 1.95 | 2.58 |

When dividing patients by age groups (age ranges: 25–40; 41–60; 60–72), statistically significant differences were observed between the youngest (25–40 years old) and oldest group (60–72 years old) of patients (MBL = 0.85mm and MBL = 0.73mm, respectively)

Figure 4, Table 3. The patient's age given in the results is the age at the time of the 7-year follow-up; patients were younger at the time of surgery.

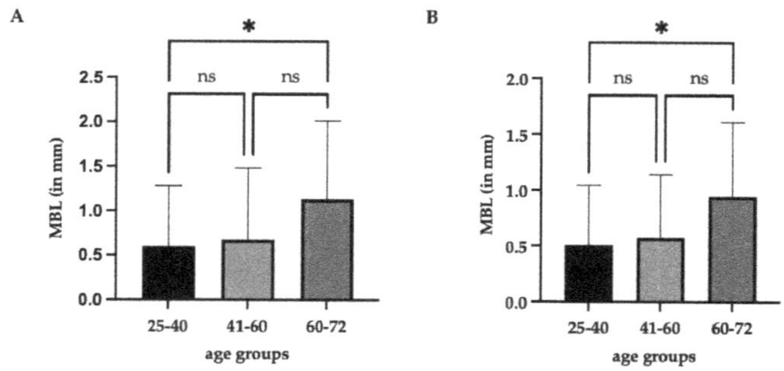


**Figure 4.** Marginal bone loss (MBL) in age groups. (**A**) all patients included in the study; (**B**) patients with peri-implantitis excluded. Error bars shown in this figure are means ± SD. The abbreviation ns is used for statistically nonsignificant, * statistically significant at $p \leq 0.05$.

**Table 3.** Marginal bone loss (MBL) in age groups. Data are means ± SD.

| All Implants | 25–40 Years Old | 41–60 Years Old | 60–72 Years Old |
|---|---|---|---|
| mean MBL (in mm) | 0.60 | 0.67 | 1.13 |
| SD | 0.68 | 0.80 | 0.88 |
| minimum | 0 | 0 | 0 |
| maximum | 2.60 | 3.97 | 3.50 |
| Excluded peri-implantitis | 25–40 years old | 41–60 years old | 60–72 years old |
| mean MBL (in mm) | 0.51 | 0.57 | 0.95 |
| SD | 0.54 | 0.57 | 0.67 |
| minimum | 0 | 0 | 0 |
| maximum | 1.95 | 2.17 | 2.58 |

### 3.4. *Soft Tissue*

The mean value of the thickness of keratinized tissue (TKT) analyzed together for both G1 and G2 was 1.87 mm. The mean values of TKT in the implant area were similar in both groups. No statistically significant differences were observed between these groups, G1 (no bone augmentation) and G2 (bone augmentation), in terms of the TKT (Figure 5, Table 4). In this case, all patients were included, including those diagnosed with peri-implantitis, and importantly, even after excluding cases of peri-implantitis, no significant differences were observed between the groups (Figure 5B).

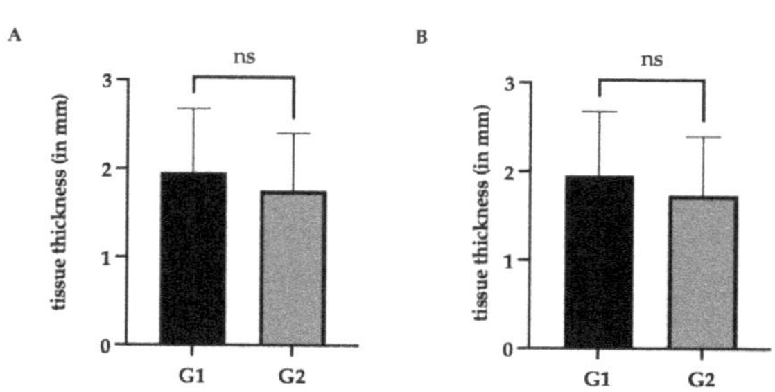


**Figure 5.** The thickness of keratinized tissue (TKT) in G1 (no bone augmentation) and G2 (bone augmentation). (**A**) all patients included in the study; (**B**) patients with peri-implantitis excluded. Error bars shown in this figure are means ± SD. The abbreviation ns is used for statistically nonsignificant, statistically significant at $p \leq 0.05$.

**Table 4.** Thickness of keratinized tissue (TKT) in studied groups of patients. Data are means ± SD.

| | G1 | G2 | G1, Excluded Peri-Implantitis | G2, Excluded Peri-Implantitis |
|---|---|---|---|---|
| mean TKT (in mm) | 1.95 | 1.74 | 1.95 | 1.73 |
| SD | 0.72 | 0.65 | 0.72 | 0.67 |
| minimum | 0.72 | 0.45 | 0.72 | 0.45 |
| maximum | 3.45 | 2.9 | 3.45 | 2.90 |

Regarding the research hypotheses:

1. The first research hypothesis was accepted. No statistically significant ($p < 0.05$) differences in terms of marginal bone loss were found between the groups with and without guided bone regeneration;
2. The second research hypothesis was accepted. No gender-related differences were found in marginal bone loss;
3. The third hypothesis was rejected. A statistically significant difference in marginal bone loss around the implant neck was found between the age group 25–40 and 60–72.

## 4. Discussion

Our aim was to evaluate the long-term effectiveness of the applied GBR procedure in correcting small peri-implant bone dehiscence using the xenogeneic deproteinized bovine bone mineral material and a xenogeneic native bilayer collagen membrane. To assess the effectiveness of treatment with the GBR method, several factors affecting long-term treatment were evaluated. Among them are the implant survival rate in augmented and nonaugmented sites, the incidence of complications (particularly peri-implantitis), and the marginal bone loss in the peri-implant area.

The implant survival rate was 100% in the 7 years of observation. However, the survival rate itself applies only to implants that have been integrated or lost and is not sufficient for a positive assessment of the treatment method.

The stability of hard and soft tissues around dental implants is believed to be a key factor for long-term implant treatment. In our study, it was found that when the guided bone regeneration with a xenogeneic bone is used for implant dehiscence treatment, it does not influence the marginal bone loss around the implant in 7 years of observation.

Taking into account the frequency of the need to perform GBR procedures presented by Cha et al. [18] who, during a retrospective evaluation of the 1512 implants, placed found that bone graft was performed in estimated that up to 50% of all dental implant procedures, among the bone grafted sites, sinus lifting with lateral approach (22.1%) and guided bone regeneration (22.7%).

An important aspect is the type of material used in the GBR procedure. Despite the widespread use of bone grafts and their substitutes, there are still limitations that remain associated with these commonly used dental surgical biomaterials. Starting with golden standard autogenous bone that needs to be obtained from intraoral and extraoral sites from the same individual. The disadvantages of autogenous bone are the lack of availability of graft tissue, associated pain, and morbidity at the site donor. Autogenous odontogenic materials are biocompatible and have the inorganic component of autogenous teeth; however, it is necessary to have and process patient teeth [19]. Then allogeneic bone provides many options for its use, ranging from guided bone regeneration of small defects to extensive reconstructions using 3D allogenic graft blocks for mandibular sagittal bone defect reconstruction, as described by Dominiak et al. [20]. Allogenic materials can be prepared in three primary forms—fresh, frozen, or freeze-dried. Fresh and frozen allograft materials possess superior osteoinductive properties, but at the same time, they carry the greatest risks risk of a host immunogenic response [21]. The further processing of allogenic material through freeze-drying can decrease the immunogenicity at the cost of decreased osteoinductive potential [21]. Animal materials are also widely used, including the deproteinized bovine bone, which is commercially available as BioOss (Bio-Oss®,

Geistlich Pharma AG, Switzerland) and was used in our study. The porous structure of deproteinized bovine bone resembles the human bone and can provide mechanical support and stimulate bone healing through osteoconduction [22–24]. The application of the bovine bone is very wide and covers most GBR indications. However, it is important to keep in mind the biggest limitation of this material, which is exclusively osteogenic potential. Referring to the systematic review and meta-analysis from the Canellas et al. group [25], it seems that xenograft materials should be considered among the best available graft materials for preserving the alveolar process after tooth extraction. A 5-year study conducted by Ozkan et al. [26] found that sufficient quality and volume of bone allows for the predictable placement of implants in the maxillary sinus augmented with bovine bone grafts. Various combinations of biomaterial combinations have been described in the literature to maximize the advantage and minimize the disadvantage of the biomaterials described above. As an example, allogenic bone can successfully be used in combination with xenografts for guided bone regeneration (GBR) in bone augmentation procedures as described by the Urban group for the technique known by the common name "the sausage technique" where a particulated autogenous bone with an organic bovine bone-derived mineral is used [27,28]. The literature also describes the possible use of bovine xenogeneic bone in GBR combined with blood derivates such as platelet-rich plasma (PRP), platelet-rich fibrin (PRF), and concentrated growth factors CGF are used in various days of dentistry to promote healing and their combination with bone graft particles is known colloquially as a sticky bone [23,29,30].

The use of xenogeneic bone to graft increases the width of the alveolar process when used in lateral augmentation [31]. Sanz-Sanches et al. found that lateral ridge augmentation procedures with implant placement can maintain peri-implant health over time [32]. Zitzmann et al. [33], in a 5-year follow-up, demonstrated that dehisced implants, if treated with GBR (membrane + grafting material), may lead to a survival rate of implants similar to that obtained in implants completely embedded in native bone. Severi et al. [34], in the latest systematic review and meta-analysis, have found that reconstructive surgical correction of peri-implant dehiscences and fenestrations with GBR is associated with a lower probability of implant dehiscences and fenestrations persistence when compared to a repositioning of a full-thickness flap without use of reconstructive techniques. The application of the xenogeneic bone material and a xenogeneic collagen membrane is considered to be a recommended, well-documented and widely used dental surgical procedure [35,36]. We have found no statistically significant differences in MBL between no GBR G1 and GBR G2; moreover, even after excluding cases of peri-implantitis, still no significant differences were observed between the groups, and the nominal differences between the groups were even smaller.

Taking into account the characteristics of the material, it seems reasonable to recommend xenogeneic bone in the case of the treatment of small peri-implant bone defects such as dehiscence.

In our material, the incidence of peri-implantitis complications was assessed, and a total of 5.3% of patients were diagnosed with peri-implantitis. Peri-implantitis is an inflammatory process that affects both the hard and soft tissues that surround dental implants. This condition is caused by a polymicrobial aggressive biofilm that colonizes the implant and abutment surface at the peri-implant crevice level [37]. According to Diaz et al. [38], as stated in a systematic review and meta-analysis, the mean prevalence of peri-implantitis is 19.53% at the patient level. Derks et al., in a 9-year observational study of randomly selected 588 patients of the Swedish population, observed 45% of all patients with peri-implantitis (bleeding on probing/suppuration and bone loss > 0.5 mm) and a moderate/severe peri-implantitis (bleeding on probing/suppuration and bone loss > 2 mm) was diagnosed in 14.5% of patients and bone loss > 2 mm) [39]. However, the reports of the prevalence of peri-implant mucositis and peri-implantitis range are relatively wide and can be dependent on the study population, as Wada et al. found in their review the population that attends dental office for regular maintenance have a lower incidence of peri-implant disease [40]. Our result of 5.3% of patients diagnosed with peri-implantitis is significantly less than the recent available literature describes. However, it should be noted that in our study, the included patients were generally healthy, heavy smokers, and patients with uncontrolled metabolic diseases were excluded. In addition, the group of patients analyzed in our study was under regular medical care from the time the implants were inserted, which, as Wada et al. [40] point out, is not insignificant for the occurrence of peri-implant inflammation. Although peri-implantitis is thought to be caused mainly by dental plaque accumulation on the implant or abutment surface, many other risk factors have been reported, including cigarette smoking, noncontrolled diabetes, osteoporosis, history of periodontitis, presence of keratinized mucosa, occlusal overload, the surface of trans gingival abutment element, and the position of implant-abutment junction [40–43]. Our results have shown a three-fold increase in peri-implantitis incidence, comparing the groups without and with bone augmentation (no GBR G1 = 2.27%, GBR G2 = 9.7%). However, the literature does not mention GBR as a risk factor for peri-implantitis [38,44]. Similarly age structure of the patient with a diagnosed peri-implant disease, in our study, there were differences found between the age groups of patients, but there are still isolated cases of peri-implantitis that are, therefore, difficult to interpret.

Proper width and thickness of the gingival connective tissue have been proven to be one of the success criteria in dental reconstructive surgery. The mean value of the thickness of keratinized tissue (TKT) analyzed together for both G1 and G2 was 1.87 mm.

According to the literature, the influence of soft tissue remains not insignificant in terms of preserving the bone around the implant. Linkevicius [45] found that the gingival tissue thickness at the alveolar crest can significantly affect marginal bone loss (MBL) around implants. A value of 2 mm has been described in the literature as necessary to maintain the proper level of bone in the area of the implant [14,45–47]. Gianfilippo et al. [48], in a recent systematic review, have found that the soft tissue thickness is correlated with MBL except in cases of platform-switching implants when implants with thin tissues and screw-retained prostheses are used. In the case of our study, platform-switching implants were used, and soft tissue thickness was similar in both groups with no GBR G1 = 1.95 and GBR G2 = 1.74 with no statistically significant difference, so it can be assumed that tissue thickness did not affect the results of our comparison between G1 without augmentation and G2 with augmentation on the MBL.

The characteristics of the dental implant have an influence on the surrounding tissue behavior among the position of the implant platform in relation to the height of the alveolar crest (supracrestal, equicrestall, subcrestal); the type of connection between the implant and the superstructure, e.g., utilizing the platform switching [49–51]. Valles et al. [52], in a systematic review, found that platform-switching implants placed in a subcrestal position seem to have less marginal bone level changes when compared with implants placed equicrestall. However, Valles et al. [52] pointed out that significant differences were only observed in animal studies. In our study, Conelog®, Camlog bone level platform switching implants were used and placed equicrestally in all cases, so it can be assumed that the position of the implants did not affect the results of the comparison between the groups.

The limitation of the presented study is its design as a retrospective study. The long-term analysis is based on the patients' medical records.

## 5. Conclusions

Within the limitations of this retrospective study, it can be concluded that the use of xenogeneic deproteinized bovine bone mineral material and a xenogeneic native bilayer collagen membrane in a GBR procedure can be recommended to correct small peri-implant bone dehiscence.

**Author Contributions:** Conceptualization, J.H.; methodology, J.H.; software, J.H.; formal analysis, M.D.; investigation, J.H. and A.B.; data curation, A.B.; writing—original draft preparation, J.H.; writing—review, J.H. and T.G.; visualization, J.H.; supervision, J.H. All authors have read and agreed to the published version of the manuscript.

**Funding:** Initial study was supported by Camlog Foundation with a grant (CF41106). This follow-up study received no external funding and was supported by the and Wroclaw Medical University SUBZ.B040.23.048.

**Institutional Review Board Statement:** All the patients in the original study were informed of the planned treatment, its possible consequences and had given their written consent for the procedure. The protocol of this retrospective study was approved by the Bioethics Committee of the Medical University of Wroclaw. The follow-up required a bioethics committee approval that was granted (registration number 861/2021).

**Informed Consent Statement:** All patients gave two written consents: the first was general consent to have dental implants placed, and the other consent involved the participation in the clinical study. The study has been conducted in full compliance with the Declaration of Helsinki.

**Data Availability Statement:** Data available on request.

**Acknowledgments:** Authors thank Monika Puzio for her involvement and participation in the first part of the study.

**Conflicts of Interest:** The authors declare no conflict of interest.

## References

1. Balshi, T.; Wolfinger, G.; Stein, B.; Balshi, S. A Long-term Retrospective Analysis of Survival Rates of Implants in the Mandible. *Int. J. Oral Maxillofac. Implant.* **2015**, *30*, 1348–1354. [CrossRef] [PubMed]
2. Chappuis, V.; Buser, R.; Brägger, U.; Bornstein, M.M.; Salvi, G.E.; Buser, D. Long-Term Outcomes of Dental Implants with a Titanium Plasma-Sprayed Surface: A 20-Year Prospective Case Series Study in Partially Edentulous Patients. *Clin. Implant Dent. Relat. Res.* **2013**, *15*, 780–790. [CrossRef] [PubMed]
3. Elgali, I.; Omar, O.; Dahlin, C.; Thomsen, P. Guided bone regeneration: Materials and biological mechanisms revisited. *Eur. J. Oral Sci.* **2017**, *125*, 315–337. [CrossRef] [PubMed]
4. Aghaloo, T.; Misch, C.; Lin, G.-H.; Iacono, V.; Wang, H.-L. Bone Augmentation of the Edentulous Maxilla for Implant Placement: A Systematic Review. *Int. J. Oral Maxillofac. Implant.* **2017**, *31*, s19–s30. [CrossRef] [PubMed]
5. Retzepi, M.; Donos, N. Guided Bone Regeneration: Biological principle and therapeutic applications. *Clin. Oral Implant. Res.* **2010**, *21*, 567–576. [CrossRef] [PubMed]
6. Soldatos, N.K.; Stylianou, P.; Koidou, P.; Angelov, N.; Yukna, R.; Romanos, G.E. Limitations and options using resorbable versus nonresorbable membranes for successful guided bone regeneration. *Quintessence Int.* **2017**, *48*, 131–147. [CrossRef] [PubMed]
7. Wickramasinghe, M.L.; Dias, G.J.; Premadasa, K.M.G.P. A novel classification of bone graft materials. *J. Biomed. Mater. Res. Part B Appl. Biomater.* **2022**, *110*, 1724–1749. [CrossRef]
8. Kao, S.T.; Scott, D.D. A Review of Bone Substitutes. *Oral Maxillofac. Surg. Clin. N. Am.* **2007**, *19*, 513–521. [CrossRef]
9. Sbricoli, L.; Guazzo, R.; Annunziata, M.; Gobbato, L.; Bressan, E.; Nastri, L. Selection of collagen membranes for bone regeneration: A literature review. *Materials* **2020**, *13*, 30786. [CrossRef]
10. Ren, Y.; Fan, L.; Alkildani, S.; Liu, L.; Emmert, S.; Najman, S.; Rimashevskiy, D.; Schnettler, R.; Jung, O.; Xiong, X.; et al. Barrier Membranes for Guided Bone Regeneration (GBR): A Focus on Recent Advances in Collagen Membranes. *Int. J. Mol. Sci.* **2022**, *23*, 14987. [CrossRef]
11. Wang, J.; Wang, L.; Zhou, Z.; Lai, H.; Xu, P.; Liao, L.; Wei, J. Biodegradable polymer membranes applied in guided bone/tissue regeneration: A review. *Polymers* **2016**, *8*, 115. [CrossRef]
12. Testori, T.; Weinstein, T.; Scutellà, F.; Wang, H.L.; Zucchelli, G. Implant placement in the esthetic area: Criteria for positioning single and multiple implants. *Periodontology 2000* **2018**, *77*, 176–196. [CrossRef]
13. Chiapasco, M.; Zaniboni, M. Clinical outcomes of GBR procedures to correct peri-implant dehiscences and fenestrations: A systematic review. *Clin. Oral Implant. Res.* **2009**, *20*, 113–123. [CrossRef]
14. Puzio, M.; Hadzik, J.; Błaszczyszyn, A.; Gedrange, T.; Dominiak, M. Soft tissue augmentation around dental implants with connective tissue graft (CTG) and xenogenic collagen matrix (XCM). 1-year randomized control trail. *Ann. Anat.* **2020**, *230*, 151484. [CrossRef]
15. Hadzik, J.; Błaszczyszyn, A.; Gedrange, T.; Dominiak, M. Soft-Tissue Augmentation around Dental Implants with a Connective Tissue Graft (CTG) and Xenogeneic Collagen Matrix (CMX)—5-Year Follow-Up. *J. Clin. Med.* **2023**, *12*, 924. [CrossRef]
16. Puzio, M.; Błaszczyszyn, A.; Hadzik, J.; Dominiak, M. Ultrasound assessment of soft tissue augmentation around implants in the aesthetic zone using a connective tissue graft and xenogeneic collagen matrix—1-year randomised follow-up. *Ann. Anat.* **2018**, *217*, 129–141. [CrossRef]

17. Berglundh, T.; Armitage, G.; Araujo, M.G.; Avila-Ortiz, G.; Blanco, J.; Camargo, P.M.; Chen, S.; Cochran, D.; Derks, J.; Figuero, E.; et al. Peri-implant diseases and conditions: Consensus report of workgroup 4 of the 2017 World Workshop on the Classification of Periodontal and Peri-Implant Diseases and Conditions. *J. Clin. Periodontol.* **2018**, *45*, S286–S291. [CrossRef]
18. Cha, H.S.; Kim, J.W.; Hwang, J.H.; Ahn, K.M. Frequency of bone graft in implant surgery. *Maxillofac. Plast. Reconstr. Surg.* **2016**, *38*, 1–4. [CrossRef]
19. Zhang, S.; Li, X.; Qi, Y.; Ma, X.; Qiao, S.; Cai, H.X.; Zhao, B.C.; Jiang, H.B.; Lee, E.S. Comparison of Autogenous Tooth Materials and Other Bone Grafts. *Tissue Eng. Regen. Med.* **2021**, *18*, 327–341. [CrossRef] [PubMed]
20. Dominiak, M.; Dominiak, S.; Targonska, S.; Gedrange, T. Three-Dimensional Bone Block Planning for Mandibular Sagittal Bone Defect Reconstruction. *J. Healthc. Eng.* **2020**, *2020*, 8829288. [CrossRef] [PubMed]
21. Zhao, R.; Yang, R.; Cooper, P.R.; Khurshid, Z.; Shavandi, A.; Ratnayake, J. Bone grafts and substitutes in dentistry: A review of current trends and developments. *Molecules* **2021**, *26*, 3007. [CrossRef] [PubMed]
22. Elnayef, B.; Porta, C.; del Amo, F.; Mordini, L.; Gargallo-Albiol, J.; Hernández-Alfaro, F. The Fate of Lateral Ridge Augmentation: A Systematic Review and Meta-Analysis. *Int. J. Oral Maxillofac. Implant.* **2018**, *33*, 622–635. [CrossRef] [PubMed]
23. Barbu, H.M.; Iancu, S.A.; Rapani, A.; Stacchi, C. Guided bone regeneration with concentrated growth factor enriched bone graft matrix (Sticky bone) vs. bone-shell technique in horizontal ridge augmentation: A retrospective study. *J. Clin. Med.* **2021**, *10*, 3953. [CrossRef] [PubMed]
24. Jain, G.; Blaauw, D.; Chang, S. A Comparative Study of Two Bone Graft Substitutes–InterOss® Collagen and OCS-B Collagen®. *J. Funct. Biomater.* **2022**, *13*, 28. [CrossRef] [PubMed]
25. Canellas, J.V.d.S.; Soares, B.N.; Ritto, F.G.; Vettore, M.V.; Vidigal Júnior, G.M.; Fischer, R.G.; Medeiros, P.J.D.A. What grafting materials produce greater alveolar ridge preservation after tooth extraction? A systematic review and network meta-analysis. *J. Cranio-Maxillofac. Surg.* **2021**, *49*, 1064–1071. [CrossRef]
26. Özkan, Y.; Akoğlu, B.; Kulak-Özkan, Y. Maxillary sinus floor augmentation using bovine bone grafts with simultaneous implant placement: A 5-year prospective follow-up study. *Implant Dent.* **2011**, *20*, 455–459. [CrossRef]
27. Urban, I.A.; Nagursky, H.; Lozada, J.L.; Nagy, K. Horizontal Ridge Augmentation with a Collagen Membrane and a Combination of Particulated Autogenous Bone and Anorganic Bovine Bone–Derived Mineral: A Prospective Case Series in 25 Patients. *Int. J. Periodontics Restor. Dent.* **2013**, *33*, 299–307. [CrossRef]
28. Arnal, H.M.; Angioni, C.D.; Gaultier, F.; Urbinelli, R.; Urban, I.A. Horizontal guided bone regeneration on knife-edge ridges: A retrospective case–control pilot study comparing two surgical techniques. *Clin. Implant Dent. Relat. Res.* **2022**, *24*, 211–221. [CrossRef]
29. Selahi, D.; Spiegel, M.; Hadzik, J.; Pitułaj, A.; Michalak, F.; Kubasiewicz-ross, P.; Dominiak, M. The Appliance of A-PRF and CGF in the Treatment of Impacted Mandibular Third Molar Extraction Sockets—Narrative Review. *Appl. Sci.* **2023**, *13*, 165. [CrossRef]
30. Pietruszka, P.; Chruścicka, I.; Duś-Ilnicka, I.; Paradowska-Stolarz, A. PRP and PRF—Subgroups and Divisions When Used in Dentistry. *J. Pers. Med.* **2021**, *11*, 944. [CrossRef]
31. Aludden, H.C.; Mordenfeld, A.; Hallman, M.; Dahlin, C.; Jensen, T. Lateral ridge augmentation with Bio-Oss alone or Bio-Oss mixed with particulate autogenous bone graft: A systematic review. *Int. J. Oral Maxillofac. Surg.* **2017**, *46*, 1030–1038. [CrossRef]
32. Sanz-Sánchez, I.; Carrillo de Albornoz, A.; Figuero, E.; Schwarz, F.; Jung, R.; Sanz, M.; Thoma, D. Effects of lateral bone augmentation procedures on peri-implant health or disease: A systematic review and meta-analysis. *Clin. Oral Implant. Res.* **2018**, *29*, 18–31. [CrossRef]
33. Zitzmann, N.U.; Schärer, P.; Marinello, C.P. Long-term results of implants treated with guided bone regeneration: A 5-year prospective study. *Int. J. Oral Maxillofac. Implant.* **2001**, *16*, 355–366.
34. Severi, M.; Simonelli, A.; Farina, R.; Tu, Y.K.; Lan, C.H.; Shih, M.C.; Trombelli, L. Effect of lateral bone augmentation procedures in correcting peri-implant bone dehiscence and fenestration defects: A systematic review and network meta-analysis. *Clin. Implant Dent. Relat. Res.* **2022**, *24*, 251–264. [CrossRef] [PubMed]
35. Avila-Ortiz, G.; Chambrone, L.; Vignoletti, F. Effect of alveolar ridge preservation interventions following tooth extraction: A systematic review and meta-analysis. *J. Clin. Periodontol.* **2019**, *46*, 195–223. [CrossRef] [PubMed]
36. Majzoub, J.; Ravida, A.; Starch-Jensen, T.; Tattan, M.; Suárez-López del Amo, F. The Influence of Different Grafting Materials on Alveolar Ridge Preservation: A Systematic Review. *J. Oral Maxillofac. Res.* **2019**, *10*, 10306. [CrossRef] [PubMed]
37. Kubasiewicz-Ross, P.; Fleischer, M.; Pitułaj, A.; Hadzik, J.; Nawrot-Hadzik, I.; Bortkiewicz, O.; Dominiak, M.; Jurczyszyn, K. Evaluation of the three methods of bacterial decontamination on implants with three different surfaces. *Adv. Clin. Exp. Med.* **2020**, *29*, 177–182. [CrossRef]
38. Diaz, P.; Gonzalo, E.; Villagra, L.J.G.; Miegimolle, B.; Suarez, M.J. What is the prevalence of peri-implantitis? A systematic review and meta-analysis. *BMC Oral Health* **2022**, *22*, 1–13. [CrossRef]
39. Derks, J.; Schaller, D.; Håkansson, J.; Wennström, J.L.; Tomasi, C.; Berglundh, T. Effectiveness of Implant Therapy Analyzed in a Swedish Population: Prevalence of Peri-implantitis. *J. Dent. Res.* **2016**, *95*, 43–49. [CrossRef] [PubMed]
40. Wada, M.; Mameno, T.; Otsuki, M.; Kani, M.; Tsujioka, Y.; Ikebe, K. Prevalence and risk indicators for peri-implant diseases: A literature review. *Jpn. Dent. Sci. Rev.* **2021**, *57*, 78–84. [CrossRef] [PubMed]
41. Skorik, Y.A.; Puppi, D.; Wiessner, A.; Wassmann, T.; Wiessner, J.M.; Schubert, A.; Wiechens, B.; Hampe, T.; Bürgers, R. In Vivo Biofilm Formation on Novel PEEK, Titanium, and Zirconia Implant Abutment Materials. *Int. J. Mol. Sci.* **2023**, *24*, 1779. [CrossRef]

42. Hadzik, J.; Kubasiewicz-Ross, P.; Gębarowski, T.; Waloszczyk, N.; Maciej, A.; Stolarczyk, A.; Gedrange, T.; Dominiak, M.; Szajna, E.; Simka, W. An Experimental Anodized Titanium Surface for Transgingival Dental Implant Elements—Preliminary Report. *J. Funct. Biomater.* **2023**, *14*, 34. [CrossRef]
43. Hadzik, J.; Kubasiewicz-Ross, P.; Simka, W.; Gębarowski, T.; Barg, E.; Cieśla-Niechwiadowicz, A.; Szajna, A.T.; Szajna, E.; Gedrange, T.; Kozakiewicz, M.; et al. Fractal Dimension and Texture Analysis in the Assessment of Experimental Laser-Induced Periodic Surface Structures (LIPSS) Dental Implant Surface-In Vitro Study Preliminary Report. *Materials* **2022**, *15*, 82713. [CrossRef] [PubMed]
44. Kordbacheh Changi, K.; Finkelstein, J.; Papapanou, P.N. Peri-implantitis prevalence, incidence rate, and risk factors: A study of electronic health records at a U.S. dental school. *Clin. Oral Implant. Res.* **2019**, *30*, 306–314. [CrossRef] [PubMed]
45. Linkevicius, T.; Apse, P.; Grybauskas, S.; Puisys, A. The influence of soft tissue thickness on crestal bone changes around implants: A 1-year prospective controlled clinical trial. *Int. J. Oral Maxillofac. Implant.* **2009**, *24*, 712–719.
46. Lissek, M.; Boeker, M.; Happe, A. How thick is the oral mucosa around implants after augmentation with different materials: A systematic review of the effectiveness of substitute matrices in comparison to connective tissue grafts. *Int. J. Mol. Sci.* **2020**, *21*, 5043. [CrossRef] [PubMed]
47. Hadzik, J.; Kubasiewicz-Ross, P.; Nawrot-Hadzik, I.; Gedrange, T.; Pitułaj, A.; Dominiak, M. Short (6 mm) and regular dental implants in the posterior maxilla–7-years follow-up study. *J. Clin. Med.* **2021**, *10*, 940. [CrossRef]
48. Gianfilippo, R.D.; Valente, N.A.; Toti, P.; Wang, H.L.; Barone, A. Influence of implant mucosal thickness on early bone loss: A systematic review with meta-analysis. *J. Periodontal Implant Sci.* **2020**, *50*, 209–225. [CrossRef]
49. Hadzik, J.; Botzenhart, U.; Krawiec, M.; Gedrange, T.; Heinemann, F.; Vegh, A.; Dominiak, M. Comparative evaluation of the effectiveness of the implantation in the lateral part of the mandible between short tissue level (TE) and bone level (BL) implant systems. *Ann. Anat.* **2017**, *213*, 78–82. [CrossRef]
50. Saleh, M.H.A.; Ravidà, A.; Suárez-López del Amo, F.; Lin, G.H.; Asa'ad, F.; Wang, H.L. The effect of implant-abutment junction position on crestal bone loss: A systematic review and meta-analysis. *Clin. Implant Dent. Relat. Res.* **2018**, *20*, 617–633. [CrossRef]
51. Makowiecki, A.; Hadzik, J.; Błaszczyszyn, A.; Gedrange, T.; Dominiak, M. An evaluation of superhydrophilic surfaces of dental implants—A systematic review and meta-analysis. *BMC Oral Health* **2019**, *19*, 79. [CrossRef] [PubMed]
52. Valles, C.; Rodríguez-Ciurana, X.; Clementini, M.; Baglivo, M.; Paniagua, B.; Nart, J. Influence of subcrestal implant placement compared with equicrestal position on the peri-implant hard and soft tissues around platform-switched implants: A systematic review and meta-analysis. *Clin. Oral Investig.* **2018**, *22*, 555–570. [CrossRef] [PubMed]

applied sciences

MDPI

Article

# Study of Elevation Forces and Resilience of the Schneiderian Membrane Using a New Balloon Device in Maxillary Sinus Elevations on Pig Head Cadavers

**Erick Rafael Fernández Castellano [1,*], Magaly Teresa Marquez Sanchez [2] and Javier Flores Fraile [1]**

1 Department of Surgery, University of Salamanca, 37007 Salamanca, Spain; j.flores@usal.es
2 Salamanca Biomedical Research Institute, 37007 Salamanca, Spain; maglymarquez77@gmail.com
* Correspondence: er.fernandez@usal.es

**Abstract: Background**: Although elevation of the sinus can be considered a predictable procedure, it is nonetheless not free of complications, for which reason there is a constant search for new tools and techniques that may reduce these complications. The present study focused on maxillary sinus lifts performed on pig heads cadavers, using a new device with the balloon technique. **Materials and Methods**: Fifteen ex vivo adult pig heads were used in this experimental study. Sinus floor elevation was performed using the new balloon elevation control system, which consists of a syringe containing latex and serum as well as a system of burs for membrane access and control. Each lift was performed within a 3 min time frame while constant pressure was applied to allow the tissue to adapt to the tension. **Results**: In 100% of cases, perforations do not occur during aperture or in the elevation of the wall. In the global sample, there was histological elevation in 73.33% compared to 26.66% non-elevation ($p$ = 0.0268). **Conclusions**: Within the limits of this study, the maxillary sinus lifts employing the new device and the balloon technique were minimally invasive procedures. The elevations achieved proved sufficient to allow future placement of implants of varying lengths and diameters without risk of perforating the membranes, even in the presence of crests of less than 1 mm.

**Keywords:** balloon elevation; sinus floor elevation; schneiderian membrane; pigs head; ex vivo

**Citation:** Fernández Castellano, E.R.; Marquez Sanchez, M.T.; Flores Fraile, J. Study of Elevation Forces and Resilience of the Schneiderian Membrane Using a New Balloon Device in Maxillary Sinus Elevations on Pig Head Cadavers. *Appl. Sci.* **2022**, *12*, 4406. https://doi.org/10.3390/app12094406

Academic Editor: Vittorio Checchi

Received: 29 March 2022
Accepted: 25 April 2022
Published: 27 April 2022



## 1. Introduction

Currently, rehabilitation with dental implants is an effective therapeutic option for the replacement of missing teeth in patients with partial or total edentulism. For this to be achieved, the success and survival of these implants must be ensured, with one crucial factor being sufficient bone availability to bear functional loads [1–3]. The loading forces which occur during chewing have been shown to require implants of sufficient length, within 8–10 mm for the premolar and molar regions in both the mandible and the maxilla, these being generally accepted as standard measurements [4,5].

Given that patients frequently present with bone defects of variable characteristics as a result of various processes such as tooth loss, which leads to an average 40–60% decrease in horizontal and vertical bone loss of the alveolar crest during the first year, periodontal disease, trauma, tumors, and cysts, the correct three-dimensional placement of implants often becomes complicated [6–10]. Because of this, various surgical techniques have been proposed, such as onlay–inlay bone grafts, distraction osteogenesis, inferior alveolar nerve transposition, split crest, guided bone regeneration (GBR), and maxillary sinus augmentation [11–15].

This last procedure, which is one of the most used in implant practice, arises from the need to rehabilitate the posterior maxillary areas which are often atrophic due to the prevalence of type IV cancellous bone and to dental extractions which cause rapid vertical and horizontal resorption, in many cases accompanied by increased pneumatization of the sinus in these areas [12–16]. This procedure was first described by Boyne et al. in 1965, becoming popular in the 1980s. In it, the Caldwell-Luc procedure was used to access the sinus. Summers, for his part, popularized the crestal approach together with the use of osteotomes and bone grafts, a procedure which is considered less invasive [16–18].

Although the sinus lift procedure can be considered clinically predictable, it is not exempt from complications such as the dispersion of graft material in the sinus cavity, wound dehiscence, hematomas, migration of implants inside the sinus, fenestrations, oroantral fistulae, epistaxis, bone sequestration, acute sinusitis, and perforations of the Scheiderian membrane [19–22]. This last complication is considered the main drawback of this procedure, occurring in 10–35% of cases where the direct method is used, with an approach through the lateral wall of the maxillary sinus [23,24]; or in 25% of cases with an indirect approach through the alveolar crest and where the initial bone height lay between 3 and 6 mm [25–28]. Elevation of the mucosa of the maxillary sinus inevitably causes stretching of the tissue which, in cases of higher elevations, may easily lead to tearing and perforation of the sinus membrane [29]. A retrospective study reported similar findings: the highest rates of perforation were correlated to higher elevations. These perforations often lead to contamination of graft tissue and to the subsequent loss of both the graft and the implants [30,31].

The present study based on maxillary sinus lifts was performed on ex vivo bisected pig heads, employing a new device for the balloon technique patented by the author. The study was justified by the need to assess the efficacy of this new system, which is proposed as both a more conservative technique for the elevation of the Schneiderian membrane, and a novel procedure which currently has no articles proving its reliability. The study aims to assess the feasibility of the device, describe the technique, and contrast its advantages and disadvantages.

## 2. Materials and Methods

An experimental study was carried out by a single operator. Fifteen ex vivo heads of adult pigs were used. The pig is well established in implant research as an animal model. The maxillary sinus of adult pigs is known to provide a volume of up to 30 $cm^3$ sufficient for the elevation procedure and a soft tissue lining comparable to that of humans. The pig heads were obtained from the local butchery immediately after slaughter. Hence, consultation with the appropriate ethics committee was not necessary. The bisected heads were sold as a base material for food processing by the slaughterhouse.

Due to the pronounced height of the alveolar crest in adult pigs, an approach to the maxillary sinus through the lateral wall of the sinus was preferred for the experiments. The lateral approach to the sinus allowed a greater control over the dissection of the membrane.

All animals were free of local and systemic diseases to prevent any bias due to pathological alterations of the tissue. The experiments were carried out within a standard 6 h post-mortem under a constant room temperature of 21 °C.

Sinus floor elevation was performed with the new elevation control system patented by the author and registered in the Spanish Official Industrial Property Gazette (patent application: 202130571). This system consists of a syringe containing stops, retaining elements, latex, and serum (see Figure 1a).

To access the sinus, a Bien-Air turbine with a 3.5 mm diameter diamond bur was used to outline the window, with abundant irrigation, followed by a donut-type bur with 20:1 reduction NSK contra-angle at 2000 rpm, 35 Ncm torque with abundant irrigation, and a 3 mm stop to prevent rupture of the membrane. The sinus was accessed at 2 cm perpendicular to the gingival margin of the maxillary first molar (see Figure 1b).

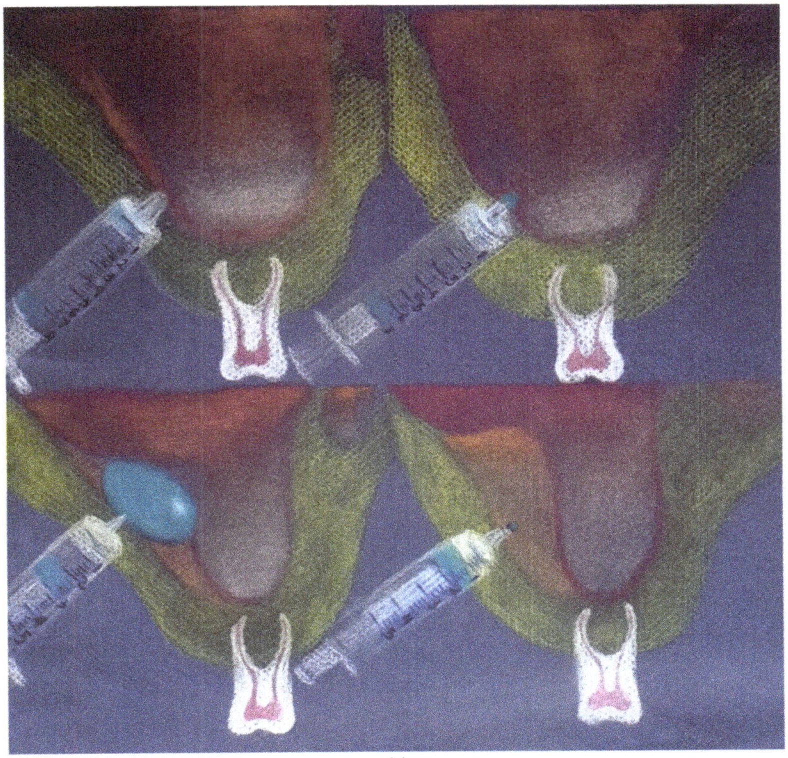

(a)

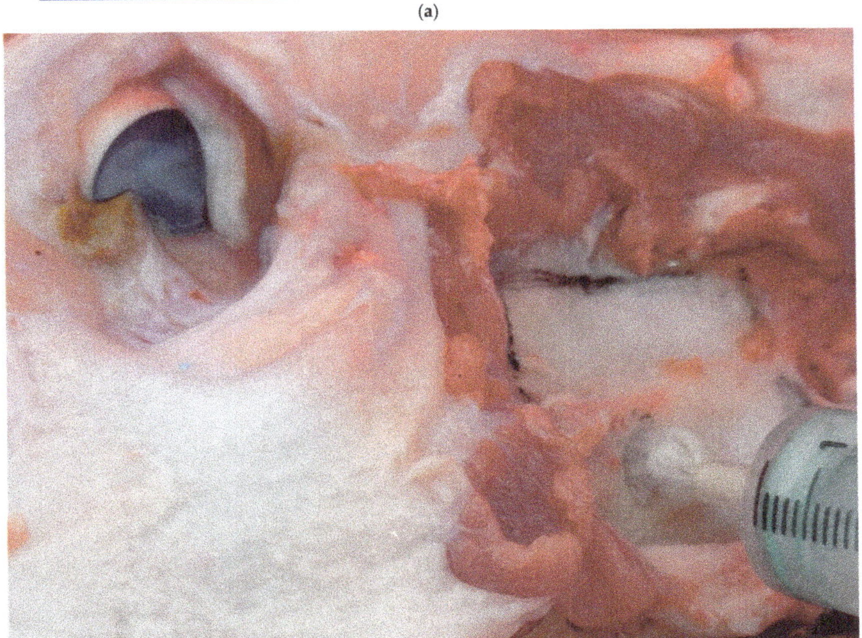

(b)

**Figure 1.** *Cont.*

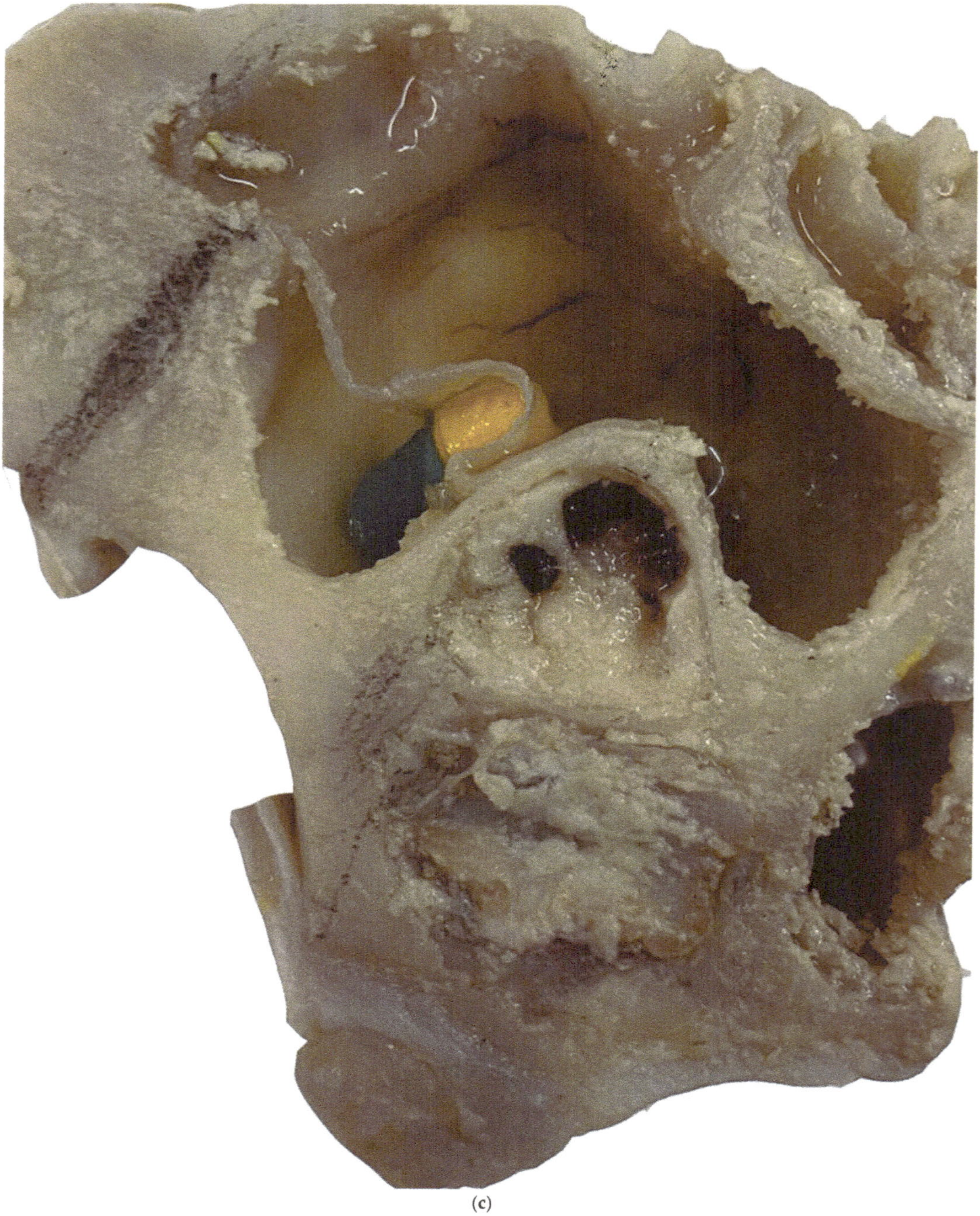

(c)

**Figure 1.** *Cont.*

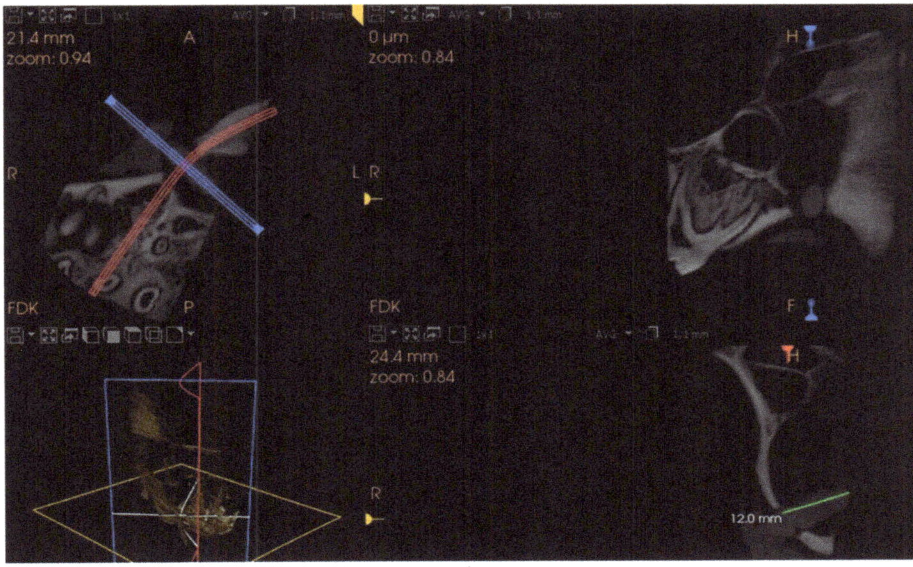


(**d**)

**Figure 1.** (**a**) New lifting device invented by the author. From left to right. Insertion of the device into the sinus, beginning of inflation, maximum pressure and inflation, deflation of the balloon after elevation. (**b**) Elevation window. (**c**) Section for histological analysis. (**d**) CBCT scans, 5 × 5. Oblique cut.

### 2.1. Measurement of Balloon Pressure and Resistance

A manometer was connected to a lateral outlet valve on the syringe, allowing maximum measurement of pressure throughout the experiment, with the aim of recording pressure changes during the separation of the sinus mucosa from the sinus floor. The pressure monitoring equipment used for this study consisted of an AZ 82152 digital pressure gauge (Resolution: Bar: 1.034 (0.001), Range: 0~15 psi, Accuracy: 0.3% FS at 25 C, Linearity/Hysteresis: 0.29~1%FS, Repeatability 0.2~0.5%FS, Combined Accuracy 1.0% FS).

The zero point of the pressure gauge was set to ambient pressure during each experiment to rule out any influence. Following insertion into the maxillary sinus as described above, the balloon was progressively filled to a target volume of 2 mL of serum, while pressure was applied. The pressure exerted during balloon filling and the resulting elevation of the mucosa were constantly monitored and recorded. Each elevation was carried out within a 3 min timeframe while constant pressure was applied to allow the tissue to adapt to the altered tension and separate from the surface of the bone. Once this time had elapsed and the elevation procedure was complete, the balloon and the syringe were removed from the sinus.

To prevent bias with regard to pressure data obtained during monitoring of the elevation, a pilot trial was required to measure the influence of wear on the balloon material, and the resistance of this material to the recorded pressure. To this end, the balloon was filled three times consecutively with 2 mL of serum and the resulting maximum pressures were recorded: 318.2, 315.3, and 320.7 mmHg, respectively, with a mean of 318.1 mmHG. This preliminary experiment was performed in ex vivo pig heads with no tissue or other material around the balloon. The acquired pressure data were interpreted as the elastic resistance of the balloon material to volumetric expansion. The pressure recorded in this pilot experiment was subtracted from the maximum pressure measured during the ex vivo elevation experiment in order to determine the force originating solely from the mucosa.

The elevation heights were obtained by carefully stretching the mucosa and introducing a standard impression material (Elite HD + Putty soft regular set, Zhermack, Rovigo, Italy) in the space below the mucosa. This material was subsequently dried and cut with a jigsaw into pieces measuring approximately 4 × 4 × 4 cm for histological study, with a safety margin sufficient to avoid accidental damage to the mucosa (see Figure 1c).

The 5 × 5 CBCT scans were then taken with a CS 8100 3D unit in order to measure the elevations obtained in the samples (see Figure 1d).

### 2.2. Histological Processing: Non-Decalcified Bone Samples Embedded in Plastic

The bone samples obtained following the slaughter of the experimental animals were preserved in formalin for fixation and conservation.

Since these bone samples were non-decalcified, they were washed in water and sawn to macroscopically delimit the study areas. The samples were then dehydrated by immersion in ethanol solutions of increasing concentration (70°, 80°, 90°, and 95°), soaking for 24 h in each solution until reaching absolute ethanol, where they remained for 2 days.

The samples were then placed for 15 days under agitation in liquid polymethyl metacrilate (PMMA) at 4 °C. After 15 days of immersion, the bone samples were transferred to glass cylinders with a base of solid PMMA and filled with liquid PMMA. The tubes were sealed with parafilm and kept in an oven at 32 °C for 5–6 until polymerization. The polymerized block with the bone sample was then cut with a microtome (Microm HM 350 S). The first sections were made with a thickness of 30 μm until reaching the study area, where 5 μm sections were cut and placed on gelatinized slides, covered with polyethylene film and pressed and dried at 60 °C for 24 h.

For histological staining, the sections were deplasticized by immersion in methyl acetate for 55 min, then washed in decreasing alcohol solutions until distilled water. The stain used was Goldner's Trichrome, which allows osteoid to be distinguished from calcified bone, as well as the study of the morphology and distribution of cells in the tissues.

Microscopic images of histological samples were captured using a Nikon Digital Sight DS-smc camera coupled to a Nikon Eclipse 90i optical microscope.

## 3. Results

Fifteen 5 × 5 scans were obtained with a CS 8100 3D unit, measuring the thickness of the sinus wall and the elevation height which was obtained (see Table 1). The mean thickness of the sinus walls studied was 1.45 mm ± 0.53, median 1.20 mm, range 0.90–2.40 mm, while the mean elevation achieved was 10.6 mm. The mean height was 10.63 mm ± 1.32, median 10.20, range 8.00–13.30 (see Tables 1 and 2 and Figure 2a).

**Table 1.** Study of sinus wall thickness and heights achieved measured with CBCT.

| Sinus | Sinus Wall Thickness (mm) | Elevation Height Measured with CBCT (mm) | Membrane Perforated during Aperture | Membrane Perforated during Elevation | Elevation of All Layers. Histological Analysis |
|---|---|---|---|---|---|
| 1 | 1 | 10.6 | No | No | Yes |
| 2 | 1.1 | 11 | No | No | No |
| 3 | 1 | 10.1 | No | No | Yes |
| 4 | 0.9 | 10.7 | No | No | Yes |
| 5 | 1.8 | 10.1 | No | No | Yes |
| 6 | 0.9 | 12.5 | No | No | No |
| 7 | 2.2 | 9.7 | No | No | Yes |
| 8 | 2.4 | 8 | No | No | Yes |
| 9 | 1.2 | 13.3 | No | No | Yes |

**Table 1.** *Cont.*

| Sinus | Sinus Wall Thickness (mm) | Elevation Height Measured with CBCT (mm) | Membrane Perforated during Aperture | Membrane Perforated during Elevation | Elevation of All Layers. Histological Analysis |
|---|---|---|---|---|---|
| 10 | 1.8 | 9.8 | No | No | No |
| 11 | 1.1 | 10.1 | No | No | No |
| 12 | 1 | 11.8 | No | No | Yes |
| 13 | 1.4 | 10.2 | No | No | Yes |
| 14 | 1.7 | 12 | No | No | Yes |
| 15 | 2.3 | 9.6 | No | No | Yes |

**Table 2.** Shows a comparison between the thickness of the sinus floor ($p = 0.000002$) and the elevation height measured with CBCT ($p = 0.0014$). There was a significant difference of 0.97 mm between sinus floor thickness groups. There were significant differences of 2.08 mm in the elevation height.

| | Sinus Floor Thickness (mm) | | Elevation Height Measured with CBCT (mm) | |
|---|---|---|---|---|
| **Men** | 1.45 | | 10.63 | |
| SD | 0.53 | | 1.32 | |
| Median | 1.20 | | 10.20 | |
| Minimum value | 0.90 | | 8.00 | |
| Maximum value | 2.40 | | 13.30 | |
| Groups | **Thickness < 1.45 mm** | **Thickness > 1.45 mm** | **Height < 10.63 mm** | **Height > 10.63 mm** |
| Mean | 1.06 | 2.03 | 9.80 | 11.88 |
| SD | 0.15 | 0.30 | 0.73 | 0.95 |
| Median | 1.00 | 2.00 | 10.10 | 11.90 |
| Minimum value | 0.90 | 1.70 | 8.00 | 10.70 |
| Maximum value | 1.40 | 2.40 | 10.60 | 13.30 |
| *p*-value T-student | 0.000002 | | 0.0014 | |

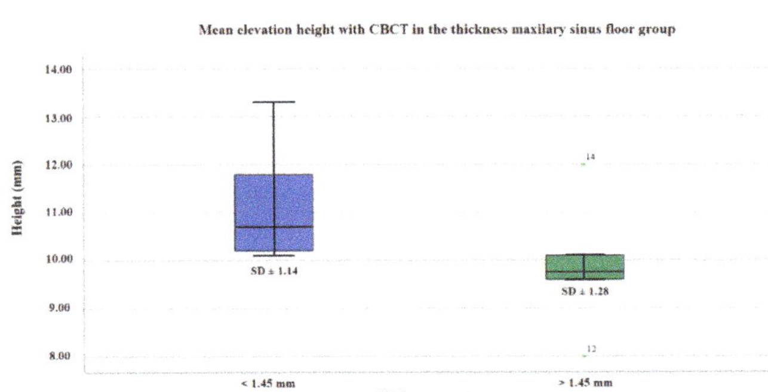


(a)

**Figure 2.** *Cont.*

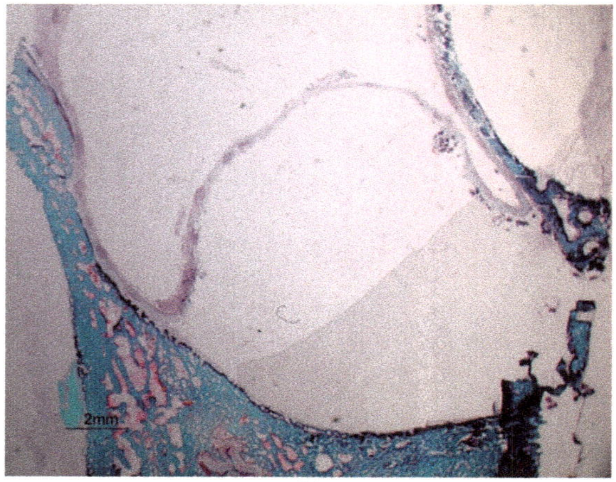


(**b**)

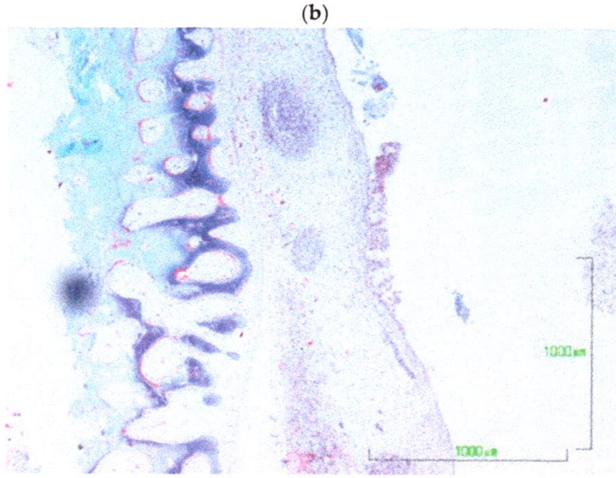

(**c**)

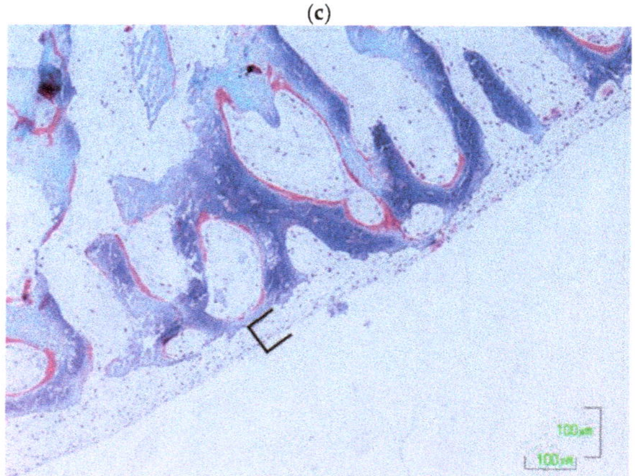

(**d**)

**Figure 2.** (**a**) Distribution of the mean elevation height with the CBCT (mm) in the maxillary sinus floor thickness groups. (**b**) Osteotomy, elevated mucosa 100 µm. (**c**) Elevation start zone 100 µm. (**d**) Periosteum 100 µm.

In 100% of cases, perforations do not occur during aperture or in the elevation of the wall. There was histological elevation in all layers in 53.33% of the >10.63 mm height group compared to 46.67% of the <10.63 mm height group ($p$ = 1.0000); there was no elevation in 86.67% of the >10.63 mm height group compared to 13.33% in the <10.63 mm height group. In the global sample, there was histological elevation in 73.33% compared to 26.66% non-elevation ($p$ = 0.0268) (see Table 3, Figure 3a,b).

**Table 3.** Distribution and comparison of membrane perforation and histology within groups for maxillary membrane height and global sample.

| | | | | | | | |
|---|---|---|---|---|---|---|---|
| | | | Global Sample | | | | |
| **Variables** | *n* | | | | % | | *p*-Value |
| Membrane perforated during aperture (no) | 15 | | | | 100.00 | | 1.000 |
| Membrane perforated during elevation (no) | 15 | | | | 100.00 | | |
| Elevation of all layers. Histological analysis (no) | 4 | | | | 26.66 | | 0.0268 |
| Elevation of all layers. Histological analysis (yes) | 11 | | | | 73.33 | | |
| **Subgroups** | **Height < 10.63 mm** | | **Height > 10.63 mm** | | **Total** | | **Fisher's Exact Test** |
| **Variables** | *n* | % | *n* | % | % | *n* | *p*-Value |
| Membrane perforated during aperture (no) | 9 | 60.00 | 6 | 40.00 | 15 | 100.00 | 0.4661 |
| Membrane perforated during elevation (no) | 9 | 60.00 | 6 | 40.00 | 15 | 100.00 | 0.4661 |
| Elevation of all layers. Histological analysis (no) | 2 | 13.33 | 13 | 86.67 | 15 | 100.00 | 0.0001 |
| Elevation of all layers. Histological analysis (yes) | 7 | 46.67 | 8 | 53.33 | 15 | 100.00 | 1.0000 |

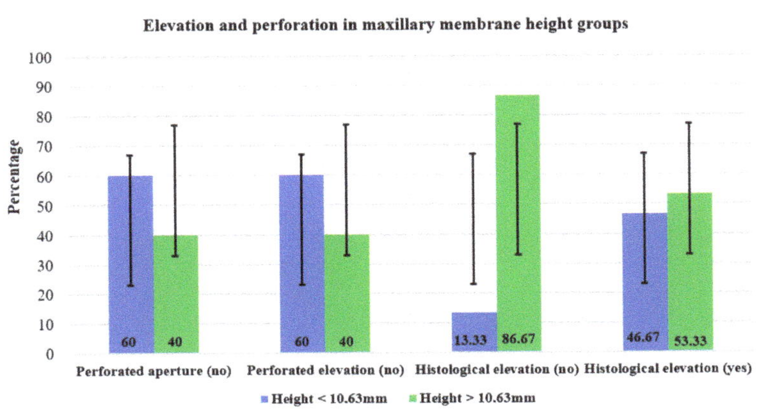


(a)

**Figure 3.** *Cont.*

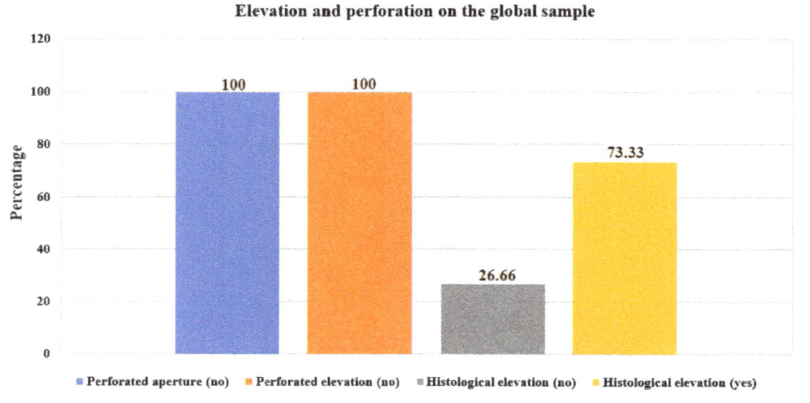


(**b**)

**Figure 3.** (**a**) Distribution of the histological elevation and the membrane perforated in the height groups, (**b**) Distribution of the histological elevation and the membrane perforated on the global sample.

Microscopic images of the histological samples did not reveal ruptures or laceration of the membranes in any of the samples. Only in four cases was it impossible to elevate all the layers, with the glandular layer left unelevated and a clearer view of the epithelium in the elevated mucous membranes. A thin layer of collagen tissue was observed in the bone, which may be interpreted as the periosteum or parts of it (see Figure 2b–d).

The mean maximum pressure obtained during the balloon experiments was 662.62 mmHg. The maximum values did not exceed 726.20 mmHg. The minimum monitored pressure was 598.80 mmHg. The pressure required to overcome the resistance of the balloon material, as determined during the pilot test, was subtracted from the maximum pressure. Therefore, the mean pressure required to elevate the maxillary bone floor mucosa was calculated to be 344.46 mmHg in this ex vivo animal model. No mucosal tearing was observed. Pressure values over time and fill volume showed a strong initial rise in pressure. In 5 of the 15 cases, there was an Underwood septum in the region where the mucosa was elevated. However, the elevation process in regions with Underwood septa (mean pressure = 368.12 mmHg) did not produce significantly different elevation forces ($p$ = 0.096) compared to sinus mucosal elevations without the presence of septa (mean pressure = 332.63 mmHg) (see Tables 4 and 5, Figure 4a–c)

**Table 4.** Pressure values in mmHg.

| | Max | Septum | Pressure on Membrane |
|---|---|---|---|
| SINUS 1 | 598.8 | NO | 280.7 |
| SINUS 2 | 620.2 | NO | 302.1 |
| SINUS 3 | 680.2 | SI | 362.1 |
| SINUS 4 | 650.7 | NO | 332.6 |
| SINUS 5 | 601.9 | NO | 283.8 |
| SINUS 6 | 630.8 | NO | 312.7 |
| SINUS 7 | 654.9 | SI | 335.8 |
| SINUS 8 | 635.4 | NO | 317.3 |
| SINUS 9 | 726.2 | SI | 408.1 |
| SISUS 10 | 659.7 | NO | 341.6 |

**Table 4.** *Cont.*

| | Max | Septum | Pressure on Membrane |
|---|---|---|---|
| SINUS11 | 704.4 | NO | 386.3 |
| SINUS 12 | 658.2 | SI | 340.1 |
| SINUS 13 | 706.8 | NO | 388.7 |
| SINUS 14 | 698.6 | NO | 380.5 |
| SINUS 15 | 712.6 | SI | 394.5 |

**Table 5.** Distribution and comparison of maximum pressures and pressures on the membrane in the global sample and in the sinuses with and without a septum.

| | Maximum Pressure mmHg | | Pressure on Membrane | |
|---|---|---|---|---|
| **Mean** | 662.62 | | 344.46 | |
| SD | 40.86 | | 40.88 | |
| Median | 658.20 | | 340.10 | |
| Minimum value | 598.80 | | 280.70 | |
| Maximum value | 726.20 | | 408.10 | |
| Groups | Without septum | With septum | Without septum | With septum |
| Media | 650.73 | 686.42 | 332.63 | 368.12 |
| SD | 50.88 | 32.00 | 40.88 | 32.24 |
| Median | 643.050 | 680.20 | 324.95 | 362.10 |
| Minimum value | 598.80 | 654.90 | 280.70 | 335.80 |
| Maximum value | 706.80 | 726.20 | 388.70 | 408.10 |
| *p*-value | 0.093 | | 0.096 | |

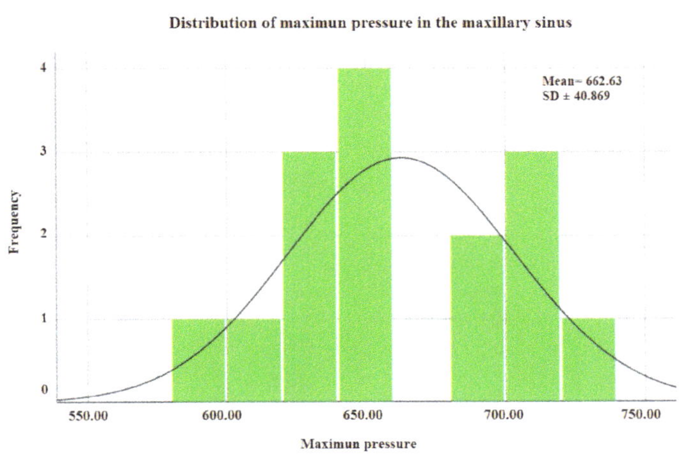


(a)

**Figure 4.** *Cont.*

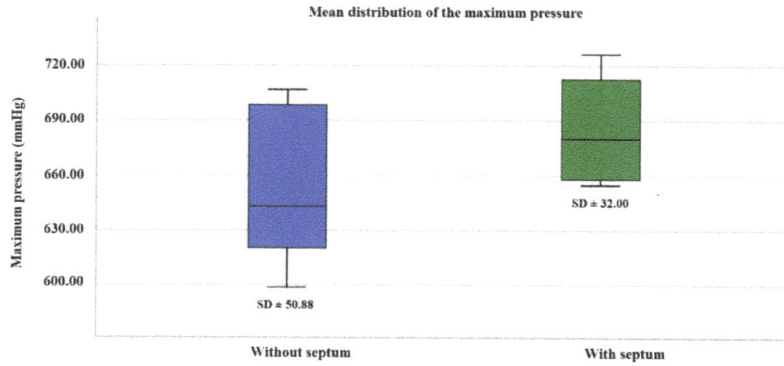


(**b**)

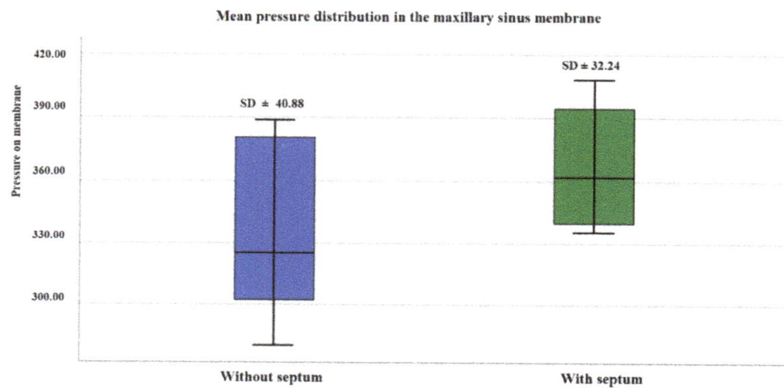


(**c**)

**Figure 4.** (**a**) General distribution of maximum pressure in the maxillary sinus. (**b**) Distribution of mean maximum pressure in the maxillary sinus with and without a septum. (**c**) Mean pressure distribution in the maxillary sinus membrane with and without a septum.

## 4. Discussion

With a mean elevation height of 10.6 mm, no membrane lacerations could be found during gross and microscopic examinations. The mean pressure during maxillary sinus augmentation was therefore assumed to be below the soft tissue tear point for this animal model. However, the results of the balloon experiment should be interpreted with caution, as they were obtained from an ex vivo animal model and changes in tissue resistance and stability due to post-mortem degradation and dehydration of proteins cannot be ruled out. Pig heads are a well-established animal model in implantology research due to their similarity with human anatomy [32–34]. Nevertheless, the mucosa of the maxillary sinus of the pig is known to be thicker than that of humans [35,36]. This can lead to increased adhesion and elastic tensile forces.

In pigs, there is a greater number of Underwood septa. However, the Underwood septa in the region of the lifting procedure did not show a significant influence ($p = 0.096$) on the lifting process or the lifting force required in this study. Therefore, it is assumed that this anatomical variation may have no influence on sinus elevation procedures where a balloon system is used. Similar results were noted by Stelzle et al. in their study of pressure and resilience with the Meisinger system [31].

Due to the pronounced crestal bone height found in this animal model, the lateral surgical approach through the maxillary sinus wall was chosen. In this area, the bone level in the pig would not exceed 2–3 mm, reflecting the situation found in a patient with an atrophied maxillary alveolar process [36,37]. All other steps of the procedure were performed and assessed analogous to a crestal approach. However, the lateral accessed may have influenced the pressure values obtained, as the thickness of the lateral sinus mucosa may be different to that of the sinus floor. The thickness of healthy sinus membrane in humans has been shown to vary depending on the region of the maxillary sinus which is being studied (0.99 to 2.58 mm), as well as between individuals [38,39].

The mean pressure needed to elevate the mucosa of the maxillary bone floor was calculated to be 344.5 mmHg, a considerably lower value than that obtained in the pressure and resilience measurement study by Stelzle et al., where the balloon elevation system (Meisinger) was used on ex vivo bisected pig heads, giving a pressure of 748 mmHg [31].

Histological images did not reveal ruptures or lacerations of the membranes in any of the samples. Thin layers of collagen were observed in the bone, which may be interpreted as periosteum or parts of it, in agreement with the study by Stelzle et al. which compared various methods of indirect elevation in an ex vivo experimental study.

Despite the above limitations, the preliminary results of this study with an experimental set-up based on the author's patented sinus floor elevation kit with an inflatable balloon demonstrate that the measuring configuration is appropriate for directly and reliably determining the pressures which occurred in the sinus during the elevation procedure. The possible transfer of this procedure to a clinical environment has therefore been proven, along with a demonstration of the general applicability of this technical configuration for future clinical trials.

## 5. Conclusions

Within the limits of this study on ex vivo bisected pig heads, maxillary sinus elevations using the new device and balloon technique were found to be minimally invasive procedures, with no membrane perforations observed in the histological analyses, even in the presence of a septum and of residual crests less than 1 mm. The heights achieved, analyzed histologically and measured with CBCT, proved sufficient to allow the future placement of implants of varying lengths and diameters.

## 6. Patents

Sinus floor elevation was performed with the new elevation control system patented by the author and registered in the Spanish Official Industrial Property Gazette (patent application: 202130571). This system consists of a syringe containing stops, retaining elements, latex, and serum.

**Author Contributions:** Conceptualization, E.R.F.C.; literature search, E.R.F.C.; data analysis, M.T.M.S.; writing—original draft preparation, E.R.F.C.; writing—review and editing, E.R.F.C. and J.F.F. All authors have read and agreed to the published version of the manuscript.

**Funding:** This research received no external funding.

**Institutional Review Board Statement:** Not applicable.

**Informed Consent Statement:** Not applicable.

**Data Availability Statement:** Not applicable.

**Conflicts of Interest:** The authors declare no conflict of interest.

## References

1. Jung, R.E.; Fenner, N.; Hämmerle, C.H.; Zitzmann, N.U. Long-term outcome of implants placed with guided bone regeneration (GBR) using resorbable and non-resorbable membranes after 12–14 years. *Clin. Oral Implants Res.* **2013**, *24*, 1065–1073. [CrossRef] [PubMed]
2. Sagheb, K.; Schiegnitz, E.; Moergel, M.; Walter, C.; Al-Nawas, B.; Wagner, W. Clinical outcome of alveolar ridge augmentation with individualized CAD-CAM-produced titanium mesh. *Int. J. Implant Dent.* **2017**, *3*, 36. [CrossRef] [PubMed]

3. Zita Gomes, R.; Paraud Freixas, A.; Han, C.H.; Bechara, S.; Tawil, I. Alveolar Ridge Reconstruction with Titanium Meshes and Simultaneous Implant Placement: A Retrospective, Multicenter Clinical Study. *BioMed Res. Int.* **2016**, *2016*, 5126838. [CrossRef]
4. Pommer, B.; Frantal, S.; Willer, J.; Posch, M.; Watzek, G.; Tepper, G. Impact of dental implant length on early failure rates: A meta-analysis of observational studies. *J. Clin. Periodontol.* **2011**, *38*, 856–863. [CrossRef] [PubMed]
5. Winkler, S.; Morris, H.F.; Ochi, S. Implant Survival to 36 Months as Related to Length and Diameter. *Ann. Periodontol.* **2000**, *5*, 22–31. [CrossRef] [PubMed]
6. Luongo, F.; Mangano, F.G.; Macchi, A.; Luongo, G.; Mangano, C. Custom-Made Synthetic Scaffolds for Bone Reconstruction: A Retrospective, Multicenter Clinical Study on 15 Patients. *BioMed Res. Int.* **2016**, *2016*, 5862586. [CrossRef] [PubMed]
7. De Avila, E.D.; Scarso Filho, J.; de Oliveira Ramalho, L.T.; Gabrielli, M.F.R.; Pereira Filho, V.A. Alveolar ridge augmentation with the perforated and nonperforated bone grafts. *J. Periodontal Implant Sci.* **2014**, *44*, 33–38. [CrossRef]
8. Gultekin, B.A.; Bedeloglu, E.; Kose, T.E.; Mijiritsky, E. Comparison of Bone Resorption Rates after Intraoral Block Bone and Guided Bone Regeneration Augmentation for the Reconstruction of Horizontally Deficient Maxillary Alveolar Ridges. *BioMed Res. Int.* **2016**, *2016*, 4987437. [CrossRef]
9. Yang, J.-W.; Park, H.-J.; Yoo, K.-H.; Chung, K.; Jung, S.; Oh, H.-K.; Kim, H.-S.; Kook, M.-S. A comparison study between periosteum and resorbable collagen membrane on iliac block bone graft resorption in the rabbit calvarium. *Head Face Med.* **2014**, *10*, 15. [CrossRef]
10. Sakkas, A.; Ioannis, K.; Winter, K.; Schramm, A.; Wilde, F. Clinical results of autologous bone augmentation harvested from the mandibular ramus prior to implant placement. An analysis of 104 cases. *GMS Interdiscip. Plast. Reconstr. Surg. DGPW* **2016**, *5*, Doc21.
11. Cucchi, A.; Vignudelli, E.; Napolitano, A.; Marchetti, C.; Corinaldesi, G. Evaluation of complication rates and vertical bone gain after guided bone regeneration with non-resorbable membranes versus titanium meshes and resorbable membranes. A randomized clinical trial. *Clin. Implant Dent. Relat. Res.* **2017**, *19*, 821–832. [CrossRef] [PubMed]
12. Dal Polo, M.R.; Poli, P.P.; Rancitelli, D.; Beretta, M.; Maiorana, C. Alveolar ridge reconstruction with titanium meshes: A systematic review of the literature. *Med. Oral Patol. Oral Y Cir. Bucal* **2014**, *19*, 639–646. [CrossRef] [PubMed]
13. Jegham, H.; Masmoudi, R.; Ouertani, H.; Blouza, I.; Turki, S.; Khattech, M. Ridge augmentation with titanium mesh: A case report. *J. Stomatol. Oral Maxillofac. Surg.* **2017**, *118*, 181–186. [CrossRef] [PubMed]
14. Poli, P.P.; Beretta, M.; Cicciù, M.; Maiorana, C. Alveolar Ridge Augmentation with Titanium Mesh. A Retrospective Clinical Study. *Open Dent. J.* **2014**, *8*, 148–158. [CrossRef]
15. Kim, Y.-K.; Ahn, K.-J.; Yun, P.-Y. A retrospective study on the prognosis of single implant placed at the sinus bone graft site. *Oral Surg. Oral Med. Oral Pathol. Oral Radiol.* **2014**, *118*, 181–186. [CrossRef]
16. Chirilă, L.; Rotaru, C.; Filipov, I.; Săndulescu, M. Management of acute maxillary sinusitis after sinus bone grafting procedures with simultaneous dental implants placement—A retrospective study. *BMC Infect. Dis.* **2016**, *16*, 94. [CrossRef]
17. Kayabasoglu, G.; Nacar, A.; Altundag, A.; Cayonu, M.; Muhtarogullari, M.; Cingi, C. A retrospective analysis of the relationship between rhinosinusitis and sinus lift dental implantation. *Head Face Med.* **2014**, *10*, 53. [CrossRef]
18. Kim, Y.-K.; Hwang, J.-Y.; Yun, P.-Y. Relationship Between Prognosis of Dental Implants and Maxillary Sinusitis Associated with the Sinus Elevation Procedure. *Int. J. Oral Maxillofac. Implants* **2013**, *28*, 178–183. [CrossRef]
19. Park, J.S.; Kim, B.C.; Choi, B.; Lee, J. ORAL SURGERY Facial skin fistula as a postoperative complication related to maxillary sinus grafting: A case report. *Quintessence Int.* **2015**, *46*, 145–149.
20. Nooh, N. Effect of schneiderian membrane perforation on posterior maxillary implant survival. *J. Int. Oral Health* **2013**, *5*, 28–34.
21. Nam, K.Y.; Kim, J.B. Treatment of dental implant-related maxillary sinusitis with functional endoscopic sinus surgery in combinationmwith an intra-oral approach. *J. Korean Assoc. Oral Maxillofac. Surg.* **2014**, *40*, 87–90. [CrossRef] [PubMed]
22. Alkan, A.; Çelebi, N.; Baş, B. Acute Maxillary Sinusitis Associated with Internal Sinus Lifting: Report of a Case. *Eur. J. Dent.* **2008**, *02*, 69–72. [CrossRef]
23. Emmerich, D.; Att, W.; Stappert, C. Sinus floor elevation using os- teotomes: A systematic review and meta-analysis. *J. Periodontol.* **2005**, *76*, 1237–1251. [CrossRef]
24. Le Gall, M.G. Localized sinus elevation and osteocompression with single-stage tapered dental implants: Technical note. *Int. J. Oral Maxillofac. Implants* **2004**, *19*, 431–437. [PubMed]
25. Ho, S.C.; Wallace, S.S.; Froum, S.J.; Tarnow, D. Influence of anatomy on Schneiderian membrane perforations during sinus elevation surgery: Three-dimensional analysis. *Pract. Proced. Aesthetic Dent.* **2001**, *13*, 160–163.
26. Shlomi, B.; Horowitz, I.; Kahn, A.; Dobriyan, A.; Chaushu, G. The effect of sinus membrane perforation and repair with Lambone on the outcome of maxillary sinus floor augmentation: A radiographic assessment. *Int. J. Oral Maxillofac. Implants* **2004**, *19*, 559–562.
27. Berengo, M.; Sivolella, S.; Majzoub, Z.; Cordioli, G. Endoscopic evaluation of the bone-added osteotome sinus floor elevation procedure. *Int. J. Oral Maxillofac. Surg.* **2004**, *33*, 189–194. [CrossRef]
28. Reiser, G.M.; Rabinovitz, Z.; Bruno, J.; Damoulis, P.D.; Griffin, T.J. Evaluation of maxillary sinus membrane response following elevation with the crestal osteotome technique in human cadavers. *Int. J. Oral Maxillofac. Implants* **2002**, *16*, 833–840.
29. Nkenke, E.; Schlegel, A.; Schultze-Mosgau, S.; Neukam, F.W.; Wiltfang, J. The endoscopically controlled osteotome sinus floor elevation: A preliminary prospective study. *Int. J. Oral Maxillofac. Implants* **2002**, *17*, 557–566.
30. Ardekian, L.; Oved-Peleg, E.; Mactei, E.E.; Peled, M. The clinical signifi-cance of sinus membrane perforation during augmentation of the maxillary sinus. *J. Oral Maxillofac. Surg.* **2006**, *64*, 277–282. [CrossRef]

31. Stelzle, F.; Rohde, M. Elevation forces and resilience of the sinus membrane during sinus floor elevation: Preliminary measurements using a balloon method on ex vivo pig heads. *Int. J. Oral Maxillofac. Implants* **2014**, *29*, 550–557. [CrossRef] [PubMed]
32. Fenner, M.; Vairaktaris, E.; Fischer, K.; Schlegel, K.A.; Neukam, F.W.; Nkenke, E. Influence of residual alveolar bone height on osseointegration of implants in the maxilla: A pilot study. *Clin. Oral Implants Res.* **2009**, *20*, 555–559. [CrossRef] [PubMed]
33. Schlegel, K.A.; Zimmermann, R.; Thorwarth, M.; Neukam, F.-W.; Klongnoi, B.; Nkenke, E.; Felszeghy, E. Sinus floor elevation using autogenous bone or bone substitute combined with platelet-rich plasma. *Oral Surg. Oral Med. Oral Pathol. Oral Radiol. Endodontol.* **2007**, *104*, e15–e25. [CrossRef] [PubMed]
34. Mueller, C.K.; Solcher, P.; Peisker, A.; Mtsariashvilli, M.; Schlegel, K.A.; Hildebrand, G.; Rost, J.; Liefeith, K.; Chen, J.; Schultze-Mosgau, S. Analysis of the influence of the macro- and microstructure of dental zirconium implants on osseointegration: A minipig study. *Oral Surg. Oral Med. Oral Pathol. Oral Radiol.* **2013**, *116*, e1–e8. [CrossRef] [PubMed]
35. Stelzle, F.; Benner, K.-U. An animal model for sinus floor elevation with great elevation heights. Macroscopic, microscopic, radiological and micro-CT analysis: Ex vivo. *Clin. Oral Implants Res.* **2010**, *21*, 1370–1378. [CrossRef] [PubMed]
36. Aimetti, M.; Massei, G.; Morra, M.; Cardesi, E.; Romano, F. Correlation between gingival phenotype and Schneiderian membrane thickness. *Int. J. Oral Maxillofac. Implants* **2009**, *23*, 1128–1132.
37. Stelzle, F.; Benner, K.-U. Evaluation of Different Methods of Indirect Sinus Floor Elevation for Elevation Heights of 10 mm: An Experimental Ex Vivo Study. *Clin. Implant Dent. Relat. Res.* **2011**, *13*, 124–133. [CrossRef]
38. Bornstein, M.M.; Wasmer, J.; Sendi, P.; Janner, S.F.; Buser, D.; Von Arx, T. Characteristics and dimensions of the Schneiderian membrane and apical bone in maxillary molars referred for apical surgery: A comparative radiographic analysis using limited cone beam computed tomography. *J. Endod.* **2012**, *38*, 51–57. [CrossRef]
39. Janner, S.F.M.; Caversaccio, M.D.; Dubach, P.; Sendi, P.; Buser, D.; Bornstein, M.M. Characteristics and dimensions of the Schneiderian membrane: A radiographic analysis using cone beam computed tomography in patients referred for dental implant surgery in the posterior maxilla. *Clin. Oral Implants Res.* **2011**, *22*, 1446–1453. [CrossRef]

*applied sciences*

MDPI

*Article*

# Relevance of the Operator's Experience in Conditioning the Static Computer-Assisted Implantology: A Comparative In Vitro Study with Three Different Evaluation Methods

**Gerardo Pellegrino [1,*], Giuseppe Lizio [1], Filippo D'Errico [1], Agnese Ferri [1], Annalisa Mazzoni [1], Federico Del Bianco [1], Luigi Vito Stefanelli [2] and Pietro Felice [1]**

1 Department of Biomedical and Neuromotor Sciences (DIBINEM), University of Bologna, 40100 Bologna, Italy
2 Department of Oral and Maxillo-Facial Sciences, Sapienza, University of Rome, 00100 Rome, Italy
* Correspondence: gerardo.pellegrino2@unibo.it; Tel.: +39-32872222127

**Abstract:** The present study aimed to evaluate the influence of manual expertise on static computer-aided implantology (s-CAI) in terms of accuracy and operative timings. After the cone-beam CT (CBCT) scanning of eleven mandibular models, a full-arch rehabilitation was planned, and two different skilled operators performed s-CAI. The distances between the virtual and actual implant positions were calculated considering the three spatial vectorial axes and the three-dimensional Euclidean value for the entry (E) and apical (A) points, along with the axis orientation differences (Ax). These values emerged from the overlapping of the pre-op CBCT to post-op CBCT data (method 1), from scanning the data from the laboratory scanner (method 2), and from the intra-oral scanner (method 3) and were correlated with the operators' expertise and operative timings. The mean values for accuracy from the three methods were: E = 0.57 (0.8, 0.45, 0.47) mm, A = 0.6 (0.8, 0.48, 0.49) mm, and Ax 1.04 (1.05,1.03,1.05) ° for the expert operator; and E = 0.8 (0.9, 0.87, 0.77), A = 0.95 (1.02, 0.95, 0.89), and Ax =1.64 (1.78, 1.58, 1.58) for the novice. The mean value of the operative timings was statistically inferior for the expert operator ($p < 0.05$), with an improved accuracy over time for both operators. A significant difference ($p < 0.05$) emerged between method 1 and methods 2 and 3 for seven of the nine variables, without differences between the evaluations from the two scanners. The support from digital surgical guides does not eliminate the importance of manual expertise for the reliability and the shortening of the surgical procedure, and it requires a learning pathway over time.

**Keywords:** clinical skill; data accuracy; dental implant; outcome assessment

**Citation:** Pellegrino, G.; Lizio, G.; D'Errico, F.; Ferri, A.; Mazzoni, A.; Bianco, F.D.; Stefanelli, L.V.; Felice, P. Relevance of the Operator's Experience in Conditioning the Static Computer-Assisted Implantology: A Comparative In Vitro Study with Three Different Evaluation Methods. *Appl. Sci.* **2022**, *12*, 9561. https://doi.org/10.3390/app12199561

Academic Editor: Bruno Chrcanovic

Received: 28 July 2022
Accepted: 20 September 2022
Published: 23 September 2022



## 1. Introduction

Standardizing a treatment to a high level of reliability and effectiveness, beyond personal human experience and capabilities, is the goal of applied Digital Science [1]. Computerized aided implantology (CAI), both static (s-CAI) and dynamic (d-CAI), allowed a more precise fixture placement than a freehand approach, reducing the surgical timing and the patient discomfort [2–6].

This procedure, however, can present criticisms due to its complexity and the number of steps as well as the competence required. The quality of the Digital Imaging and Communications in Medicine (DICOM) from cone-beam CT (CBCT) and Standard Tessellation Language (STL) data and the reliability of the digital algorithm in merging these files condition the virtual planning [4,7–10]. Furthermore, in s-CAI, the computer-aided manufacturing (CAM) process [11] and the structural features of the surgical guide are relevant to the final result [2,4,12].

Assuming the integrity of the digital planning and guide printing, it appears helpful to verify whether, and how much, the personal operator's ability can interfere in the final surgical phase, improving the precision of the implant placement and shortening the surgical timing.

Conflicting outcomes have emerged in in vitro and in vivo trials about the relevance of human expertise, not only as a freehand implantologist, but also whether there is competence in using s-CAI, and whether there is a learning curve. No relevance of the s-CAI expertise for skilled implantologists has been recorded [13], and better accuracy by novices under senior control has emerged compared to expert operators [14]. Significant deviations from the planned and the actual positions have been attributed to improper use of the handle piece, the conditioning of the action of the drills in the sleeves [15], and to the positioning of the guide into the patient's mouth [13]. The presence of improvement over time for experienced implantologists has been excluded, at least for edentulous patients [16]. In the most recent literature reviews on s- CAI, the operator's experience has not emerged as influencing the accuracy of the procedure. Nevertheless, the variability and unreliability of the assessment methods adopted by the studies considered were highlighted, due to the difficulty in performing meta-analyses [6,7,12,17].

Concerning the methods of accuracy evaluation, the degree of digital superimposition for the postoperative with the virtually planned implant positions—the matching of the pre- and post-CT DICOM data—has been ratified and shared as an accuracy parameter in the literature. The shifting of the coronal and apical portion of the fixture and its tilting and deepening were considered geometrical reference points [18]. Optical scanners introduced an alternative to the previous analysis, but the same factors affecting the registration process in the planning phase with these tools also conditioned the assessment method [19–22]. No study has investigated the influence of operator skill on reducing the operative timing.

The primary objective of the present study was to understand the relevance of the operator's expertise in conditioning implant placement accuracy with the s-CAI approach and to determine if accuracy improved over time for experts and novices (learning curve).

The secondary objective was to understand if the operator's expertise could influence the operative time in the s-CAI approach.

Three methods of superimposition data evaluation were adopted and compared to each other: CBCT (pre and post), CBCT (pre) and laboratory scanning (post), and CBCT (pre) and intraoral scanning (post).

## 2. Materials and Methods

### 2.1. Digital and Operative Flow-Chart

Eleven acrylic resin models, reproducing completely edentulous mandibles with different alveolar shapes, were scanned with a CBCT. The models reproduced typical situations to be managed without grafting techniques to avoid dehiscence or fenestrations. DICOM data were imported in a dedicated software (B&B Dent SL GS, B&B Dental Implant Company, Bologna, Italy). The placement of eight implants 4 mm wide and 11 mm long (Duravit 3P, B&B Dental implant company, Bologna, Italy) in each model, uniformly distributed in posterior and anterior locations, was planned for a fixed full-arch rehabilitation according to the bone volumes and shapes simulated by the models. The virtual implant position was identified through the DICOM data, which were then converted into STL-files for the models' segmentation and the guide design and printing, according to the implant positions. The first dentist (GP), the more experienced operator, accomplished the planning phase in collaboration with the digital designer.

The surgical guides were projected according to the supporting bone modality. Since there was no occlusal correlation with an opposite maxilla, the plan could not start from actual prosthetic demands. Three vestibular fixing pins to stabilize the guides and eight sleeves of 4.2 and 5 mm in diameter and length, respectively, were designed. The sleeves were made in poly-ether-ether-ketone (PEEK), instead of using metallic ones, to avoid friction and overheating during the implant site preparation. Five models and a half, with the applied guides, were randomly assigned to each of the two operators and fixed to the dental chair headboard to simulate the clinical ergonomics (Figure 1). The guides were fixed to all the models by the more experienced operator (GP), who was unaware of the subsequent casual operator's assignment.

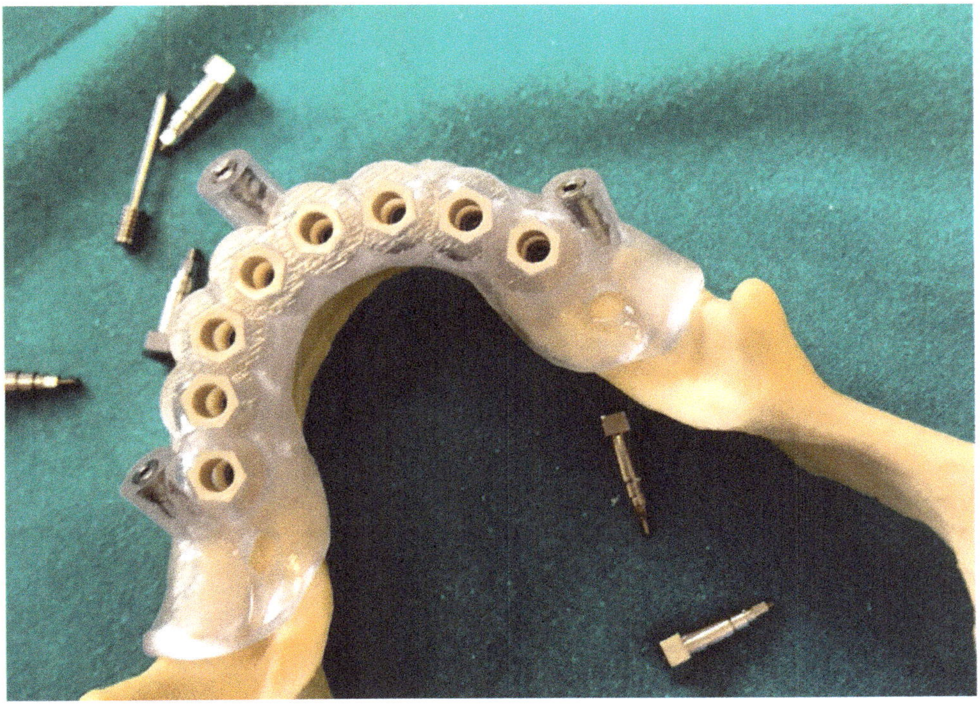

**Figure 1.** Surgical guide fixed to the acrylic resin model.

The first dentist (GP) had had more than fifteen years of experience in freehand implantology and more than ten years of experience in s-CAI. The second one (FD) was a post-graduate dentist, an utter novice in general dental practice. The implants were placed independently in different sittings dedicated to accomplishing each model procedure, and the time taken was recorded. For each model a new kit of burs was used to eliminate the bias of the tool's wear. The operative timings were recorded in seconds and statistically elaborated.

After that, the implanted models were CBCT scanned once again, and the DICOM data was imported in the same software mentioned above (method n.1). The "image substitution analysis" matched the pre- and post-CT session without the segmentation of the implants and the STL data conversion.

Optical scanning of the resin models was taken with a laboratory scanner (EGS dscan3) and an intra-oral scanner (3 Shape Trios, Copenhagen, Denmark) after connecting the scan bodies with the implants as in methods n.2 and n.3.

The flow-chart is shown in Figure 2.

The data relating to the external surface of the resin clones from the three techniques, exported as STL data, were volumetrically analyzed, and the pre- and postoperative virtual models and implants were aligned by the *GOM inspect* software. The alignment of the pre- and postoperative surfaces was singularly exported and loaded onto *Meshmixer* software, which was able to remove the superimposing surfaces of the resin copies while maintaining those of the implants (Figure 3).

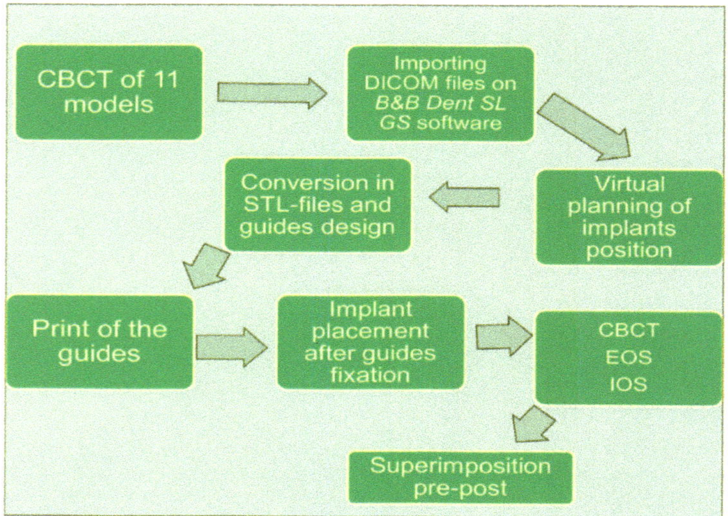


**Figure 2.** The scheme of the flow-chart.

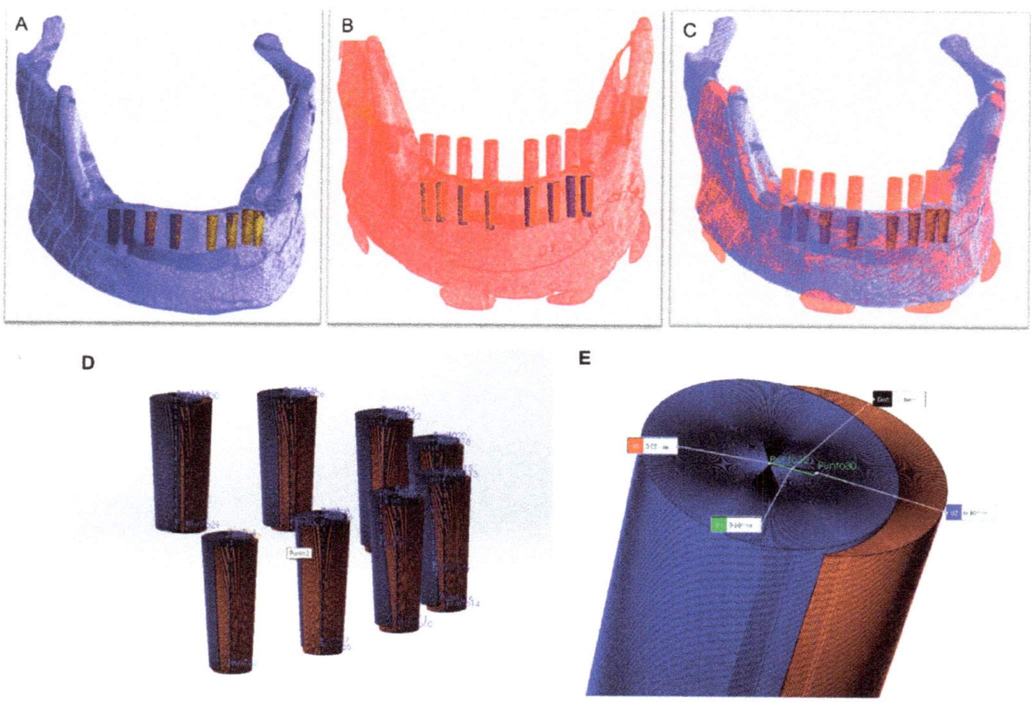


**Figure 3.** Pre- (**A**) and post- (**B**) operative virtual models and their alignment superimposing the external surfaces (**C**). Planned (**D**) and actual (**E**) implant positions after removing the models' superimposing surface.

### 2.2. Measurement Parameters for Accuracy Analysis

For each pre-and postoperative implant surface, the *entry point* (E) and the *apical point* (A) were identified as the most coronal and apical points, respectively, obtained from the geometric intersection of the symmetric line of the fixture and its surface. The distance between these two points was divided into three vectorial components, *vestibular-lingual* (x), *mesiodistal* (y), and *apical-coronal* (z), and assumed to be deviation values from the planned positions in the respective implant portions (*Edx, Edy, Edz; Adx, Ady, and Adz*). The three-dimensional Euclidean distance was calculated to have a single entry (*Ed*) and an apical (*Ad*) point. The angular discrepancy (*Ang*), expressed in grades, was further calculated from the longitudinal axes of the pre- and postoperative implants. The more the spread from the "zero" value, the more the inaccuracy amount.

These calculations were performed for the five groups derived from matching each operator with the three analysis methods.

### 2.3. Measurement Parameters for Operative Timing Analysis

The time counter was managed by an external assessor (FDB), and the counting started when the motor switched on and off for each site preparation and implant placement. Every phase time was added to the subsequent with a total value calculated for every implant site management. A mean value for each model timing was reported on the ten simulators excluding the shared one, on a total number of 80 implants.

### 2.4. Statistical Analysis

A descriptive analysis was performed, presenting continuous variables as mean $\pm$ standard deviations (SDs) and giving minimum and maximum values. An inferential analysis compared the groups in terms of the mean values of all the accuracy variables (the Friedman test was used since the data were not normally distributed).

The significance level was set at 0.05. All the analyses were performed using Stata, version 15 (Stata Corp LP, College Station, TX, USA).

The sample size was calculated considering an alpha error of 0.05, a power of 0.80, and an f-effect size of 0.40, taking the literature data into consideration.

A double-tailed *t*-test evaluated the significant difference between the two operators regarding implant placement velocity.

## 3. Results

### 3.1. Accuracy

An overall number of 88 implant positions were compared with the relative pre-operative planned ones.

An overall significant level of accuracy resulted for the first operator, compared to the second, from the mean values from the three evaluation methods ($p < 0.05$) (Table 1).

According to the method nr.1, $Ed = 0.8 \pm 0.43$ mm, $Ad = 0.85 \pm 0.39$ mm, and $Ang = 1.05 \pm 0.53°$ were reached by the first operator; and $Ed = 0.91 \pm 46$, $Ad = 1.02 \pm 0.45$, and $Ang = 1.78 \pm 1.12°$ by the second one. The overall mean values were: $Ed = 0.86 \pm 44$, $Ad = 0.93 \pm 43$, and $Ang = 1.41 \pm 0.95°$. Considering each vectorial component, the second operator obtained more minimal values than the first one for all the variables except the *Ay* one, all compensated by the higher maximum data.

According to the method nr.2, $Ed = 0.45 \pm 0.23$ mm, $Ad = 0.48 \pm 0.24$ mm, and $Ang = 1.03 \pm 0.47°$ were reached by the first operator; and $Ed = 0.87 \pm 45$, $Ad = 0.95 \pm 0.42$, and $Ang = 1.58 \pm 0.97°$ by the second one, with $Ed = 0.66 \pm 41$, $Ad = 0.72 \pm 42$, and $Ang = 1.31 \pm 0.81°$ as the mean values between each of them.

**Table 1.** Pairwise ANOVA analysis (Tukey HSD test) correlating the dependent variables with the three methods'.

| Parameters of Evaluation | Three Methods Results Mean Values | | Means Values' Differential between the Operators | HSD-Test | *p* Value |
|---|---|---|---|---|---|
| | Operator 1 | Operator 2 | | | |
| *Ed* point | 0.5728 | 0.8505 | 0.2777 | 16.2522 * | >0.0001 |
| *Edx* | 0.1489 | 0.1983 | 0.0494 | 6.1613 * | 0.0031 |
| *Edy* | 0.2655 | 0.4597 | 0.1942 | 11.7764 * | >0.0001 |
| *Edz* | 0.3980 | 0.5842 | 0.1862 | 7.7265 * | 0.0002 |
| *Ad* point | 0.6084 | 0.9533 | 0.3449 | 20.4794 * | >0.0001 |
| *Adx* | 0.1671 | 0.2436 | 0.0765 | 8.8757 * | 0.0002 |
| *Ady* | 0.3035 | 0.5516 | 0.2481 | 14.1916 * | >0.0001 |
| *Adz* | 0.4028 | 0.5721 | 0.1693 | 6.9093 * | 0.001 |
| *Ang* | 1.0424 | 1.6463 | 0.6039 | 21.6030 * | >0.0001 |

* Means results for each operator.

The second operator obtained more minimal deviations than the first one, but for fewer variables, e.g., *Ed, Adx, Ady, and Ang*, than in method nr.1. According to method nr.3, $Ed = 0.47 \pm 0.27$ mm, $Ad = 0.49 \pm 0.25$ mm;, and $Ang = 1.05 \pm 0.57°$ were reached by the first operator; and $Ed = 0.77 \pm 34$, $Ad = 0.89 \pm 0.36$, and $Ang = 1.58 \pm 0.83°$ by the second one, with $Ed = 0.62 \pm 34$, $Ad = 0.69 \pm 37$, and $Ang = 1.31 \pm 0.76°$ as the mean values between each of them. An identical value of *Edx*, $0.15 \pm 0.1$, was identified for both operators. The second operator's minimal deviations, as reported above with the previous methods, regarded the *Edx, Ed,* and *Ad* variables (Table 2).

**Table 2.** Means, SDs (Standard Deviations), and extreme values for each operator from the three methods of evaluation.

| Methods of Evaluation | Operator | Parameters | *Edx* | *Edy* | *Edz* | *Ed* | *Adx* | *Ady* | *Adz* | *Ad* | *Ang* |
|---|---|---|---|---|---|---|---|---|---|---|---|
| n.1 | 1 | mean | 0.14 | 0.16 | 0.74 | 0.8 | 0.15 | 0.25 | 0.76 | 0.85 | 1.05 |
| | | SD | 0.10 | 0.13 | 0.45 | 0.43 | 0.10 | 0.21 | 0.44 | 0.39 | 0.53 |
| | | minimum | 0.00 | 0.01 | 0.08 | 0.22 | 0.17 | 0.00 | 0.03 | 0.36 | 0.24 |
| | | maximum | 0.34 | 0.61 | 1.92 | 1.92 | 0.41 | 1.15 | 1.92 | 1.93 | 2.13 |
| | 2 | mean | 0.28 | 0.31 | 0.75 | 0.91 | 0.28 | 0.43 | 0.77 | 1.02 | 1.78 |
| | | SD | 0.19 | 0.22 | 0.49 | 0.46 | 0.22 | 0.3 | 0.5 | 0.45 | 1.12 |
| | | minimum | 0.41 | 0.01 | 0.00 | 0.19 | 0.00 | 0.01 | 0.01 | 0.24 | 0.13 |
| | | maximum | 0.83 | 0.76 | 2.02 | 2.15 | 0.88 | 1.11 | 1.96 | 2.27 | 4.13 |
| n.2 | 1 | mean | 0.15 | 0.3 | 0.22 | 0.45 | 0.18 | 0.32 | 0.22 | 0.48 | 1.03 |
| | | SD | 0.12 | 0.2 | 0.19 | 0.23 | 0.13 | 0.25 | 0.18 | 0.24 | 0.47 |
| | | minimum | 0.00 | 0.01 | 0.01 | 0.16 | 0.02 | 0.01 | 0.01 | 0.21 | 0.11 |
| | | maximum | 0.5 | 0.71 | 0.92 | 1.18 | 0.63 | 1.07 | 0.84 | 1.36 | 2.19 |
| | 2 | mean | 0.16 | 0.58 | 0.52 | 0.87 | 0.23 | 0.57 | 0.53 | 0.95 | 1.58 |
| | | SD | 0.13 | 0.36 | 0.41 | 0.45 | 0.19 | 0.43 | 0.45 | 0.42 | 0.97 |
| | | minimum | 0.01 | 0.07 | 0.07 | 0.13 | 0.01 | 0.01 | 0.07 | 0.24 | 0.04 |
| | | maximum | 0.49 | 1.23 | 1.65 | 1.77 | 0.64 | 1.5 | 1.78 | 1.79 | 3.62 |
| n.3 | 1 | mean | 0.15 | 0.33 | 0.23 | 0.47 | 0.17 | 0.34 | 0.23 | 0.49 | 1.05 |
| | | SD | 0.1 | 0.27 | 0.15 | 0.27 | 0.14 | 0.25 | 0.15 | 0.25 | 0.57 |
| | | minimum | 0.01 | 0.01 | 0.00 | 0.09 | 0.00 | 0.01 | 0.01 | 0.06 | 0.21 |
| | | maximum | 0.4 | 0.86 | 0.65 | 1.04 | 0.55 | 0.89 | 0.63 | 1.06 | 2.66 |
| | 2 | mean | 0.15 | 0.49 | 0.48 | 0.77 | 0.22 | 0.65 | 0.41 | 0.89 | 1.58 |
| | | SD | 0.11 | 0.32 | 0.33 | 0.34 | 0.17 | 0.42 | 0.27 | 0.36 | 0.83 |
| | | minimum | 0.01 | 0.03 | 0.02 | 0.07 | 0.01 | 0.04 | 0.02 | 0.3 | 0.08 |
| | | maximum | 0.43 | 1.24 | 1.05 | 1.44 | 0.63 | 1.65 | 1.01 | 1.77 | 3.19 |

A statistically significant difference ($p < 0.05$) resulted between method n.1 and both the methods n.2 and n.3, except for the *Adx* and *Ang* values, with no differences between the n.2 and n.3 optic scanner evaluations for all the variables (Table 3).

**Table 3.** Pairwise ANOVA analysis (Tukey HSD test) correlating the single dependent variables mean results from the two operators for each evaluation method.

| Parameters of Evaluation | Evaluation Methods' Comparison | Operators' Mean Values' for Each Method | | Mean Values' Difference | HSD-Test | *p* Value |
|---|---|---|---|---|---|---|
| *Ed* | n.1 vs n.2 | 0.8564 | 0.6209 | 0.1987 | 9.4939 * | >0.05 |
| | n.1 vs. n.3 | 0.8564 | 0.6209 | 0.2355 | 11.2534 * | >0.05 |
| | n.2 vs. n.3 | 0.6577 | 0.1560 | 0.0368 | 1.7594 | <0.05 |
| *Edx* | n.1 vs. n.2 | 0.2147 | 0.1501 | 0.0586 | 5.9700 * | >0.05 |
| | n.1 vs. n.3 | 0.2147 | 0.1501 | 0.0646 | 6.5715 * | >0.05 |
| | n.2 vs. n.3 | 0.1560 | 0.4414 | 0.0059 | 0.6015 | <0.05 |
| *Edy* | n.1 vs. n.2 | 0.2345 | 0.4120 | 0.2069 | 10.2443 * | >0.05 |
| | n.1 vs. n.3 | 0.2345 | 0.4120 | 0.1776 | 8.7926 * | >0.05 |
| | n.2 vs. n.3 | 0.4414 | 0.3717 | 0.0293 | 1.4518 | <0.05 |
| *Edz* | n.1 vs. n.2 | 0.7485 | 0.3532 | 0.3768 | 12.7676 * | >0.05 |
| | n.1 vs. n.3 | 0.7485 | 0.3532 | 0.3953 | 13.3953 * | >0.05 |
| | n.2 vs. n.3 | 0.3717 | 0.7185 | 0.0185 | 0.6277 | <0.05 |
| *Ad* | n.1 vs. n.2 | 0.9335 | 0.6905 | 0.2150 | 10.4235 * | >0.05 |
| | n.1 vs. n.3 | 0.9335 | 0.6905 | 0.2431 | 11.7842 * | >0.05 |
| | n.2 vs. n.3 | 0.7185 | 0.2019 | 0.0281 | 1.3607 | <0.05 |
| *Adx* | n.1 vs. n.2 | 0.2166 | 0.1974 | 0.0147 | 1.3931 | <0.05 |
| | n.1 vs. n.3 | 0.2166 | 0.1974 | 0.0193 | 1.8236 | <0.05 |
| | n.2 vs. n.3 | 0.2019 | 0.4486 | 0.0045 | 0.4305 | <0.05 |
| *Ady* | n.1 vs. n.2 | 0.3387 | 0.4952 | 0.1099 | 5.1349 * | >0.05 |
| | n.1 vs. n.3 | 0.3387 | 0.4952 | 0.1565 | 7.3113 * | >0.05 |
| | n.2 vs. n.3 | 0.4486 | 0.3759 | 0.0466 | 2.1763 | <0.05 |
| *Adz* | n.1 vs. n.2 | 0.7626 | 0.3239 | 0.3867 | 12.8877 * | >0.05 |
| | n.1 vs. n.3 | 0.7626 | 0.3239 | 0.4387 | 14.6223 * | >0.05 |
| | n.2 vs. n.3 | 0.3759 | 1.3059 | 0.0520 | 1.7346 | <0.05 |
| *Ang* | n.1 vs. n.2 | 1.4127 | 1.3144 | 0.1068 | 3.1201 | <0.05 |
| | n.1 vs. n.3 | 1.4127 | 1.3144 | 0.0983 | 2.8712 | <0.05 |
| | n.2 vs. n.3 | 1.3059 | 0.6577 | 0.0085 | 0.2489 | <0.05 |

* Statistic insignificance.

The mean values from the three methods were 0.57 mm (*Ed*), 0.60 mm (*Ad*), and 1.04° (*Ang*) for the first, and 0.85 mm (*Ed*), 0.95 mm (*Ad*), and 1.64° (*Ang*) for the second operator. Figure 4 contains the box plots comparing the two operators relative to the mean values of the three methods.

**Table 4.** Double-tailed *t*-test verifying a significant difference between the two operators in terms of implant placement velocity.

| Operator | Obs | Mean | SD | [Intervallo Conf. 95%] | | *t* | *p* Value |
|---|---|---|---|---|---|---|---|
| 1 | 5 | 14.24 | 3.91 | 9.38 | 19.1 | −3.9 | 0.0046 |
| 2 | 5 | 25.48 | 5.13 | 19.1 | 31.86 | | |
| combined | 10 | 19.86 | 7.32 | 14.62 | 25.1 | | |
| differents | | −11.24 | | −17.89 | −4.59 | | |

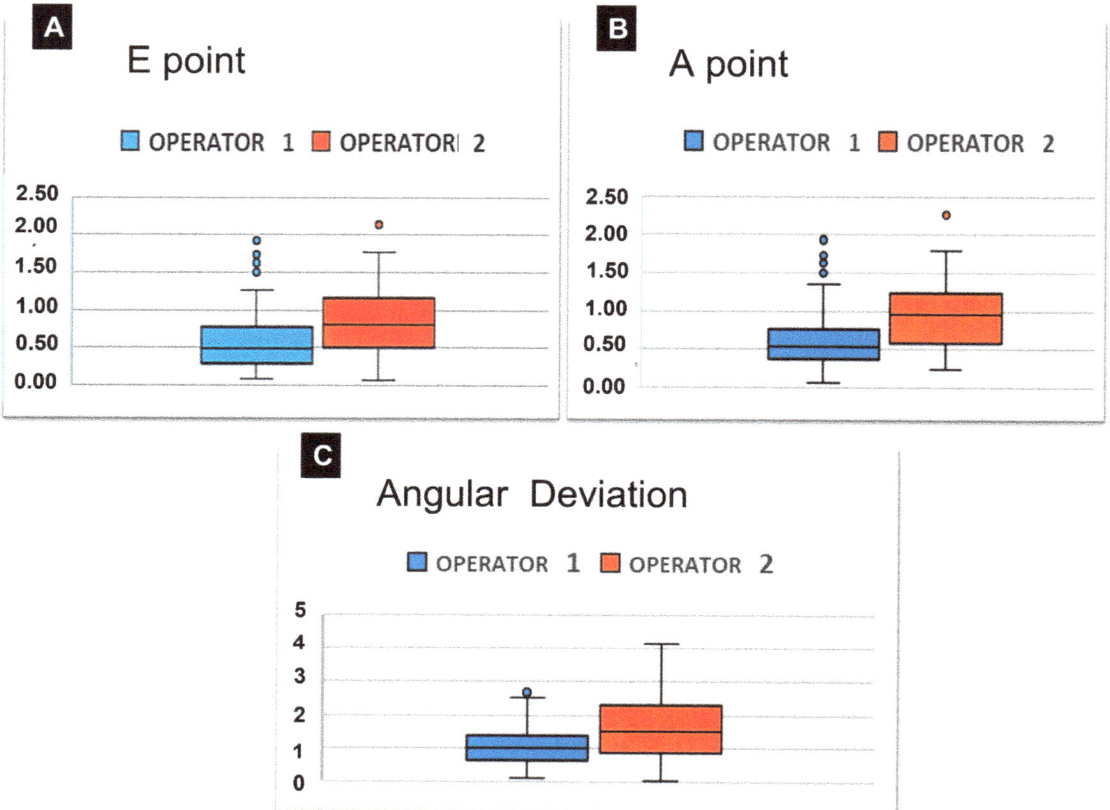


**Figure 4.** Box-plots showing the comparison of the two operators relative to the mean values from the three methods evaluation for E point (**A**), A point (**B**), and angular deviation (**C**).

A positive correlation resulted between the number of progressively implanted models and the implant placement accuracy, although this result was statistically significant for the second operator only (Table 4).

### 3.2. *Operative Timings*

The first operator accomplished the implant seating with a mean time of 14.24 min for each model, which was less than 25.48 min taken by the second operator, and this difference was statistically significant ($p < 0.05$) (Table 5).

**Table 5.** Linear regression model for the correlation of the sequence of the model preparation and the operator error in implant placement.

| Operator | Coef | Standard Error | *t* | [Intervallo Conf. 95%] | | *p* Value |
|---|---|---|---|---|---|---|
| 1 | −1.271402 | 0.29 | −4.42 | −2.19 | −0.36 | 0.021 |
| 2 | −1.30442 | 0.47 | −2.80 | −2.79 | 0.18 | 0.068 |

## 4. Discussion

Freehand dental implantology depends on the manual skills of the operator, particularly for the axial implant shifting to what is prosthetically required [23]. An average angular deviation of 3.04° (ranging from 0.4–6.3°) and 7.03° (ranging from 0.7–21.3°) has been reported for s-CAI and traditional treatment, respectively [24]. Younes et al. reported that 19.2% of the freehand-placed implants were bearing cement-retained prostheses compared to 100% of screw-retained super-structures on fixtures inserted with digital guides [6]. An overall accuracy value with s-CAI systems has been reported as ≤1 mm for all linear evaluations and ≤5° for angular shifting [4,25]. Provided there is the correct procedure for realizing the digital template, the principal reason for the higher precision of the s-CAI could be that the human error is reduced. The present study tried to investigate the possible relevance of human expertise intended to enhance the accuracy and reduce the operative timing as derived from the repetition of a specific practical activity over time. The method followed aimed to eliminate, as much as possible, the factors interfering with the univocal interpretation of the data. Since the present study was undertaken "in vitro", it was not affected by the variables of clinical practice that would not have been reduced by using an operative guide and allowed a novice operator to carry out the procedure independently. The models used in this trial reproduced similar edentulous mandibular situations with the same complexity level. The flowchart for guide manufacturing was simplified to minimize the risk of procedural mistakes and a bone-supported device was planned without an opposite dental arcade and the soft tissues feature. Since the guides' application to the model was performed by the expert dentist and accurately controlled, the possible bias related to an error in this phase was prevented. The present trial results are, on the other hand, poorly attributable to flapless approaches where soft tissue scanning is mandatory.

The major accuracy for the expert operator recorded reported in this study confirms what has been reported in in vitro trials [2,26–28] while clinical studies are inconsistent [29,30]. One study reported more accuracy with the guided digital system than with the free-hands systems when used by novices [2]. An average of 1.12 mm and a maximum value of 4.5 mm at the entry point, an average of 1.39 mm and a maximum value of 7.1 mm at the apex point, and an average axis shifting of 3.89°, and a maximum value of 21.16° were recorded in in vivo studies reported in a literature review [4]. Naeini et al. reported 1.00 mm, 1.23 mm, and 3.13° for coronal, apical, and angular deviations respectively, in another clinical literature review about the flapless technique [7]. Cuhna et al. recorded, in vivo, a mean angular deviation of 2.04 degrees and mean coronal, central, and apical linear deviations of 0.68 mm, 0.72 mm, and 0.82 mm, respectively [29]. The present study's overall deviations were lower than those in the literature studies with patients, particularly for angular shifting, both for expert and inexpert operators, regardless of evaluation methods.

Strictly correlated with the experience is the learning curve concept, which expresses that there are a progressive number of attempts needed to reach a repeatable level of precision. The awareness of this data helps standardize and optimize the method of training. With reference to the d-CAI, e.g., Block et al., in a clinical trial, reported the presence of a learning curve, and set the twentieth attempt as the initial plateau case [30]. Cassetta et al. did not find a learning curve for s-CAI after analyzing the results from two different implantologists, both experts in the freehand procedure but inexpert with the s-CAI, who were working on totally edentulous patients. At the same time, a significant correlation between coronal and angular deviation and the progressive number of treated cases over time, emerged for partially edentulous subjects [16]. Nevertheless, the authors accept that a reduced sample size and the absence of the operative timing evaluation are limits of their trial. No in vitro studies have correlated the accuracy of implant placement with the progressive number of operative performances.

Even if a real learning curve reaching the same accuracy level plateau was not identified, a continuous enhancement of accuracy for both operators over time resulted in the present survey.

The habit of managing the physical opposition of the bone during the implant placement phases by keeping a steady position of the handle-piece, has maintained its importance [7,15]. Nevertheless, the reported deviations in the present study were so low that the differences between the two operators did not compromise the final results of the procedure. The major reliability of s-CAI with respect to the freehand approach was confirmed. On the basis that the fitting between the sleeves and the drills is considered crucial for implant placement accuracy, the adopted device's characteristics may have positively affected the outcomes. The present study adopted specific disposable poly-ether-ether-ketone (PEEK) sleeves, as used in another similar trial [31]. This innovation, proposed for the same purposes in orthopedics [32], should give less rigidity to the system while keeping a good fitting with the drills, thanks to the thermoplastic properties of the PEEK. The templates with tunnels directly printed according to the digital project appear more customized than those with standard metallic sleeves inserted subsequently in the device at the designed positions.

Nevertheless, particularly in partial edentulism with five residual teeth at least, these devices reached a similar level of accuracy [33,34].

Before the advent of optical scanners, the way for evaluating the superimposition of virtually placed with actually placed implants was through the comparison of the pre-and postoperative CT scans [35,36]. The "indirect" methods, with the EOS or IOS, avoid a second x-ray exam for the patient, but are prone to the above-cited shortcomings in the phase of imaging data acquisition. Impression distortions and related cast imprecisions for EOS, intraoral conditions, and the movements of the patients or erroneous device movements during IOS, can affect the accuracy of STL data [20,34] along with causing an imprecise connection with the scanning pins for both techniques. Furthermore, the quality of the 3D planning software algorithms for matching DICOM and STL files affects the absolute reliability of the s-CAI using optical scanners [35]. Regarding in vitro surveys, Stefanelli et al. reported a minimal discrepancy between a new type of IOS with improved scan bodies and the EOS [37]; and Franchina et al. did not find a significant difference between the outcomes from radiographic, EOS, and IOS methods of accuracy evaluation as compared to free-hand implantology, s-CAI, and d-CAI methods,, as accomplished by a relevant expert in each [31]. A notable discrepancy among the outcomes of scanning and radiologic evaluation methods emerged in the literature [19,20,34,37]. Since a gold standard has not yet been stated, it was declared that cross-validation using both direct and indirect methods should be recommended [7,11,16]. The present trial adopted and compared the results from three assessment methods to eliminate the evaluation bias highlighted by several papers.

A recent literature review on clinical studies revealed that a pre-and postoperative comparison of CT images, a scanned post-surgical model, and intraoral optical scanning were adopted for accuracy evaluation in eight, two, and four studies, respectively [35].

The average values between the expert and the novice operators for the three methods were 0.2 mm, 0.3 mm, and 0.6° for the *Ed, Ad,* and *Ang* parameters, confirming the apex orientation and the implant inclination as the most critical points. Skjerven et al. reported in vivo studies showing a significant difference between the deviation measurements for coronal and apex points with pre-and postoperative CBCT and pre-op CBCT and post-op IOS [19].

In particular, the overall mean angular deviation value from the three methods, i.e., 1.04° and 1.64° for the expert and the novice operators respectively, were both lower than those reported by a similar study in vitro: i.e., 3.23 $\pm$ 1.00°, as an average of radiological and optical scanning analysis. In addition, a lower deviation resulted when comparing our angular results by method n.1: i.e., 1.05 $\pm$ 0.53° and 1.78 $\pm$ 1.12° for experienced and novice operators, respectively, with the 2.60 $\pm$1.25°, and the 3.96 $\pm$ 1.64° results of Cushen & Turkyilmaz, who adopted only the CBCT pre-and post- superimposition data as analysis [28]. In any case, an exhaustive comparison within the different trials is challenging due to many variables related to data importing, matching, and the elaboration processes, even in the same method adopted.

## 5. Conclusions

The present trial confirmed, by all three analysis methods, that there was an impressive level of accuracy for novice and skilled implantologists with s-CAI, which was undoubtedly superior to the free-hand approach. The starting experience and the improvement in precision over time was significantly relevant to implementing the implant placement reliability.

**Author Contributions:** Conceptualization: G.P. and F.D.; methodology: G.P., A.F. and G.L.; software: F.D., L.V.S. and G.P.; validation: A.M., F.D.B. and P.F.; formal analysis: A.F., G.L., G.P. and F.D.B.; resources: G.P.; data curation: P.F., A.M. and G.P.; writing—original draft preparation: G.L.; writing—review and editing: G.L.; visualization: P.F. and G.P.; supervision: G.P. and L.V.S.; project administration: G.P.; funding acquisition: G.P. All authors have read and agreed to the published version of the manuscript.

**Funding:** This research received no external funding.

**Institutional Review Board Statement:** Not applicable.

**Informed Consent Statement:** Not applicable.

**Conflicts of Interest:** The authors declare no conflict of interest.

## References

1. Pellegrino, G.; Lizio, G.; Ferri, A.; Marchetti, C. Flapless and bone-preserving extraction of partially impacted mandibular third molars with dynamic navigation technology. A report of three cases. *Int. J. Comput. Dent.* **2021**, *24*, 253–262.
2. Abduo, J.; Lau, D. Accuracy of static computer-assisted implant placement in long span edentulous area by novice implant clinicians: A cross-sectional in vitro study comparing fully-guided, pilot-guided, and freehand implant placement protocols. *Clin. Implant Dent. Relat. Res.* **2021**, *23*, 361–372. [CrossRef]
3. Pellegrino, G.; Bellini, P.; Cavallini, P.F.; Ferri, A.; Zacchino, A.; Taraschi, V.; Marchetti, C.; Consolo, U. Dynamic Navigation in Dental Implantology: The Influence of Surgical Experience on Implant Placement Accuracy and Operating Time. An in Vitro Study. *Int. J. Environ. Res. Public Health* **2020**, *17*, 2153. [CrossRef]
4. Tahmaseb, A.; Wu, V.; Wismeijer, D.; Coucke, W.; Evans, C. The accuracy of static computer-aided implant surgery: A systematic review and meta-analysis. *Clin. Oral Implants Res.* **2018**, *29* (Suppl. S16), 416–435. [CrossRef]
5. Younes, F.; Eghbali, A.; De Bruyckere, T.; Cleymaet, R.; Cosyn, J. A randomized controlled trial on the efficiency of free-handed, pilot-drill guided and fully guided implant surgery in partially edentulous patients. *Clin. Oral Implants Res.* **2019**, *30*, 131–138. [CrossRef]
6. Vermeulen, J. The Accuracy of Implant Placement by Experienced Surgeons: Guided vs. Freehand Approach in a Simulated Plastic Model. *Int. J. Oral Maxillofac. Implants* **2017**, *32*, 617–624. [CrossRef]
7. Naeini, E.N.; Atashkadeh, M.; De Bruyn, H.; D'Haese, J. Narrative review regarding the applicability, accuracy, and clinical outcome of flapless implant surgery with or without computer guidance. *Clin. Implant Dent. Relat. Res.* **2020**, *22*, 454–467. [CrossRef]
8. Joda, T.; Derksen, W.; Wittneben, J.G.; Kuehl, S. Static computer-aided implant surgery (s-CAIS) analysing patient-reported outcome measures (PROMs), economics and surgical complications: A systematic review. *Clin. Oral Implants Res.* **2018**, *29* (Suppl. S16), 359–373. [CrossRef]
9. Vercruyssen, M.; Laleman, I.; Jacobs, R.; Quirynen, M. Computer-supported implant planning and guided surgery: A narrative review. *Clin. Oral Implants Res.* **2015**, *26* (Suppl. S11), 69–76. [CrossRef]
10. Elliott, T.; Hamilton, A.; Griseto, N.; Gallucci, G.O. Additively Manufactured Surgical Implant Guides: A Review. *J. Prosthodont.* **2022**, *31* (Suppl. S1), 38–46. [CrossRef]
11. Anadioti, E.; Kane, B.; Zhang, Y.; Bergler, M.; Mante, F.; Blatz, M.B. Accuracy of Dental and Industrial 3D Printers. *J. Prosthodont.* **2022**, *31* (Suppl. S1), 30–37. [CrossRef]
12. Derksen, W.; Wismeijer, D.; Flügge, T.; Hassan, B.; Tahmaseb, A. The accuracy of computer-guided implant surgery with tooth-supported, digitally designed drill guides based on CBCT and intraoral scanning. A prospective cohort study. *Clin. Oral Implants Res.* **2019**, *30*, 1005–1015. [CrossRef]
13. Cassetta, M.; Bellardini, M. How much does experience in guided implant surgery play a role in accuracy? A randomized controlled pilot study. *Int. J. Oral Maxillofac. Surg.* **2017**, *46*, 922–930. [CrossRef]
14. Van de Wiele, G.; Teughels, W.; Vercruyssen, M.; Coucke, W.; Temmerman, A.; Quirynen, M. The accuracy of guided surgery via mucosa-supported stereolithographic surgical templates in the hands of surgeons with little experience. *Clin. Oral Implants Res.* **2015**, *26*, 1489–1494. [CrossRef]
15. Van Assche, N.; Quirynen, M. Tolerance within a surgical guide. *Clin. Oral Implants Res.* **2010**, *21*, 455–458. [CrossRef]

16. Cassetta, M.; Altieri, F.; Giansanti, M.; Bellardini, M.; Brandetti, G.; Piccoli, L. Is there a learning curve in static computer-assisted implant surgery? A prospective clinical study. *Int. J. Oral Maxillofac. Surg.* **2020**, *49*, 1335–1342. [CrossRef]
17. Bover-Ramos, F.; Viña-Almunia, J.; Cervera-Ballester, J.; Peñarrocha-Diago, M.; García-Mira, B. Accuracy of Implant Placement with Computer-Guided Surgery: A Systematic Review and Meta-Analysis Comparing Cadaver, Clinical, and In Vitro Studies. *Int. J. Oral Maxillofac. Implants* **2018**, *33*, 101–115. [CrossRef]
18. Verhamme, L.M.; Meijer, G.J.; Boumans, T.; Schutyser, F.; Bergé, S.J.; Maal, T.J.J. A clinically relevant validation method for implant placement after virtual planning. *Clin. Oral Implants Res.* **2013**, *24*, 1265–1272. [CrossRef]
19. Skjerven, H.; Olsen-Bergem, H.; Rønold, H.J.; Riis, U.H.; Ellingsen, J.E. Comparison of postoperative intraoral scan versus cone beam computerised tomography to measure accuracy of guided implant placement—A prospective clinical study. *Clin. Oral Implants Res.* **2019**, *30*, 531–541. [CrossRef]
20. Park, J.H.; Hwang, C.J.; Choi, Y.J.; Houschyar, K.S.; Yu, J.-H.; Bae, S.-Y.; Cha, J.-Y. Registration of digital dental models and cone-beam computed tomography images using 3-dimensional planning software: Comparison of the accuracy according to scanning methods and software. *Am. J. Orthod. Dentofac. Orthop.* **2020**, *157*, 843–851. [CrossRef]
21. Kessler, A.; Le, V.; Folwaczny, M. Influence of the tooth position, guided sleeve height, supporting length, manufacturing methods, and resin E-modulus on the in vitro accuracy of surgical implant guides in a free-end situation. *Clin. Oral Implants Res.* **2021**, *32*, 1097–1104. [CrossRef]
22. Schnutenhaus, S.; Edelmann, C.; Rudolph, H. Does the macro design of an implant affect the accuracy of template-guided implantation? A prospective clinical study. *Int. J. Implant Dent.* **2021**, *7*, 42. [CrossRef]
23. Jemt, T.; Olsson, M.; Renouard, F.; Stenport, V.; Friberg, B. Early Implant Failures Related to Individual Surgeons: An Analysis Covering 11,074 Operations Performed during 28 Years. *Clin. Implant Dent. Relat. Res.* **2016**, *18*, 861–872. [CrossRef]
24. Varga, E., Jr.; Antal, M.; Major, L.; Kiscsatári, R.; Braunitzer, G.; Piffkó, J. Guidance means accuracy: A randomized clinical trial on freehand versus guided dental implantation. *Clin. Oral Implants Res.* **2020**, *31*, 417–430. [CrossRef]
25. Jorba-García, A.; González-Barnadas, A.; Camps-Font, O.; Figueiredo, R.; Valmaseda-Castellón, E. Accuracy assessment of dynamic computer-aided implant placement: A systematic review and meta-analysis. *Clin. Oral Investig.* **2021**, *25*, 2479–2494. [CrossRef]
26. Fernández-Gil, Á.; Gil, H.S.; Velasco, M.G.; Vázquez, J. An In Vitro Model to Evaluate the Accuracy of Guided Implant Placement Based on the Surgeon's Experience. *Int. J. Oral Maxillofac. Implants* **2017**, *32*, 515–524. [CrossRef]
27. Pettersson, A.; Kero, T.; Söderberg, R.; Näsström, K. Accuracy of virtually planned and CAD/CAM-guided implant surgery on plastic models. *J. Prosthet. Dent.* **2014**, *112*, 1472–1478. [CrossRef]
28. Cushen, S.E.; Turkyilmaz, I. Impact of operator experience on the accuracy of implant placement with stereolithographic surgical templates: An in vitro study. *J. Prosthet. Dent.* **2013**, *109*, 248–254. [CrossRef]
29. Cunha, R.M.; Souza, F.A.; Hadad, H.; Poli, P.P.; Maiorana, C.; Carvalho, P.S.P. Accuracy evaluation of computer-guided implant surgery associated with prototyped surgical guides. *J. Prosthet. Dent.* **2021**, *125*, 266–272. [CrossRef]
30. Block, M.S.; Emery, R.W.; Lank, K.; Ryan, J. Implant Placement Accuracy Using Dynamic Navigation. *Int. J. Oral Maxillofac. Implants* **2017**, *32*, 92–99. [CrossRef]
31. Franchina, A.; Stefanelli, L.V.; Maltese, F.; Mandelaris, G.A.; Vantaggiato, A.; Pagliarulo, M.; Pranno, N.; Brauner, E.; Angelis, F.D.; Carlo, S.D. Validation of an Intra-Oral Scan Method Versus Cone Beam Computed Tomography Superimposition to Assess the Accuracy between Planned and Achieved Dental Implants: A Randomized In Vitro Study. *Int. J. Environ. Res. Public Health* **2020**, *17*, 9358. [CrossRef]
32. Choi, D.; Yoon, Y.S.; Hwang, D. Evaluation of sleeved implant fixation using a rat model. *Med. Eng. Phys.* **2011**, *33*, 310–314. [CrossRef] [PubMed]
33. Kiatkroekkrai, P.; Takolpuckdee, C.; Subbalekha, K.; Mattheos, N.; Pimkhaokham, A. Accuracy of implant position when placed using static computer-assisted implant surgical guides manufactured with two different optical scanning techniques: A randomized clinical trial. *Int. J. Oral Maxillofac. Surg.* **2020**, *49*, 377–383. [CrossRef] [PubMed]
34. Tallarico, M.; Xhanari, E.; Kim, Y.J.; Cocchi, F.; Martinolli, M.; Alushi, A.; Baldoni, E.; Meloni, S.M. Accuracy of computer-assisted template-based implant placement using conventional impression and scan model or intraoral digital impression: A randomised controlled trial with 1 year of follow-up. *Int. J. Oral Implantol.* **2019**, *12*, 197–206.
35. Putra, R.H.; Yoda, N.; Astuti, E.R.; Sasaki, K. The accuracy of implant placement with computer-guided surgery in partially edentulous patients and possible influencing factors: A systematic review and meta-analysis. *J. Prosthodont. Res.* **2022**, *66*, 29–39. [CrossRef]
36. Pyo, S.W.; Lim, Y.J.; Koo, K.T.; Lee, J. Methods Used to Assess the 3D Accuracy of Dental Implant Positions in Computer-Guided Implant Placement: A Review. *J. Clin. Med.* **2019**, *8*, 54. [CrossRef]
37. Stefanelli, L.V.; Franchina, A.; Pranno, A.; Pellegrino, G.; Ferri, A.; Pranno, N.; Di Carlo, S.; De Angelis, F. Use of Intraoral Scanners for Full Dental Arches: Could Different Strategies or Overlapping Software Affect Accuracy? *Int. J. Environ. Res. Public Health* **2021**, *18*, 9946. [CrossRef]

*applied sciences*

MDPI

*Hypothesis*

# Reverse Guided Bone Regeneration (R-GBR) Digital Workflow for Atrophic Jaws Rehabilitation

**Pietro Felice [1], Giuseppe Lizio [1,*], Carlo Barausse [1], Lorenzo Roccoli [1], Lorenzo Bonifazi [1], Roberto Pistilli [2], Massimo Simion [3] and Gerardo Pellegrino [1]**

1 Department of Biomedical and Neuromotor Sciences (DIBINEM), University of Bologna, 40125 Bologna, Italy
2 Unit of Oral and Maxillofacial Surgery, San Camillo Hospital, 00152 Rome, Italy
3 Department of Biomedical, Surgical and Dental Sciences, University of Milan, 20122 Milano, Italy
* Correspondence: giuseppe.lizio2@unibo.it

**Abstract: Background**: Treating extended alveolar defects is challenging for their irregular shape and lack of hard and soft tissues. Virtual planned guided bone regeneration (GBR) with customized meshes aims to optimize the treatment by reducing the risk of dehiscence. The mucosa characteristics are crucial in preserving the bone graft covering and vitality. **Methods**: Two three-dimensional and extended defects, a mandibular posterior and anterior maxillary atrophy were reconstructed with a particulate graft and a digitally customized scaffold. The workflow entailed merging the pre-operatory clinical related data from intra-oral scanning with the radiologic ones from cone beam-CT. A final ideal prediction of the soft tissue relationship with the implant-borne prosthesis was virtually elaborated, conditioning the design of the titanium membrane fitting the bone defects. **Results**: A good matching between the scaffold and the bone surface was intra-operatory noted; no complications were registered in the first months of healing with complete integrity of the soft tissues above the graft. **Conclusions**: A careful evaluation of the soft tissues and a forecast of their final relationship with the implant and prosthesis can improve digital mesh/membrane manufacturing with a suitable healing process up to implant placement and loading, favoring peri-implant tissue stability over time.

**Keywords:** virtual planning; GBR; titanium meshes; digital workflow

**Citation:** Felice, P.; Lizio, G.; Barausse, C.; Roccoli, L.; Bonifazi, L.; Pistilli, R.; Simion, M.; Pellegrino, G. Reverse Guided Bone Regeneration (R-GBR) Digital Workflow for Atrophic Jaws Rehabilitation. *Appl. Sci.* **2022**, *12*, 9947. https://doi.org/10.3390/app12199947

Academic Editors: Giuliana Muzio and Bert Müller

Received: 19 July 2022
Accepted: 26 September 2022
Published: 3 October 2022



## 1. Introduction

Guided bone regeneration (GBR) with titanium meshes enabled clinicians to treat three-dimensional and extended defects due to the stiffness of their structure, which contains in situ the particulate graft and contrasts the collapse of the overlying soft tissues [1–3]. Digital technology improved this approach, allowing the design and printing of a scaffold that fits the defect to be reconstructed, correlating the bone grafting to what is needed to support the fixtures and reducing surgical timings and discomfort [1,4–6]. Hence, the dehiscence, the significant shortcoming of this technique, seems to be lowered [4,6,7], with >80% bone volume regeneration predictability of what was virtually planned [4,7–9]. Nevertheless, some doubts about the actual standardization of this approach were raised, and the reliability of the digital systems in realizing what is virtually planned is still unclear [2,4]. Indeed, the literature is scarce on patients and the methodology of the studies, with 97–100% implant survival rate up to 30 months of mean follow-up after implant loading [2,4,7]. When the exposure complication is manageable, appearing after about a month since the intervention and without signs of infection, the CAD/CAM GBR approach is reliable in fulfilling what was pre-operatively planned, homogenizing the outcomes [2].

The precision of the virtual project, comparing the starting clinical situation with the ideal prediction of the final result, is a crucial issue. The forecasting of peri-implant mucosa thickness and shape, and its interaction with the abutment and crowns to be reached at the end of treatment, can allow for predicting the surgical or prosthetic correction of the soft tissues before or after the bone reconstruction with a more accurate implant positioning [10]. Static computer-aided implantology (s-CAI) entails coupling the tissue surfaces data from intra- or extra-oral scanning with the radiographic hard tissues information from the CT to guide the seating of the fixtures. This approach obtained better results regarding insertion accuracy than the free-hand one [11]. The starting bone defect extension and the soft tissue characteristics were crucial in conditioning the GBR with membranes and no customized titanium meshes [12], even with a customized protocol [2,13]. Atrophic sites present an impaired mucosa, raising the muscle insertions toward the residual bone ridge and losing keratinized epithelium. The soft tissues can be irregular with different thicknesses, scars due to previous lesions and treatment, or particularly thin and fragile. A correct soft tissue evaluation can condition the flap design, reducing the exposure rate [13]. Furthermore, the passivation of the flap to cover the graft after the muscle detachment and the periosteum releasing cuts entails a vestibule reduction and a lifting of the mouth pavement with the necessity of soft tissue grafting procedures to obtain keratinized peri-implant marginal tissues [2,4,13]. According to a so-called fully digital protocol, two mono-edentulous sites were treated with implant insertion contextual to the bone reconstruction after pre-surgical planning of the ideal soft tissue architecture [14,15]. Another clinical case was managed by evaluating the vestibular mucosa thickness to resolve the horizontal deficit of an edentulous site with surgical soft tissue modification in combination with prosthetics tricks [10].

This paper proposes a modified workflow for manufacturing a mesh/membrane to reconstruct two different extended alveolar defects. This protocol was called "reverse" since the operative phase started after the digital prediction of the final ideal relationship between dental crowns and gingiva, adding the pre-operative clinical situation.

## 2. Materials and Methods

Two male patients were referred for a fixed prosthetic rehabilitation of their edentulous areas. The general health condition of both subjects did not contraindicate oral surgical procedures.

The clinical intra-oral exam of the first patient showed a left posterior mandible without premolars and molars, lost more than ten years before due to an untreated severe periodontal disease (Figure 1).

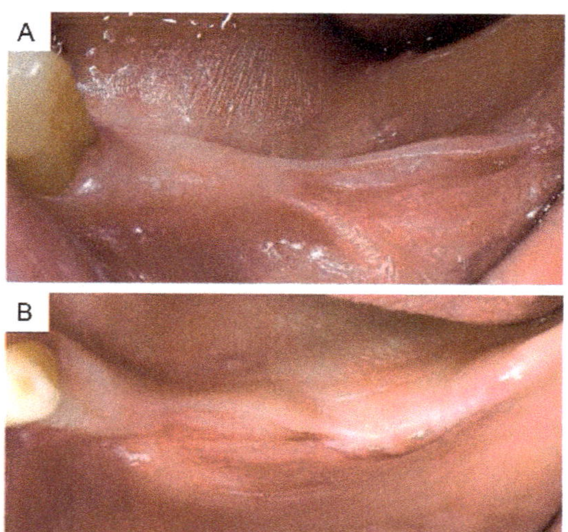


**Figure 1.** The pre-operative clinical situation of the first patient. Vestibular (**A**) and occlusal (**B**) point of view.

The edentulous lacuna of the second patient corresponded to the upper right pre-molars, canine and incisor area, including the left first incisor, lost for trauma and dental caries and temporarily rehabilitated with a removable residual teeth-supported prosthetic device. The mandibular arch, lacking the first molars, did not present other dental diseases (Figure 2).

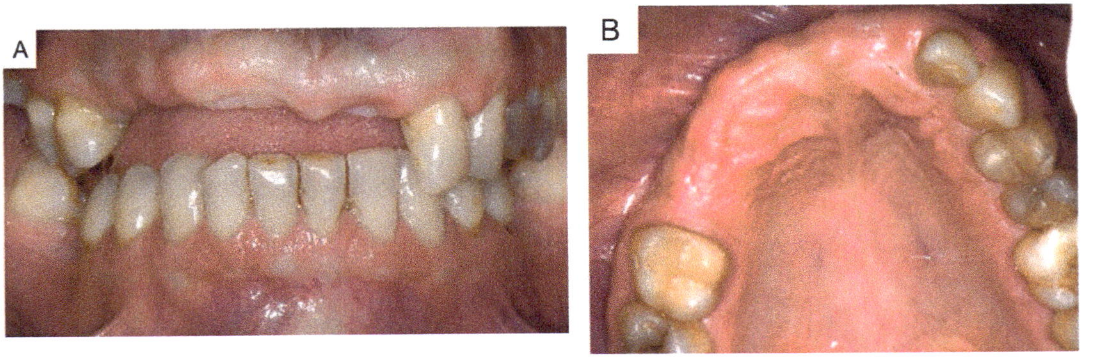


**Figure 2.** The pre-operative clinical situation of the second patient. Vestibular (**A**) and occlusal (**B**) point of view.

After taking a cone-beam CT (My Ray, Cefla, Imola, Italy), patients underwent scanning of the mouth with an intra-oral scanner (IOS) (iTero Element 2, Align Technology, CA, USA). The DICOM data relative to the bone status were coupled with the standard tessellation language (STL) files relative to the soft tissue characteristics. A virtual wax-up for the correct position of the dental crowns was performed according to the occlusal demands with the opposite dental arch; the crowns were subsequently superimposed to the bone and mucosa representation to identify the discrepancies between the prosthetic and anatomical issues. A simulation of the correct soft tissue final profile was set up, configuring the dimensions and shape of the papillae, and the implants were virtually positioned. The prediction of the bone reconstruction to provide the fixtures with sufficient support came after. The membrane was designed according to the hard tissue volume, position planned and the location of fixation screws. In the first case, it was planned to seat two standard implants in the second pre-molar and second molar location, sustaining a five-crown screw-retained fixed bridge. Implant placement in the canine position was considered after extracting the correspondent mobile tooth. This prosthetic solution entailed a vertical and horizontal bone regeneration of about 8 and 11 mm, respectively, in the molar zone and about 10 mm of thickness in correspondence to the second pre-molar location showing a knife-edge bone ridge (Figures 3 and 4).

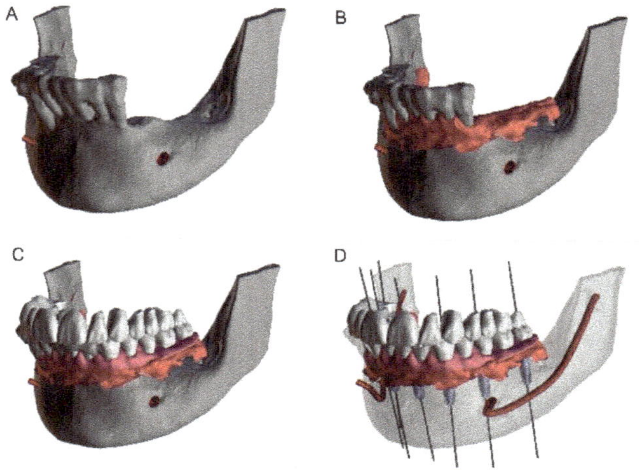


**Figure 3.** Virtual planning of the first case (phase 1). Bone defect after segmentation from pre-operative CBCT data (**A**); matching with the pre-operative soft tissue profile from the intra-oral scanning (**B**); superimposition of the digital wax-up and set up of the final ideal gingival architecture (**C**); virtual positioning of the fixtures (**D**).

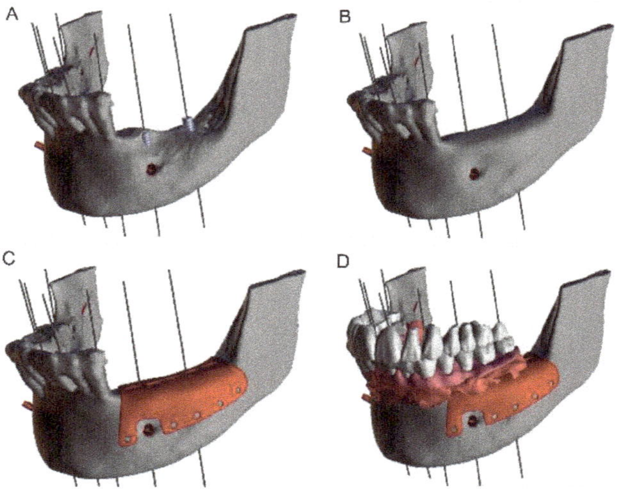


**Figure 4.** Virtual planning of the first case (phase 2). Ideal choice of the fixtures position and dimensions (**A**); simulation of the bone volume regeneration according to the final result prediction (**B**) and titanium membrane design (**C**,**D**).

The second case showed a vertical and horizontal bone deficit, with a residual bone ridge defining an extended fenestration. The digital wax-up for the correct crown position, the soft tissue ideal profile and the consequent implant locations guided the bone volume assessment and the relative mesh dimensions and shape (Figure 5).

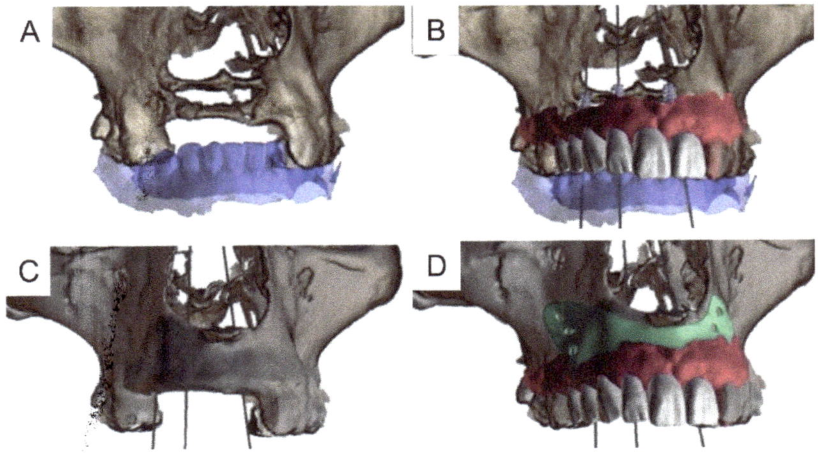


**Figure 5.** Virtual planning of the second case. Bone status after segmentation from pre-operative CBCT data coupled with the inferior arcade profile from STL data (**A**); the final prediction of rehabilitation according to the simulated ideal prosthetic and gingival profile (**B**); simulation of the necessary bone volume (**C**); the membrane design according to bone volume and final mucosal and prosthetic result (**D**).

Three standard implants were planned to be seated in the second premolar, right lateral and left central incisors location, supporting a six-crown screw-retained fixed bridge with a required bone reconstruction of about 4 mm and 8 mm in height and width, respectively. The virtual mesh/membrane, saved in STL format, was 3D-printed using digital machine laser sintering (DMLS) without macropores and a few fissures in correspondence to its coronal portion.

The same oral surgeon performed the surgical procedures in a dental office under local anesthesia. The bone defects were completely exposed after carefully raising a full-thickness trapezoidal buccal flap after a mid-crestal, two vertical releasing incisions and the detachment of a lingual/palatal flap. The flaps were coronally elongated by releasing incisions and dissection of the periosteum to obtain a complete passive closure on the mesh. Subsequently, bone chips from the buccal surface of the bone close to the defect were scraped with a bone collector. The autologous bone was mixed with a freeze-dried heterologous one (Osteobiol, Gen-Oss, Tecnoss, Turin, Italy) in a 70/30 ratio. The particulate graft was put to fill the deficit above the mesh (3DiFiC, Perugia, Italy) until its perfect stability and unity with the defect's borders. A suitable membrane fitting to the defect was noted without shifting before and after the graft placement. Three titanium mini-screws (Global D, Brignais, France) buccally stabilized the device in the mandibular defect. Two mini-screws in correspondence with the left lateral wall of the nose and the right molar pillar were inserted in the maxillary case. The flaps, coronally advanced before the graft application, were carefully sutured. Amoxicillin was assumed by the patient (two grams a day for six days) together with a non-steroidal analgesic (ibuprofen). The patients were instructed to avoid brushing on the surgical site, follow a soft diet for three weeks and maintain appropriate oral hygiene, including twice-daily rinsing with 0.2% chlorhexidine.

## 3. Results

During the post-operative healing period, patients were monitored monthly without complications until now (Figures 6 and 7).

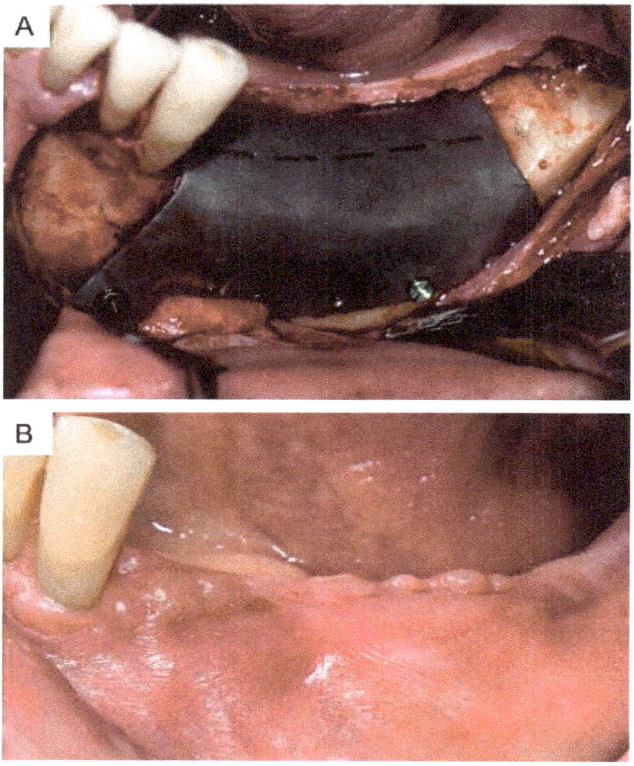

Figure 6. The intra-operatory vision of the fixed membrane (A) and clinical situation a month after surgery (B) relative to the first case.

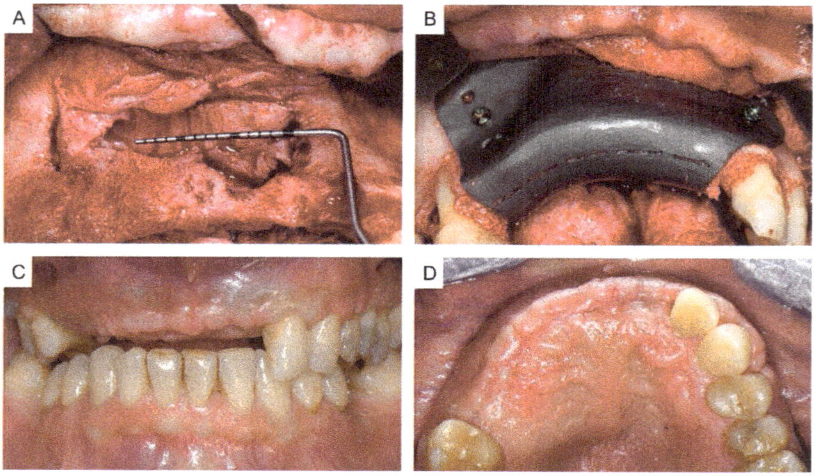

Figure 7. The intra-operatory clinical vision of the defect (A), the membrane fixed (B) and clinical situation a month after surgery (C,D).

A new cone-beam CT was taken to verify the bone augmentation and the mesh position after one month of healing, showing a good healing process without the membrane shifting (Figures 8 and 9).

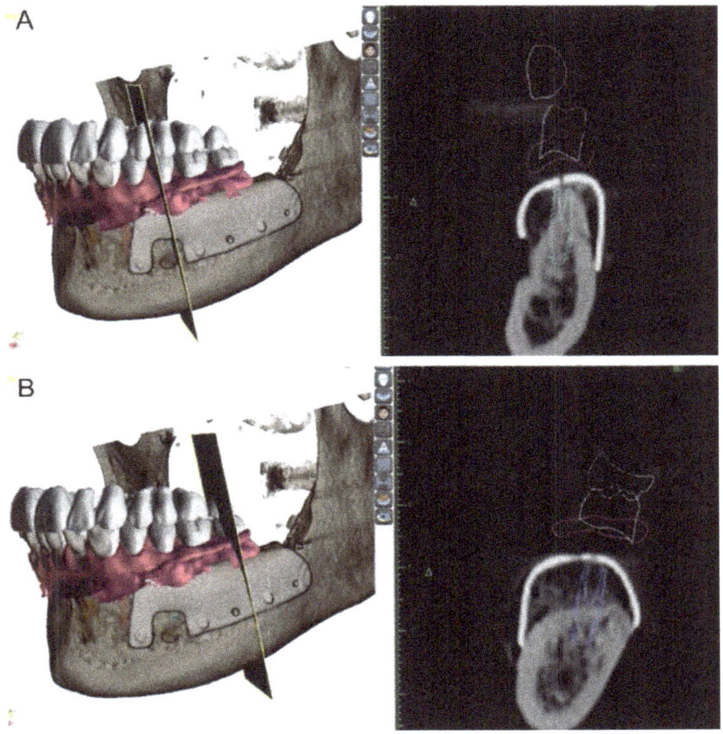


**Figure 8.** The cross–section CBCT images relative to the second premolar (**A**) and second molar implant location (**B**) in the first case after a month of healing.

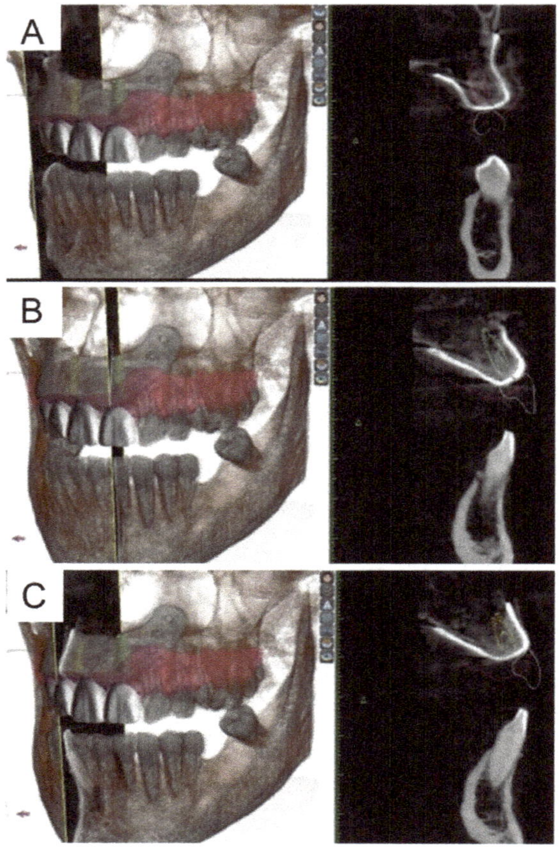


**Figure 9.** The cross−section CBCT images relative to the second premolar (**A**), right lateral (**B**) and left central incisors (**C**) location in the second case after a month of healing.

## 4. Discussion

The importance of soft tissues in conditioning a pre-implant reconstructive procedure was widely stated, protecting from infections and supplying nutrients and cells [16–21]. The relationship between the soft and hard tissues and their features conditions the choice of a bone augmentation technical approach or, otherwise, renouncing to it and accepting a prosthetic compromise.

The final prevision of the correct soft tissue profile with the prosthetic crowns can be particularly useful in managing complex alveolar defects with anatomic alterations and wrong occlusal interactions. Hence, the discussion between prosthodontists and patients allows for deciding the more suitable solution for each case. Screw-retained prostheses are today the fixed available solutions for partial edentulous atrophies with aesthetic, functional and hygienic demands [22]. The fixed bridge, without false gingiva and directly connected to the fixtures, requires a precise evaluation of the final soft tissue profile, particularly in the aesthetic zone.

The GBR technique is the most versatile approach, since the particulate graft, maintained by a scaffold, is adaptable to every defect shape. The use of titanium meshes enables the management of more critical defects with fewer infective complications than those with non-resorbable membranes, albeit a 0–68.9% of the reported exposure range [17,18,23].

The literature reports 89.9% implant success up to three years of follow-up [2]. The digital manufacturing of the titanium mesh should have homogenized the final complications and implant success results. However, a considerable variation of reported outcomes poses a few questions. Chiapasco et al. and Cucchi et al. recorded only 11 out of 53 and 1 out of 10 cases of dehiscences [4,7], while Ciocca et al. reported 66% post-operative exposure morbidity in nine patients [1]. Two authors reported 25% exposures, 16% minimal, 7% "like one tooth width" and 1.5% complete, without finding any correlation between these and the soft tissue management, thickness or mesh size [13]. Hartman et al. (2019), on 70 dis-homogeneous treated sites, reported 37% exposures [24]. Sumida et al. did not find a significant difference in mucosal dehiscence and infection between custom mesh and conventional [6]. The mean vertical bone gain reported by studies adopting linear measurements ranges from 3.9 mm [1] to 6.5 mm [25], with a maximum of 8.9 mm [4]. The width augmentation goes from 5.5 [25] to 6.35 [4] with a maximum of 11.5. These data were not compared with the virtually planned ones. Similar results were obtained with the no-digital technique, with a linear vertical augmentation mean range of 3.7–5.4 mm in combined defects [26]. Regarding the percentage of regenerated bone volume concerning the planned one, the values go from 65% [2] to 91.9% [4]. Such discrepancies can relate mainly to the different extension and morphology of the treated defects [12], often considered together in the same trial, or to the operators' experience in surgically managing the soft tissues, or, on the other hand, the precision and reliability of the digital systems and the confidence of the operator in using such a technology. Treating a homogeneous cohort of nineteen extended three-dimensional atrophies, Lizio et al. obtained five complete failures due to early infection and graft loss; nevertheless, once passed the first critical six weeks, the reliability of the technique in terms of osseous regeneration came to 88% [2].

The operator's surgical skill seems to maintain its importance, albeit, with the digital approach, a single expert surgeon obtained a lower exposure level (10–25%) [7,13] than in the two trials with more operators (52.3–66%) [1,2]. Hartman and Seiler adopted different flap designs, attributing the low rate of early exposure obtained to proper management of the mucosa. These authors warned about scars from inflammation processes or previous surgeries [13].

Regarding the reliability in reproducing what is virtually planned, Li et al. recorded +19.3% regenerated bone volume under the mesh compared with what was digitally planned, probably due to an upward shifting of the device. In addition, the same authors referred to a mean value of $0.59 \pm 0.47$ mm of mesh border deviation among the virtual and the post-GBR situation, up to a 3.4 mm maximum discrepancy [8]. Lizio et al. reported 82% matching between the digital mesh position and the surgical one from the post-operative CT data, confirming a statistically significant mesh fitting to the bone defect independent from the operator but with a relevant range (53.3% to 100%) of incongruity [2]. No other objective evaluation of this issue was reported, even if, in general, the project resulted in the number, dimensions and positions of the fixtures and prosthetic finalization [1,4,7–9,13].

From all the above considerations comes the necessity to enhance digital workflow by controlling as many elements as possible to optimize the amount and distribution of bone reconstruction. It is worth noting that a digital customization flowchart reduces the operation times and the number of fixation screws. However, it is more expensive than the traditional procedure and does not allow intra-operative correction [2,13]. In our opinion, the two reported cases required particular attention to the highly correlated risk of failure. The posterior mandibular site, difficult because of the presence of the mental foramen and the mylohyoid muscle on the lingual side, and the maxillary one, with critical aesthetic implications, forced us not to consider only the bone tissue alteration.

The mesh design in the present report did not contemplate macropores, apart from a few fissures in the portion of the device in contact with the most coronal ridge of the residual crest. This particular structure, contrasting with the recent tendency, aims to reduce the fibrotic tissue's invasion of the regenerative space with a minimal periosteum-like tissue formation. This fibrosis, helpful in preventing the graft from infection in case of dehiscence [17], reduces bone formation and complicates the mesh removal in the implant placement phase. Accurate planning of the regenerative space starting from the ideal prosthetic finalization could better reduce the risk of exposures and, consequently, the relevance of the fibrotic tissue protecting role, whose unpredictable amount and structural characteristics complicate the virtual plan fulfilment.

Indeed, no trial adopted a "titanium membrane" without holes. Apart from a few hypotheses [27], the design, thickness, pore dimensions and numbers and the treatment of the meshes surface are not demonstrated to condition the procedure. Recently, an in vivo study reported that the microporous structure of titanium mesh enhanced angiogenesis from periosteum in vertical ridge augmentation better than macro, associated with enhanced vascular permeability and osteoconductive capabilities [28]. Van Steenberghe et al. reported that about ten consecutive patients had undergone GBR with an occlusive titanium barrier, allowing the insertion of 33 fixtures to bear a fixed prosthesis. The peri-implant bone level was stable for up to 5 years of follow-up. Animal and clinical data showed the great potential of an occlusive titanium barrier, which further underlines the importance of soft tissue evaluation and surgical management [29].

In addition to the CBCT-related data quality and the printing system, this approach depends on the STL files' accuracy and the precision of the software in coupling them [11,30,31]. The precision of the extra- or intra-oral scanners was reported in different trials [32–34]. The patient clinical situation and the operator's technical skill condition the intraoral scanning, while impression distorts the reliability of extra-oral scanner data [34]. Eventually, the manufacturing process and the structure of the membrane are relevant in reproducing what is planned [11]. Several studies on s-CAI reported a greater accuracy in implant placement compared with the free-hand procedure, with a reduction in the importance of operative expertise [30,31,34]. This outcome appears more interesting in flapless procedures, where soft tissue thickness and superficial characteristics are more important [35]. A fully computerized procedure appears to be more precise than a partially computerized one [34]. Hence, the present case report aims to stimulate the research toward more and more precise customization of the titanium barrier to improve the reconstructive approach, particularly in hugely atrophic sites. The following evaluation step will be the superimposition of the data related to the pre-implant CBCT to the pre-operative project to digitally verify the membrane fitting with the surgical site beyond the surgeon's perception. According to the outcomes obtained over time with the presented cases, at least for the pre-prosthetic phase, a survey will be accomplished after the final approval of the ethics committee.

## 5. Conclusions

This preliminary reported protocol enabled surgically managing two complex and extended alveolar defects without intra-operatory complications, a perfect fitting of the mesh and reduced operative timings and no complications up to one month after surgery. The completion of the treatment will confirm the goodness of this fully planned digital approach.

**Author Contributions:** Conceptualization: P.F., M.S. and G.P.; methodology: P.F., C.B. and L.B.; software: L.R.; investigation: R.P., M.S. and L.R.; writing—original draft preparation: G.L.; writing—review and editing: G.L.; supervision: G.P., P.F. and C.B. All authors have read and agreed to the published version of the manuscript.

**Funding:** This research received no external funding.

**Institutional Review Board Statement:** The study was conducted in accordance with the Declaration of Helsinki. Ethical review is not applicable as preliminary cases report with a validated technique.

**Informed Consent Statement:** Written informed consent has been obtained from the patients to publish this paper.

**Data Availability Statement:** Not applicable.

**Conflicts of Interest:** The authors declare no conflict of interest.

## Abbreviations

| | |
|---|---|
| GBR | Guided Bone Regeneration |
| 3D | Three-Dimensional |
| CAD/CAM | Computer-Aided Design/Computer-Aided Manufacturing |
| CBCT | Cone-Beam Computerized Tomography |
| CT | Computerized Tomography |
| STL | Standard Tessellation Language |
| CA (s-CAI; d-CAI) | Computer-Aided Implantology (static and dynamic) |
| DMLS | Digital Machine Laser Sintering |

## References


1. Ciocca, L.; Lizio, G.; Baldissara, P.; Sambuco, A.; Scotti, R.; Corinaldesi, G. Prosthetically CAD-CAM–Guided Bone Augmentation of Atrophic Jaws Using Customized Titanium Mesh: Preliminary Results of an Open Prospective Study. *J. Oral Implant.* **2018**, *44*, 131–137. [CrossRef] [PubMed]
2. Lizio, G.; Pellegrino, G.; Corinaldesi, G.; Ferri, A.; Marchetti, C.; Felice, P. Guided bone regeneration using titanium mesh to augment 3-dimensional alveolar defects prior to implant placement. A pilot study. *Clin. Oral Implant. Res.* **2022**, *33*, 607–621. [CrossRef] [PubMed]
3. Maiorana, C.; Santoro, F.; Rabagliati, M.; Salina, S. Evaluation of the use of iliac cancellous bone and anorganic bovine bone in the reconstruction of the atrophic maxilla with titanium mesh: A clinical and histologic investigation. *Int. J. Oral Maxillofac. Implant.* **2001**, *16*, 427–432.
4. Chiapasco, M.; Casentini, P.; Tommasato, G.; Dellavia, C.; Del Fabbro, M. Customized CAD/CAM titanium meshes for the guided bone regeneration of severe alveolar ridge defects: Preliminary results of a retrospective clinical study in humans. *Clin. Oral Implant. Res.* **2021**, *32*, 498–510. [CrossRef] [PubMed]
5. Ciocca, L.; Ragazzini, S.; Fantini, M.; Corinaldesi, G.; Scotti, R. Work flow for the prosthetic rehabilitation of atrophic patients with a minimal-intervention CAD/CAM approach. *J. Prosthet. Dent.* **2015**, *114*, 22–26. [CrossRef]
6. Sumida, T.; Otawa, N.; Kamata, Y.; Kamakura, S.; Mtsushita, T.; Kitagaki, H.; Mori, S.; Sasaki, K.; Fujibayashi, S.; Takemoto, M.; et al. Custom-made titanium devices as membranes for bone augmentation in implant treatment: Clinical application and the comparison with conventional titanium mesh. *J. Cranio-Maxillofac. Surg.* **2015**, *43*, 2183–2188. [CrossRef]
7. Cucchi, A.; Bianchi, A.; Calamai, P.; Rinaldi, L.; Mangano, F.; Vignudelli, E.; Corinaldesi, G. Clinical and volumetric outcomes after vertical ridge augmentation using computer-aided-design/computer-aided manufacturing (CAD/CAM) customized titanium meshes: A pilot study. *BMC Oral Health* **2020**, *20*, 219. [CrossRef]
8. Li, L.; Wang, C.; Li, X.; Fu, G.; Chen, D.; Huang, Y. Research on the dimensional accuracy of customized bone augmentation combined with 3D -printing individualized titanium mesh: A retrospective case series study. *Clin. Implant Dent. Relat. Res.* **2020**, *23*, 5–18. [CrossRef]
9. Li, S.; Zhang, T.; Zhou, M.; Zhang, X.; Gao, Y.; Cai, X. A novel digital and visualized guided bone regeneration procedure and digital precise bone augmentation: A case series. *Clin. Implant Dent. Relat. Res.* **2021**, *23*, 19–30. [CrossRef]
10. Aslan, S.; Tolay, C.; Gehrke, P. Computer-aided planning of soft tissue augmentation with prosthetic guidance for the establishment of a natural mucosal contour in late implant placement. *J. Esthet. Restor. Dent.* **2019**, *31*, 553–560. [CrossRef]
11. Tahmaseb, A.; Wu, V.; Wismeijer, D.; Coucke, W.; Evans, C. The accuracy of static computer-aided implant surgery: A systematic review and meta-analysis. *Clin. Oral Implant. Res.* **2018**, *29* (Suppl. 16), 416–435. [CrossRef] [PubMed]
12. Miyamoto, I.; Funaki, K.; Yamauchi, K.; Kodama, T.; Takahashi, T. Alveolar ridge reconstruction with titanium mesh and autogenous particulate bone graft: Computed tomography-based evaluations of augmented bone quality and quantity. *Clin. Implant. Dent. Relat. Res.* **2012**, *14*, 304–311. [CrossRef] [PubMed]
13. Hartmann, A.; Seiler, M. Minimizing risk of customized titanium mesh exposures—A retrospective analysis. *BMC Oral Health* **2020**, *20*, 36. [CrossRef]
14. Tallarico, M.; Ceruso, F.M.; Muzzi, L.; Meloni, S.M.; Kim, Y.-J.; Gargari, M.; Martinolli, M. Effect of Simultaneous Immediate Implant Placement and Guided Bone Reconstruction with Ultra-Fine Titanium Mesh Membranes on Radiographic and Clinical Parameters after 18 Months of Loading. *Materials* **2019**, *12*, 1710. [CrossRef]
15. Tallarico, M.; Park, C.-J.; Lumbau, A.I.; Annucci, M.; Baldoni, E.; Koshovari, A.; Meloni, S.M. Customized 3D-Printed Titanium Mesh Developed to Regenerate a Complex Bone Defect in the Aesthetic Zone: A Case Report Approached with a Fully Digital Workflow. *Materials* **2020**, *13*, 3874. [CrossRef] [PubMed]
16. Cucchi, A.; Chierico, A.; Fontana, F.; Mazzocco, F.; Cinquegrana, C.; Belleggia, F.; Rossetti, P.; Soardi, C.M.; Todisco, M.; Luongo, R.; et al. Statements and Recommendations for Guided Bone Regeneration: Consensus Report of the Guided Bone Regeneration Symposium Held in Bologna, October 15 to 16, 2016. *Implant. Dent.* **2019**, *28*, 388–399. [CrossRef] [PubMed]
17. Lizio, G.; Corinaldesi, G.; Marchetti, C. Alveolar ridge reconstruction with titanium mesh: A three-dimensional evaluation of factors affecting bone augmentation. *Int. J. Oral Maxillofac. Implant.* **2014**, *29*, 1354–1363. [CrossRef]
18. Poomprakobsri, K.; Kan, J.Y.; Rungcharassaeng, K.; Lozada, J. Exposure of Barriers Used in GBR: Rate, Timing, Management, And Its Effect on Grafted Bone. A Retrospective Analysis. *J. Oral Implantol.* **2021**, *48*, 27–36. [CrossRef]

19. Urban, I.A.; Saleh, M.H.A.; Ravidà, A.; Forszter, A.; Wang, H.; Barath, Z. Vertical bone augmentation utilizing a titanium-reinforced PTFE mesh: A multi-variate analysis of influencing factors. *Clin. Oral Implant. Res.* **2021**, *32*, 828–839. [CrossRef]
20. De Bruyckere, T.; Cosyn, J.; Younes, F.; Hellyn, J.; Bekx, J.; Cleymaet, R.; Eghbali, A. A randomized controlled study comparing guided bone regeneration with connective tissue graft to re-establish buccal convexity: One-year aesthetic and patient-reported outcomes. *Clin. Oral Implant. Res.* **2020**, *31*, 507–516. [CrossRef]
21. Avila-Ortiz, G.; Couso-Queiruga, E.; Pirc, M.; Chambrone, L.; Thoma, D.S. Outcome measures and methods of assessment of soft tissue augmentation interventions in the context of dental implant therapy: A systematic review of clinical studies published in the last 10 years. *Clin. Oral Implant. Res.* **2022**. [CrossRef] [PubMed]
22. Fortin, Y.; Sullivan, R.M. Terminal Posterior Tilted Implants Planned as a Sinus Graft Alternative for Fixed Full-Arch Implant-Supported Maxillary Restoration: A Case Series with 10- to 19-Year Results on 44 Consecutive Patients Presenting for Routine Maintenance. *Clin. Implant. Dent. Relat. Res.* **2017**, *19*, 56–68. [CrossRef] [PubMed]
23. Pieri, F.; Corinaldesi, G.; Fini, M.; Aldini, N.N.; Giardino, R.; Marchetti, C. Alveolar ridge augmentation with titanium mesh and a combination of autogenous bone and anorganic bovine bone: A 2-year prospective study. *J. Periodontol.* **2008**, *79*, 2093–2103. [CrossRef]
24. Hartmann, A.; Hildebrandt, H.; Schmohl, J.U.; Kämmerer, P.W. Evaluation of Risk Parameters in Bone Regeneration Using a Customized Titanium Mesh: Results of a Clinical Study. *Implant. Dent.* **2019**, *28*, 543–550. [CrossRef] [PubMed]
25. Sagheb, K.; Schiegnitz, E.; Moergel, M.; Walter, C.; Al-Nawas, B.; Wagner, W. Clinical outcome of alveolar ridge augmentation with individualized CAD-CAM-produced titanium mesh. *Int. J. Implant Dent.* **2017**, *3*, 36. [CrossRef]
26. Briguglio, F.; Falcomatà, D.; Marconcini, S.; Fiorillo, L.; Briguglio, R.; Farronato, D. The Use of Titanium Mesh in Guided Bone Regeneration: A Systematic Review. *Int. J. Dent.* **2019**, *2019*, 9065423. [CrossRef]
27. Xie, Y.; Li, S.; Zhang, T.; Wang, C.; Cai, X. Titanium mesh for bone augmentation in oral implantology: Current application and progress. *Int. J. Oral Sci.* **2020**, *12*, 37. [CrossRef]
28. Senoo, M.; Hasuike, A.; Yamamoto, T.; Ozawa, Y.; Watanabe, N.; Furuhata, M.; Sato, S. Comparison of Macro-and Micro-porosity of a Titanium Mesh for Guided Bone Regeneration: An In Vivo Experimental Study. *In Vivo* **2021**, *36*, 76–85. [CrossRef]
29. Van Steenberghe, D.; Johansson, C.; Quirynen, M.; Molly, L.; Albrektsson, T.; Naert, I. Bone augmentation by means of a stiff occlusive titanium barrier. *Clin. Oral Implant. Res.* **2003**, *14*, 63–71. [CrossRef]
30. Abduo, J.; Lau, D. Accuracy of static computer-assisted implant placement in long span edentulous area by novice implant clinicians: A cross-sectional in vitro study comparing fully-guided, pilot-guided, and freehand implant placement protocols. *Clin. Implant. Dent. Relat. Res.* **2021**, *23*, 361–372. [CrossRef]
31. Derksen, W.; Wismeijer, D.; Flügge, T.; Hassan, B.; Tahmaseb, A. The accuracy of computer-guided implant surgery with tooth-supported, digitally designed drill guides based on CBCT and intraoral scanning. A prospective cohort study. *Clin. Oral Implant. Res.* **2019**, *30*, 1005–1015. [CrossRef] [PubMed]
32. Franchina, A.; Stefanelli, L.V.; Maltese, F.; Mandelaris, G.A.; Vantaggiato, A.; Pagliarulo, M.; Pranno, N.; Brauner, E.; De Angelis, F.; Di Carlo, S. Validation of an Intra-Oral Scan Method Versus Cone Beam Computed Tomography Superimposition to Assess the Accuracy between Planned and Achieved Dental Implants: A Randomized In Vitro Study. *Int. J. Environ. Res. Public Health* **2020**, *17*, 9358. [CrossRef] [PubMed]
33. Monaco, C.; Arena, A.; Corsaletti, L.; Santomauro, V.; Venezia, P.; Cavalcanti, R.; Di Fiore, A.; Zucchelli, G. 2D/3D accuracies of implant position after guided surgery using different surgical protocols: A retrospective study. *J. Prosthodont. Res.* **2020**, *64*, 424–430. [CrossRef] [PubMed]
34. Putra, R.H.; Yoda, N.; Astuti, E.R.; Sasaki, K. The accuracy of implant placement with computer-guided surgery in partially edentulous patients and possible influencing factors: A systematic review and meta-analysis. *J. Prosthodont. Res.* **2022**, *66*, 29–39. [CrossRef] [PubMed]
35. Frizzera, F.; Calazans, N.N.N.; Hooper Pascoal, C.; Elen Martins, M.; Mendonça, G. Flapless Guided Implant Surgeries Compared with Conventional Surgeries Performed by Nonexperienced Individuals: Randomized and Controlled Split-Mouth Clinical Trial. *Int. J. Oral Maxillofac. Implants* **2021**, *36*, 755–761. [CrossRef] [PubMed]

*applied sciences*

MDPI

*Review*

# Preclinical Evaluation of Bioactive Scaffolds for the Treatment of Mandibular Critical-Sized Bone Defects: A Systematic Review

**Jana Desnica [1], Sanja Vujovic [1], Dragana Stanisic [1], Irena Ognjanovic [1], Bojan Jovicic [2], Momir Stevanovic [1,*] and Gvozden Rosic [3,*]**

1 Department of Dentistry, Faculty of Medical Sciences, University of Kragujevac, Svetozara Markovića 69, 34000 Kragujevac, Serbia; jana.desnica@gmail.com (J.D.); sanja.994@live.com (S.V.); stanisic92@yahoo.com (D.S.); irena.ognjanovic@gmail.com (I.O.)

2 Dental Clinic, Military Medical Academy, University of Defence, Crnotravska 17, 11000 Belgrade, Serbia; jovicicdrbojan@gmail.com

3 Department of Physiology, Faculty of Medical Sciences, University of Kragujevac, Svetozara Markovića 69, 34000 Kragujevac, Serbia

* Correspondence: momirstevanovic7@gmail.com (M.S.); grosic@medf.kg.ac.rs (G.R.)

**Abstract:** This systematic review evaluated current in vivo research on regenerating critical-sized mandibular defects and discussed methodologies for mandibular bone tissue engineering. Out of the 3650 articles initially retrieved, 88 studies were included, and all studies that used a scaffold reported increased bone formation compared to negative controls. Combining scaffolds with growth factors and mesenchymal stem cells improved bone formation and healing. Bone morphogenic proteins were widely used and promoted significant bone formation compared to controls. However, discrepancies between studies exist due to the various methodologies and outcome measures used. The use of scaffolds with bioactive molecules and/or progenitor cells enhances success in mandibular bone engineering. Scaffold-based mandibular bone tissue engineering could be introduced into clinical practice due to its proven safety, convenience, and cost-effectiveness.

**Keywords:** bone regeneration; growth factors; mandible; mesenchymal stem cells; scaffold; tissue engineering

**Citation:** Desnica, J.; Vujovic, S.; Stanisic, D.; Ognjanovic, I.; Jovicic, B.; Stevanovic, M.; Rosic, G. Preclinical Evaluation of Bioactive Scaffolds for the Treatment of Mandibular Critical-Sized Bone Defects: A Systematic Review. *Appl. Sci.* **2023**, *13*, 4668. https://doi.org/10.3390/app13084668

Academic Editor: Vittorio Checchi

Received: 15 March 2023
Revised: 4 April 2023
Accepted: 5 April 2023
Published: 7 April 2023



## 1. Introduction

The reconstruction of mandibular bone defects following traumatic injuries, postoperative defects from tumor removal, or infection treatment is the most common reconstructive procedure in oral and maxillofacial surgery. Due to the significant impact of the craniofacial area on patients' well-being and quality of life, the proper reconstruction of defects represents a significant challenge for surgeons [1]. The reconstruction or augmentation of craniofacial bones is one of the most frequent surgical procedures in oral and maxillofacial surgery. Special consideration of mandible reconstruction exists in cases of critical-sized defects where a high quantity of bone is lost and intrinsic regeneration is not possible [1].

Standard bone augmentation procedures comprise the clinical use of autografts, allografts, and xenografts. Alloplastic materials, such as titanium load-bearing plates, were widely used as reconstruction plates to reestablish mandibular segmental defects. Still, numerous studies on titanium reconstruction plates have reported high failure rates of up to 52% due to the resorption and infection of the bone [1]. Microvascular bone grafts harvested from the fibula, scapula, radial bone, and iliac crest are currently used as standard grafts to reconstruct extensive mandibular bone defects. However, the use of autografts is complex and requires a second surgical intervention, causing donor-site morbidity and possible graft rejection [1]. To overcome these limitations, extensive research on bone tissue engineering (BTE) using bioactive and biocompatible bone substitutes has been performed in recent years. The techniques for mandibular BTE should be adjusted to certain features that are unique to mandible physiology. Firstly, materials for regeneration may come into contact with saliva and intraoral pathogens, leading to inflammation and infection. Secondly, materials used for mandibular BTE must withstand significant forces of mastication (200–400 N). Thirdly, the BTE of the mandible should restore the contour of the bone in order to ensure proper patients' appearance. Fourthly, the restored bone should be available for dental implant placement. Techniques for mandibular bone tissue engineering may be categorized into scaffolds, bioactive substances, and cell therapy [2].

Scaffolds used as synthetic or autologous bone substitutes act as matrices mimicking the artificial extracellular matrix (ECM) to promote bone healing until they are partially or wholly replaced by newly formed bone [3]. Biomaterials are mainly categorized into natural and synthetic materials. Synthetic materials are classified into polymers, bioceramics, metals, and composite scaffolds. Numerous studies reported a range of advantages and disadvantages for each scaffold type [4,5]. Natural polymeric scaffolds have excellent biocompatibility and controlled biodegradation, but their weak mechanical properties are their major drawback as bone scaffold materials [1]. Synthetic polymeric scaffolds are biocompatible, biodegradable, easily fabricated into different shapes, and provide mechanical support and a controlled degradation time. Their use in bone engineering is limited because of their decreased mechanical strength due to their rapid degradation in vivo and immune reaction to acidic degradation products [1]. Bioceramic scaffolds with excellent biocompatibility and bioactivity are extensively used in bone tissue engineering. They have high compressive strength and osteogenic properties but a low tensile strength and toughness, fabrication hitches, brittleness, and slow resorption rate [2]. Metals have been used in manufacturing biomimetic scaffolds, fixation plates, screws, pins, wires, and stents. Biodegradable metals have a variety of properties that are essential for bone regeneration scaffolds, including biodegradability properties, mechanical strength, formability, osteogenic capacity, and antibacterial properties. The term "biomimetic" refers to the process of designing materials, structures, or systems that mimic natural biological processes or structures. In the context of scaffolds for bone regeneration, biomimetic scaffolds are designed to mimic the extracellular matrix (ECM) of natural bone tissue, both in terms of its chemical composition and its physical structure [2]. Even though metallic materials are not superior to other material combinations because of the increased number of failure cases demanding revision procedures, they are still utilised in some developing countries due to their reasonable cost and availability [6]. Composite scaffolds of bioceramics with polymers have been extensively used as materials for bone repair studies. The natural bone matrix is a combination of organic/inorganic composites; thus, the composite scaffolds for bone regeneration are designed by combining the advantages of both components. The most common composite scaffolds for bone substitution are bioceramic and polymer scaffolds [4,5].

Bioactive molecules such as bone morphogenetic proteins (BMPs) promote bone healing, usually in combination with a scaffold as a carrier. Several commercial products are based on recombinant human bone morphogenetic proteins (rhBMPs) and are used for alveolar bone augmentation, sinus lift procedures, and periodontal defects [7]. The direct administration of growth factors into the bone defect is considered an excellent strategy for bone tissue regeneration. The critical point when using bioactive molecules is selecting a suitable scaffold carrier system to tailor the localized and sustained release of these molecules [8]. Stem cells (SCs) therapy is an up-and-coming technique for BTE. In BTE, SCs have been used due to their ability to produce and differentiate into osteoblasts. SCs have several advantages, including the ability to differentiate directly into osteoblasts, modulate immune responses, promote angiogenesis, and exhibit plasticity. [9]. Various scaffolds are used to mimic native ECM for SCs seeding, providing a conducive framework for the attachment and growth of cells [10]. The common sources from which SCs can be obtained are bone marrow, dental pulp, embryo, and adipose tissue [10].

### 1.1. Role of Scaffolds in BTE

The capacity of bone to regenerate represents a unique feature, influenced by various factors, but spontaneous healing is not possible in cases of bone damage with a critical shape [11]. Scaffolds are porous 3D structures that simulate native ECM features; thus, their functions are similar to those of ECM in natural tissues. They are a fundamental component of BTE, alongside SCs and growth factors, as their role is to provide structural and mechanical support for tissue formation and regeneration [12]. By producing different biophysical and chemical signals, scaffolds create a stimulative microenvironment for multiple processes, including the adhesion, migration, proliferation, and differentiation of osteoblast progenitors [13]. In such a functional three-dimensional space, bone development can occur. They may also serve as a reservoir for various growth factors required for successful bone regeneration. The main goal of scaffold-based tissue engineering is to fabricate a biomimetic structure that can prompt the directed growth of cells toward an organ-like formation [14].

### 1.2. Properties of an Ideal Scaffold for Bone Regeneration

Bone is a natural composite consisting of inorganic components, mainly calcium apatite, and organic components, mainly collagen type I. Bone has a complex architecture to withstand diverse mechanical, biological, and chemical functions. The specialized structure involves the complex arrangement of macrostructures (proportion of medullar and cortical bone), microstructures (arrangement of osteons and trabeculae), and nanostructures (collagen fibers and apatite mineral crystals) [4,5,15,16]. Scaffolds are 3D structures that imitate the in vivo environment and stimulate the formation of new tissue [12]. They promote SCs' adhesion, proliferation, and differentiation by creating a suitable microenvironment [13]. Porous scaffolds with optimal 3D architecture serve as artificial bone ECM with osteoconductive properties to promote bone healing. A scaffold should possess good biological properties, including (Table 1):

- Biocompatibility;
- Mechanical stability;
- Architecture;
- Biodegradability;
- Bioactivity [4,5,15,16].

In order to promote natural bone healing, an equilibrium between the biological properties of the scaffold, osteoprogenitor cells, and signaling molecules must exist [17,18]. The ideal 3D scaffold for bone regeneration should be composed of a biocompatible, biodegradable material with similar mechanical properties to bone ECM to provide enough mechanical support to the host cells [4,5,15,16]. Scaffolds should mimic the bone ECM to facilitate the osteogenic host cells to deposit natural ECM and replace the scaffold material. Thus, the rate of scaffold resorption should be controlled, complementing host cells' ingrowth. This is particularly important for bone regeneration, where mechanical stability of the scaffold is expected, especially in the load-bearing areas [17,18]. The 3D architecture of the scaffold should be highly porous with a high index of porosity (number of interconnected pores/$mm^2$) to allow for osteoprogenitor cell ingrowth and nutrient migration [19]. The scaffold surface should also be optimized to promote cell attachment, mainly its wettability and roughness. A high number of interconnected pores allows for the diffusion of nutrients and oxygen into the avascular scaffold. The size of the pores is essential, as well as the proportion of nano-, micro-, and macropores in the scaffold. Pores greater than 300 nm promote osteogenesis due to the ingrowth of osteoprogenitor cells and angiogenesis [19]. Micro- and nanopores with a size <10 nm increase the scaffold's overall surface, enabling protein attachment and improving cell–scaffold binding. The porous 3D architecture of the scaffold allows for the incorporation of growth factors such as BMPs, vascular endothelial growth factor (VEGF), transforming growth factor β (TGF-β), and insulin-like growth factor 1 (IGF-1) [4,17].

**Table 1.** Ideal properties of the scaffold to promote bone regeneration.

| Scaffold Property | Desirable Properties |
|---|---|
| Biocompatibility | • Non-toxic breakdown products;<br>• Non-inflammatory scaffold components;<br>• Without immune rejection;<br>• Non-carcinogenic. |
| Biodegradability | • Controlled degradation complementing tissue ingrowth and allowing host cells to produce extracellular matrix;<br>• Sufficient support to the newly formed tissue;<br>• Degradable by host biological processes. |
| Mechanical stability | • Enough compressive, elastic and fatigue strength for osteogenic cell migration;<br>• Scaffold material allows easy surgical manipulation;<br>• Material adaptive to the individual bone defect. |
| Bioactivity | • Scaffold material should interact and bind to the host tissuel<br>• Osteoconductive properties;<br>• Stimulation of cell ingrowth, attachment and differentiation;<br>• Stimulation of neoangiogenesis. |
| Architecture | • Macroporosity to allow cell migration and angiogenesis;<br>• Microporosity to increase surface area for cell–scaffold connections;<br>• High porosity index and interconnected pores allow for diffusion of nutrients and cell migration;<br>• Adequate pore size for osteogenic cells. |
| Surface of the scaffold | • Hydrophilicity and surface roughness of the scaffold surface enhances protein adsorption and host cell binding. |
| Sterilibility | • Sterilibility without loss of bioactivity. |

The most significant advantage of scaffolds is their ease of production, enabling researchers to modify numerous materials and combine them into composite grafts [17,18,20]. Thus, it is crucial that the scaffold material allows for easy surgical manipulation and is composed of a material that is adaptive to the individual bone defect. The mechanical properties of the scaffold should be comparable to the compressive strength of the cortical bone (100–250 MPa) to withstand physiological mechanical forces on the bone [20].

Previous systematic reviews of the literature concluded that preclinical in vivo studies demonstrated the clinical potential of scaffolds as an alternative to autogenous bone grafting [21,22]. Boysuni et al. [21] performed a systematic review investigating the results of mandibular BTE in animal studies. This review reported a constant increase in the frequency of publications regarding mandibular BTE, reflecting the growing interest in the field. Despite promising results in bone regeneration, clinical translation is still impossible due to a lack of understanding of the biological interplay between scaffolds, biomolecules, exogenous cells, and host immune reactions. In addition, a qualitative and quantitative comparison of outcomes between the animal and clinical studies was impossible due to the significant differences between the studies regarding the methodology, definition of critical-sized defects, follow-up period, and evaluation of outcomes. Still, there is much controversy regarding defining what constitutes a critical-sized defect. In general, a "critically-sized" defect is regarded as one that would not heal spontaneously despite surgical stabilization and requires further surgical intervention, such as autologous bone grafting [12]. Differences among studies using the same animal models for mandibular bone defects allow for an objective comparison of outcomes. The clinical evaluation of scaffolds for mandibular bone regeneration is limited to case reports or single-center case series with limited follow-up periods and questionable results. This review aimed to evaluate current research on the regeneration of mandibular defects and discuss the further development of mandibular BTE methodologies, focusing on a better understanding of the clinical use of different scaffold types in the BTE process to overcome mandibular defects. Furthermore, the goal was to compare the result of scaffold-based BTE in conjunction with various SCs and growth factors in bone reconstruction to aid reconstructive surgeons in determining the most suitable scaffolds for mandibular bone reconstruction.

## 2. Materials and Methods

The systematic review of the BTE concepts for the reconstruction of critical-size mandibular defects was conducted according to the guidelines of the Preferred Reporting Items for Systematic Reviews and Meta-Analyses (PRISMA) Statement.

### 2.1. Hypothesis

**Hypothesis 0 (H0).** *There is no significant difference between the various scaffold types, stem cells (SCs), and growth factors in bone reconstruction for critical-sized mandibular defects.*

**Hypothesis 1 (H1).** *There is a significant difference between the various scaffold types, SCs, and growth factors in bone reconstruction for critical-sized mandibular defects.*

### 2.2. Research Question

The research question for this review was: "What are the characteristics and the results of the existing studies on the use of biomimetic scaffolds in the reconstruction of critical-sized mandibular bone defects?".

### 2.3. Search Strategy

In November 2022, electronic searches were conducted in the following databases: PubMed (National Library of Medicine), Web of Science (Clarivate Analytics), and Scopus (Elsevier). These comprised both MeSH and free-text terms. The following search strategy was applied: (("bone tissue engineering" [MeSH Terms] OR ("tissue" [All Fields] AND "engineering" [All Fields] AND "mandible" [All Fields]) OR "bone tissue engineering" [All Fields]) OR ("tissue scaf-folds" [MeSH Terms] OR ("tissue" [All Fields] AND "scaffolds" [All Fields]) OR "tissue scaffolds" [All Fields] OR ("tissue" [All Fields] AND "scaffold" [All Fields]) OR "tissue scaffold" [All Fields]) OR ("mandible reconstruction" [MeSH Terms AND "engineer-ing" [All Fields]] OR ("reconstructive" [All Fields] AND "surgical" [All Fields] AND "pro-cedures" [All Fields]) OR "mandible reconstruction" [All Fields] OR "reconstruction" [All Fields]) OR ("bone morphogenetic proteins" [MeSH Terms] OR ("bone" [All Fields] AND "morphogenetic" [All Fields] AND "proteins" [All Fields]) OR "bone morphogenetic pro-teins" [All Fields] OR ("bone" [All Fields] AND "morphogenetic" [All Fields] AND "pro-tein" [All Fields]) OR "bone morphogenetic protein" [All Fields]) OR ("bone marrow cells" [MeSH Terms] OR ("bone" [All Fields] AND "marrow" [All Fields] AND "cells" [All Fields]) OR "bone marrow cells" [All Fields]) OR ("intercellular signaling peptides and proteins" [MeSH Terms] OR ("intercellular" [All Fields] AND "signaling" [All Fields] AND "peptides" [All Fields] AND "proteins" [All Fields]) OR ("growth" [All Fields] AND "factors" [All Fields]) OR "growth factors" [All Fields])) AND (("mandible" [MeSH Terms] OR "mandible" [All Fields]) OR (("mandible" [MeSH Terms] OR "mandible" [All Fields] OR "mandibular" [All Fields]) AND ("critical sized defect" [All Fields]) AND defect [All Fields])). The retrieved references were exported to the EndNote software 20.5 (Windows) (Clarivate Analytics, Philadelphia, PA, USA) to identify the duplicates.

Searches were limited to studies in the English language. The reference lists of the articles identified from the initial search were screened for further relevant studies. No restrictions were imposed on the date or the type of publication.

### 2.4. Eligibility Criteria

Only full-text papers that reported original data from in vivo studies on the regeneration of mandibular critical size defects in animal models were included. Animal in vivo studies presenting macroscopical, histological, or histomorphometric data on the amount of bone-defect bridging, bone ingrowth, results of biomechanical testing, histological or histomorphometric data of scaffold degradation, and radiographic evidence of restoration of mandibular continuity were included. The following inclusion criteria were applied: 1. research papers presenting in vivo animal data; 2. critical-sized defects; 3. reconstructive technique clearly described; 4. follow-up and healing period clearly stated; 4. the animal model used clearly described; 5. clearly presented data on bone regeneration and the methods for the evaluation of bone growth. Conference abstracts, review papers, letters to the editor, opinion pieces, and studies on animal or human tissues in vitro were excluded. Papers investigating periodontal regeneration, dental implants' osseointegration, distraction osteogenesis, autologous bone grafts or free flaps, and treatment of fracture healing were also excluded.

### 2.5. Data Extraction

Retrieved references were read for titles and abstracts by all authors. If the title/abstract met the inclusion criteria, the article was included for a full article reading. If the full text of the article was not available, the paper was not included. After the evaluation of full texts, the references that met the eligibility criteria were included. All authors performed the quality assessment and evaluated the published data. Any disagreements in judgment were resolved by a final discussion. If the published data were insufficient, the study was excluded. The data extracted for review included: study characteristics and setting (sample size, design, animal species, type and mechanism of bony defect), method of bone engineering (scaffolds, bioactive factors, and cell therapy), and outcome measures.

## 3. Results

A total of 3872 articles were initially identified using the search algorithm. After the screening of the titles and abstracts, 265 full texts were retrieved, and a total of 88 studies were included (Figure 1) [22–109]. An overview of the included trials is depicted in Supplementary Table S1.

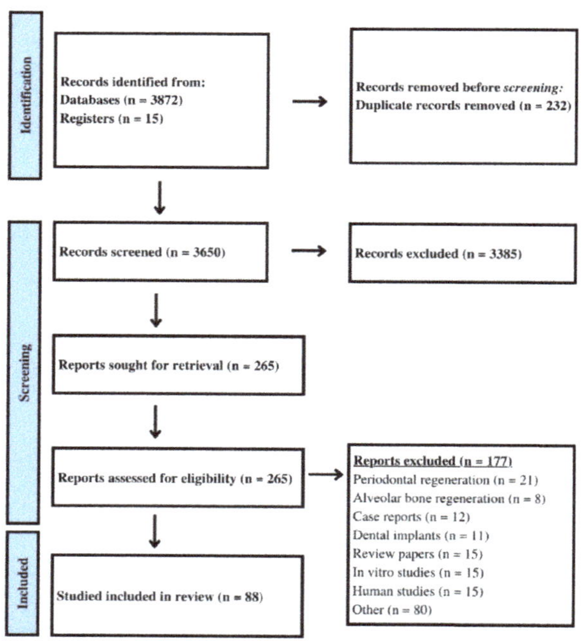


**Figure 1.** PRISMA flow diagram of studies included in the systematic review.

### 3.1. Study Design

The review included studies with critical-size mandibular defects. Regeneration modalities were categorized into tissue scaffolds, cell therapies, and bioactive substances. Most studies comprised a combination of these modalities (Figure 2). Most reported a combined use of scaffold with bioactive substances. Animal models included dogs, mini-pigs, non-human primates (nHPs), swine, rabbits, rats, sheep, and mice, which were used in 15, 7, 6, 2, 23, 26, 8, and 1 study, respectively (Table 2).

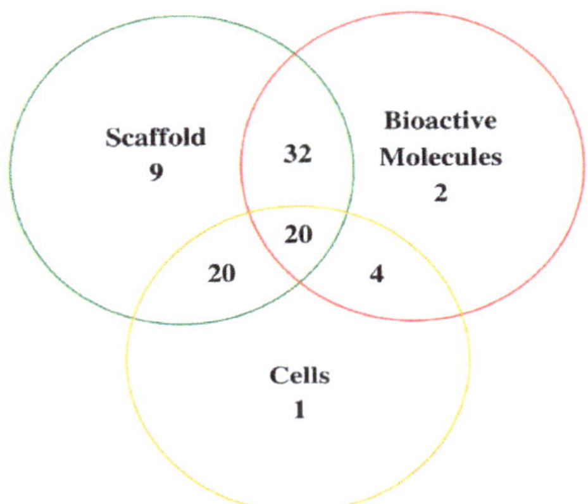


**Figure 2.** Diagram indicating the number of studies that investigated each component of the regenerative triad (bioactive molecules, scaffolds, and cells).

**Table 2.** Overview of the animal models.

| Animals | Number of Studies (%) | Critical-Sized Defect (mm) Mean (SD) | Follow Up (Weeks) Mean (SD) | References |
|---|---|---|---|---|
| Rats | 26 (29.5) | 4.76 (0.3) | 10.1 (5.8) | [24,30,39–41,49–54,56–58,60–62,65,77,80,83,87,91,95,99,104] |
| Rabbits | 23 (26.1) | 17.2 (5.3) | 12.4 (4.1) | [22,23,25–29,32,33,44,59,69,71,75,76,79,85,98,100–102,105,108] |
| Dogs | 15 (17) | 25.3 (7.8) | 27.1 (24.5) | [31,37,38,46,67,78,81,82,86,88,90,96,97,106,107] |
| Sheep | 8 (9.1) | 34.3 (4.6) | 22.1 (16.3) | [47,64,72–74,84,89,94] |
| Mini-pigs | 7 (8) | 33.5 (6.9) | 34.6 (12.9) | [34,35,48,63,92,93,109] |
| nHPs * | 6 (6.8) | 29.1 (12.2) | 43.2 (34.5) | [45,55,66,68,70,103] |
| Swine | 2 (2.3) | 24.3 (5.6) | 10.0 (4.4) | [36,43] |
| Mice | 1 (1.1) | 10.0 | 4.0 | [42] |

* nHPs—non-human primates.

The duration of follow-up (the time at which the mandibles were analyzed for bone regeneration—either using radiographic imaging of the animal or at the time of sacrifice) varied widely depending on the animal model used (Table 2). The size of the critical defect was not uniform, not even within a single animal model.

The diagnostic modalities used for characterizing the new bone formation included micro-CT examination, histology, radiography, immunohistochemistry, real-time PCR, fluorescence microscopy, biomechanical testing, and scanning electron microscopy (Table 3). The most common diagnostic modalities used were micro-CT or other X-ray modalities (computed tomography) and histological analysis.

**Table 3.** Overview of diagnostic modalities used to characterize new bone formation.

| Characterization Approach | Number of Studies (%) | References |
| --- | --- | --- |
| Micro-CT | 35 (39.8) | [24,27,30,33,35,39–41,43–45,47,49–51,62,65,69,76–80,83–86,88,90,93,99–102,107] |
| Histology | 79 (89.8) | [22,23,25–39,41–46,48–73,75–87,90–92,94–107] |
| Radiography | 38 (43.2) | [22,23,25,26,28,32,34,35,37–39,43,46,48,56,60–63,65–68,70,71,75,79,89,91–94,97,98,102,103,105,106] |
| Immunohistochemistry | 28 (31.8) | [30,35,36,41,46–50,52,57,60,61,64,67,72,73,76,83,86,88,92,93,96,97,101,102,106] |
| RT-PCR [1] (mRNA quantification) | 6 (6.8) | [23,57,80,88,92,106] |
| Fluorescence microscopy | 4 (4.5) | [53,54,72,109] |
| Biomechanical testing | 11 (12.5) | [24,28,37,38,42,63,73,74,92,102,103] |
| SPECT [2] | 1 (1.1) | [109] |
| SEM [3] | 10 (11.3) | [37,38,59,64,82,83,86,90,107,108] |
| CBCT [4] | 4 (4.5) | [36,59,71,96] |

[1] RT-PCR—reverse transcriptase polymerase chain reaction; [2] SPECT—single-photon-emission computed tomography; [3] SEM—scanning electron microscopy; [4] CBCT—cone beam computed tomography.

### 3.2. *Scaffolds*

Scaffolds were used in 81 studies, either as the primary variable of investigation or as delivery vectors for bioactive molecules and cell seeding (Table 4). Most studies used synthetic 3D porous scaffolds of a synthetic polymer, such as beta-tricalcium phosphate, PLGA, PCL, or their combination, to create composite scaffolds.

**Table 4.** Overview of scaffold types used for mandibular bone regeneration.

| Scaffold | Number of Studies (%) | References |
| --- | --- | --- |
| Natural polymers | | |
| Hyaluronic-acid-based | 3 (3.4) | [52,53,77] |
| Collagen | 23 (26.1) | [22,24,39,45,52,54,55,63–65,68,72–74,79–81,88,90,97,100–102] |
| Chitosan-based | 6 (6.8) | [49,59,76,87,99,100] |
| Synthetic polymers | | |
| PLGA [1] | 15 (17) | [26,33,35,36,40,41,43,46,47,50,51,66,70,103,108] |
| PLA-based | 3 (3.4) | [32,60,96] |
| PDLLA/$CaCO_3$ [2] | 2 (2.3) | [56,57] |
| <PEI [3] | 1 (1.1) | [36] |
| PCL [4] | 7 (8) | [27,59,82,85,98,106,107] |
| PTFE membrane [5] | 1 (1.1) | [94] |
| PU [6] | 1 (1.1) | [93] |
| Bioceramics | | |
| βTCP-based [7] | 12 (13.3) | [30,35,43–45,69,78,85,86,90,93,107] |
| HAP [8] | 16 (18.2) | [23,26–28,36,42,45,52,54,78,86,90,96,101,102,104] |
| Autologous (any tissue) | 3 (3.4) | [34,67,84] |
| Xenogenic graft (any tissue) | 3 (3.4) | [36,83,109] |

When a conjugate scaffold was used, references are placed under both categories for completion. [1] PLGA—poly(lactide-co-glycolic acid); [2] PDLLA/$CaCO_3$—poly-dl-lactic acid/calcium carbonate; [3] PEI—polyethylenimine; [4] PCL—polycaprolactone; [5] PTFE—polytetrafluoroethylene; [6] PU—polyurethane; [7] TCP—tricalciumphosphate; [8] HAP—hydroxyapatite.

### 3.3. Bioactive Substances

Bioactive molecules were used in 58 studies (66%), either alone or in combination with a scaffold or cell therapy (Table 5). The most common growth factor was BMP-2, which was used alone in 31 studies and in combination with other growth factors in 8 studies. The growth factor dosage depended on the graft size and the animal model. Several studies reported using various concentrations of growth factors for bone regeneration.

**Table 5.** Overview of bioactive molecules.

| Bioactive Molecules | Number of Studies (%) | References |
|---|---|---|
| BMP-2 | 31 (35.2) | [22,23,27,30,40,45,46,49,51,52,55–57,60,61,66,68,70,76–79,86,87,93,95,97,100,103,107,108] |
| BMP-7 | 5 (5.6) | [28,71,72,74,75] |
| BMP–4 | 1 (1.1) | [29] |
| BMP-2 + BMP-4 | 1 (1.1) | [53] |
| BMP-2 + phenamil | 1 (1.1) | [41] |
| BMP-2 + VEGF | 3 (3.4) | [43,88,92] |
| BMP-6 + VEGF | 1 (1.1) | [50] |
| BMP-2 + FGF | 3 (3.4) | [25,58,105] |
| FGF | 1 (1.1) | [80] |
| TGF1 + IGF-1 | 1 (1.1) | [91] |
| Insulin | 1 (1.1) | [33] |
| L-PRF | 1 (1.1) | [47] |
| rHOP-1 | 4 (4.5) | [63,65,73,109] |
| Dipyridamole | 1 (1.1) | [69] |
| CGF | 2 (2.3) | [101,102] |
| SDF 1α | 1 (1.1) | [24] |

BMP—bone morphogenetic protein; VEGF—vascular endothelial growth factor; FGF—fibroblast growth factor; TGF—transforming growth factor; IGF-1—insulin-like growth factor 1; L-PRF—leucocyte and platelet-rich fibrin; rHOP-1—recombinant human osteogenic protein 1; CGF—concentrated growth factor; SDF 1α—stromal-derived factor 1α.

### 3.4. Cell Therapy

Cell therapies were used for mandibular regeneration in 45 studies (51%). Bone marrow stem cells (BMSCs) were mostly used to promote bone regeneration. Regarding SCs, adipose-derived stem cells (ADSCs), stem cells derived from human exfoliated deciduous teeth (SHED), and dental-pulp-derived stem cells (DPSCs) were used in 7, 1, and 1 study, respectively (Table 6). Other cell therapies included lipid-free dedifferentiated fat cells (DFAT) and alveolar osteoblasts (AOB).

**Table 6.** Overview of cell therapies.

| Cell Therapy | Number of Studies (%) | References |
|---|---|---|
| BMSCs | 22 (25) | [23,25,29–31,33,34,37,38,42,43,48,61,68,70,71,77,80,84,95,98,105] |
| DPSCs | 1 (1.1) | [26] |
| ADSCs | 7 (8) | [35,40,49,62,99,104,106] |
| MSCs | 11 (12.5) | [28,41,50,67,75,79,82,85,94,100,101] |
| SHED | 1 (1.1) | [81] |
| DFAT | 1 (1.1) | [39] |
| Osteoblasts/osteocytes | 2 (2.3) | [65,83] |

BMSCs—bone-marrow-derived stem cells; DPSCs—dental pulp derived stem cells; ADSCs—adipose-tissue-derived stem cells; MSCs—mesenchymal stem cells; SHED—stem cells from human exfoliated deciduous teeth; DFAT—dedifferentiated adipocyte-derived progeny cells.

## 4. Discussion

Bone healing is a complex process, where there is a temporospatial interaction between the ECM, growth factors, and osteogenic cells, resulting in bone regeneration. During natural bone healing, the body generates a natural scaffold on which MSCs differentiate into osteoblasts under the influence of growth factors to regenerate bone tissue [3]. Nonetheless, critical-sized defects that cannot heal spontaneously within a patient's lifetime impair this process. In these cases, it is necessary to provide biomimetic scaffolds to bridge the defect and provide the repair site with sufficient osteogenic progenitor cells or growth factors in a suitable carrier to ensure osteoblastic differentiation [2]. The present review evaluated current therapeutic approaches regarding the BTE of critically sized mandibular defects. BTE is a promising alternative in mandibular regeneration based on in vivo studies; however, translation to clinical use is to be performed. The results of in vivo trials should be taken with caution because, for successful mandibular bone regeneration, specific clinical problems unique to the mandible should be considered. These issues include the contact between materials and saliva and intraoral pathogens, which may lead to inflammation and infection, significant forces of mastication in load-bearing locations, restoration of the normal contour of the bone for the esthetic appearance of the patient, and dental implant placement.

### *4.1. Scaffolds*

Based on the results of the present review, the use of scaffolds in mandibular bone regeneration, alone or in combination with bioactive molecules and/or cell therapies, resulted in improved osteogenesis of critical-sized mandibular defects in various animal models. The most promising results in mandibular bone regeneration were observed with composite scaffolds. Scaffolds for BTE can be classified into four classes: polymeric, ceramic, composite, and metallic scaffolds.

Natural polymeric scaffolds have excellent biocompatibility and controlled biodegradation [20]. Natural biopolymers are used for maxillofacial bone regeneration because they mimic the structure, chemical composition, and biochemical properties of the natural ECM bone organic matrix and have osteoinductive and osteoconductive properties. This was demonstrated by their ability to induce bone regeneration in mandibular bone defects. The major drawbacks of natural polymers are their poor mechanical properties, which do not approach those of natural bone tissue, and the high degradation rate of natural polymers, since they are naturally metabolizable [110]. The most commonly used natural polymeric scaffolds implemented for mandibular bone regeneration were hyaluronic-acid-based and collagen. Due to their excellent biological properties, natural polymers are extensively studied in composite scaffolds for bone repair. Several investigations have indicated that incorporating inorganic components, such as hydroxyapatite (HAP), or tricalcium phosphate (TCP), into hybrid hyaluronic-acid-based (HA) scaffolds results in enhanced osteoinductivity, osteoconductivity, and improved mechanical properties [111,112]. Natural polymers are versatile, encapsulating bioactive osteogenic factors (growth factors, drugs, hormones, peptides, nucleic acids, and cells) via a cross-linking reaction [112–114]. Recent studies reported excellent the bone regeneration of rabbit mandibular bone defects using nano-hydroxyapatite/collagen (nHAC) scaffolds with concentrated growth factors (CGF). The results of these studies showed degradation of the scaffold within 24 weeks, a high rate of new bone formation, and higher compressive strength and elastic modulus on biomechanical tests of the nHAC/CGF group compared to those of the nHAC group [99,100].

Synthetic polymers are aliphatic polyesters, and their copolymers are commonly utilized polymers in bone tissue engineering due to their mechanical properties. They are biocompatible, biodegradable, easily fabricated into different shapes, and provide mechanical support and a controlled degradation time. Their use in bone engineering is limited due to their decrease in mechanical strength due to rapid degradation in vivo and immune reaction to acidic degradation products. The chemical modification of synthetic polymers allows for the incorporation of bioactive molecules to produce biocompatible and functional materials to enhance osteogenesis. One of the major advantages of synthetic polymers is that they can be mass-produced and fabricated for individual bone sites. The traditional preparation methods of synthetic-polymer-based bone scaffolds include particle leaching, phase separation, gas forming, and fiber bonding. The 3D printing technology produces porous scaffolds by managing the arrangement of the scaffold, the thickness of each layer, and the porosity [115]. The 3D-printed scaffolds achieved better cell adhesion, proliferation, and differentiation while possessing suitable mechanical properties and a sufficiently long degradation time [116]. Recent studies have developed grafts for the mandible, skull, femoral head, tibia, fibula, and others [117].

Poly(lactic-co-glycolic acid) (PLGA), a linear copolymer of lactic acid and glycolic acid monomers, was the most widely used biodegradable polymer. PLGA was investigated as a single scaffold biomaterial for several reasons: it posesses excellent biocompatibility, non-toxic metabolites that can be safely eliminated from the metabolic cycle, and excellent processability; the degradation time of PLGA can be controlled to be consistent with bone regeneration; PLGA has suitable mechanical strength to adequately support the defect area at the early stage; grafts can be loaded with a variety of bioactive factors, such as SCs, growth factors, and drugs, to promote the regeneration of bone defects [118–120]. Inflammation is one of the main reasons for bone graft resorption. Synthetic porous polymers can be loaded with anti-inflammatory medicines (such as ibuprofen) and growth factors to reduce inflammatory reactions and enhance bone regeneration [121]. In the present review, we found that the application of synthetic polymer scaffolds, alone or in combination with bioactive molecules and/or mesenchymal SCs, resulted in improved bone regeneration.

The bioceramic scaffolds have high compressive strength, excellent biocompatibility and stability, bioactivity, and osteogenic properties. The mechanical strength of ceramics is superior to polymers, but is still inferior to natural bones, especially in terms of tensile and torsional strength [9]. Disadvantages include low tensile strength and toughness, fabrication hitches, brittleness, and slow resorption rate. Hydroxyapatite (HAP) ($Ca_{10}(PO_4)_6(OH)_2$) is the main mineral component of bone tissue and, as a scaffold, it is a bioactive ceramic material of high biocompatibility because it forms direct chemical connections with bone tissue. It has excellent bioactive, and bioresorbable properties and can be synthesized in various forms, such as ceramic plates, blocks, granules, and powder for various bone tissue applications [122,123]. In the bone tissue, HAP is deposited around and within the collagen fibers in the form of thin slabs and sticks (length 20–40 nm, width 15 nm, and thickness of 1.5–3 nm) in regular spaces [122,123]. Synthetic HAP is similar to a natural mineral apatite in bones and is widely used for bone repairs. Its structural composition is the same as natural bone, with a nominal stoichiometric Ca/P atomic ratio of 1:67 [122,123]. Still, mechanical properties are very low compared to natural bone [41,42]. Due to brittleness and fragility, HAP is commonly mainly used in the form of composite scaffolds with polymer materials [124,125]. Numerous studies have shown, that after applying a HAP scaffold, the rapid activation and binding of osteoblasts to the scaffold surface occurred due to the rapid deposition of the biological carbonate HAP, which is the primary substrate for binding of the osteoprogenitor cells [126]. The osteoprogenitor cells are known to better bond to rough surfaces than smooth surfaces. For this purpose, in addition to good biological characteristics, the topography of the HAP scaffold has an impact on cell adhesion, proliferation, and differentiation [127]. Cells on rough surface show phenotypes that are similar to osteoblasts and release pro-osteoblastic mediators such as prostaglandins and LTGF-β. In vitro research showed that osteoprogenitor cells do not differ in terms of the surface of synthetic and biological HAP [127,128].

Combining the advantages of two or more different scaffold materials into a composite scaffold has been a matter of research in many previous trials [129,130]. Composite scaffolds of bioceramics with synthetic polymers have been used in the majority of studies, either as a single regenerative therapy or as a carrier of bioactive molecules or SCs. These scaffolds mimic the natural bone matrix, a combination of organic/inorganic composites. Composite scaffolds combine the excellent biological activity of HAP and mechanical properties and 3D architecture of synthetic polymers. The HAP/PLGA scaffold was extensively studied for bone regeneration. Jokanovic et al. [110] examined the PLGA/HAP scaffold for critical-sized calvaria defects and found numerous biological advantages compared to commercially available xenograft, which were reflected mainly by the lower number of giant cells surrounding implanted material and a higher degree of mineralization in newly formed bone. Micic et al. [114] evaluated the nHAP/PLGA coating scaffold for large segmental defects in the rabbit's ulna. The authors reported almost complete bone regeneration and excellent histological parameters: new bone formation with both endochondral and endosomal types of ossification, high concentrations of BMPs, osteocalcin, and osteopontin within the newly formed bone. Zhang et al. [108] evaluated the HAP/PLGA scaffold for the repair of large segmental defects of rabbit radius and exhibited rapid and strong mineralization and osteoconductivity. Previous studies have shown that both the biocompatibility and mandibular bone regeneration performance of composite polymer/bioceramic scaffolds are enhanced compared to polymeric or bioceramic scaffolds [32]. Regarding mandible reconstruction, Stevanovic et al. [36] investigated the HAP/PLGA and HAP/PEI scaffolds for mandibular bone regeneration in a swine model and demonstrated improved biological behavior compared to conventional xenograft in the treatment of swine's mandibular defects in terms of bone density and bone tissue histological characteristics. An interesting finding in this study was the significant activation of osteocalcin, the most abundant noncollagenous protein in bone tissue, produced by osteoblasts in the HAP/PEI cohort. Osteocalcin is an important molecule for the regulation of bone mineral deposition, and its expression can serve as a marker of mineralized matrix formation [36]. Therefore, the ability of composite scaffolds to induce osteoblasts to produce more osteocalcin may be an interesting feature of these biomaterials.

Biodegradable metals (BMs) have a variety of properties that are essential for bone regeneration scaffolds, including biodegradability properties, mechanical strength, formability, osteogenic capacity, and antibacterial properties [131]. The most representative BMs are Mg-based, Zn-based, and Fe-based. These materials have been used in manufacturing biomimetic scaffolds, fixation plates, screws, pins, wires, and stents [131]. Mg-based biomaterials are widely used because of their elastic modulus, which is similar to human bones, biosafety, and biodegradability. Fe-based biomaterials have a relatively low degradation rate and insoluble degradation products, which greatly limit their application [132]. Zn-based biomaterials possess a moderate degradation rate and excellent mechanical properties for orthopedic and cardiovascular applications [51]. Critical-sized mandibular defects imply the use of load-bearing tissue scaffolds due to significant masticatory forces. Bioresorbable metallic scaffolds may potentially be used to overcome the mechanical properties of conventional tissue scaffolds. Magnesium and its alloys have outstanding mechanical and biological properties for bone regeneration, including mechanical properties and Young's modulus close to that of cortical bone [133–136]. Magnesium stimulates bone growth due to the formation of bone-apatite-like HAP crystals [136]. In vitro studies showed excellent mechanical properties of porous magnesium scaffolds with a modified Young's modulus to adjust to one of the cancellous bones (0.01–2.0 Gpa) [134,135]. The use of Mg-based bone scaffolds may be a promising strategy in future research on mandibular bone regeneration.

### 4.2. Bioactive Molecules

Bioactive molecules and the cell therapies incorporated in the scaffolds significantly improved bone regeneration in comparison to the scaffold alone in the majority of studies. Scaffolds with BMPs significantly promoted bone regeneration in a dose-dependent manner [22,24,31,46,51,56,57,83,84]. BMPs activate MSCs differentiation during bone formation through the activation of the Smad-dependent signaling pathway or the MAPK pathway [10]. The protracted slow release of BMP-2 using microspheres resulted in a better bone quality compared to the early deleterious effect of the supraphysiological dose of BMP [2]. The timing of the application of BMP-2 is important, especially for critical-sized defects, due to the initial burst release of rhBMP-2 and the insufficient number of SCs from the boundary of the bone defect in such cases [137]. Kim et al. [79] found the application of BMP-2 to the mandibular defect one week after surgery, compared with admixing with a hyaluronic acid scaffold before the operation, resulted in significant increases in the mineral density, total volume, and trabecular volume of bone. Çakır-Özkan et al. [92] found that the combined use of VEGF + BMP-2 with the PLLA/PEG scaffold for rabbit mandibular defect resulted in increased osteoblastic activity and neovascularization when compared with the use of BMP-2 or VEGF alone. Similarly, the combined use of FGF + BMP-2 with PLGA/PCL/nHA scaffold for rabbit mandibular defect resulted in significantly promoted proliferation and osteogenic differentiation of BMSCs and osteogenesis than when BMP-2 and FGF were used alone [25]. In a study on sub-human primates of different ages, the host recipient tissue had the same capacity to respond to BMP-2 induction regardless of the subject's age [55]. In addition, previous studies have shown good bone regeneration of scaffolds with BMP-7 or BMP-6 factors [50,63,109]. Das et al. [83] found that the combined use of VEGF + BMP-6 with the PLGA scaffold for rat mandibular defects resulted in significantly enhanced bone repair through the enhancement of angiogenesis and the differentiation of endogenously recruited MSCs into the bone repair site.

Despite the encouraging results of BMPs for bone regeneration in the maxillofacial area for the bridging and ingrowth of bone, the results of biomechanical testing were not uniform. The mechanical tests performed in previous papers showed that the regeneration in the mandibular critical-size defects reconstructed with BMP-7 and BMP-2 showed a wide range of mechanical properties due to the varied proportions of woven and lamellar bone formation that were histologically shown, as well as possible variations in the concentration of BMPs within the grafts [73–75].

A study with porous nHAP/collagen/PLGA scaffolds with incorporated insulin-loaded microspheres showed a higher bone restoration capacity than the defects that were filled with nHAC scaffolds [33]. This finding may be important in the bone regeneration of patients diagnosed with diabetes.

Several studies investigated the use of concentrated growth factor (CGF), a third-generation platelet concentrate extracted from blood, featuring a wide range of sources, low cost, absorbability, lack of immunogenicity, and bone inducibility [101,102]. Zhu et al. [102] investigated the HAP/collagen scaffold in combination with CGF to repair mandibular rabbit defects. The results showed a higher rate of new bone formation, better bone quality, higher osteocalcin and BMP-2 expression, and higher compressive strength and elastic modulus of the nHAC/CGF cohort.

Due to the positive influence of BMPs on mandibular bone regeneration in in vivo studies, several case reports and case series reported the human application of BMPs [138–146]. Moghadam et al. [138] successfully used a BMP bioimplant for the primary reconstruction of a 6 cm mandibular critical-size defect after the segmental resection of ameloblastoma. Warnke et al. [139] used a titanium mesh cage filled with bone mineral blocks, recombinant human BMP-7, and the patient's bone marrow implanted in the *latissimus dorsi* muscle for the growth of the grafted bone. The graft was successfully transplanted as a free bone–muscle flap to reconstruct the mandibular defect. A similar study was performed by Heliotis et al. [140], who used a vascularized pedicled bone flap created with a HAP/BMP-7 composite implant; however, an unfavorable outcome was achieved due to graft failure occurring five months after the transplantation due to MRSA infection. Herford and Boyne [141] reported successful results in 14 patients treated with BMP-2 in a collagen carrier for various mandibular defects. Chao et al. [142] reported successful mandibular reconstruction with BMP-2, applied with collagen sponge and granules of 85% TCP and 15% HAP, following a hemimandibulectomy due to aggressive juvenile ossifying fibroma in a 9-year-old boy.

### 4.3. Cell Therapy

Seeding scaffolds with biologically active cells in order to promote bone regeneration directly at the implant site is a commonly employed bone tissue engineering strategy. All the studies with scaffolds serving as carriers for MSCs reported an increased bone formation compared to scaffold-only cohorts [23,26,34,39,71,81,82,85,98,99,106]. Scaffolds can function as a substitute for native ECM for the conduction, attachment, and growth of encapsulated MSCs cells and prevent anoikis, a form of apoptosis [10]. Furthermore, scaffolds are optimized to protect against host immune attack and induce major cellular processes that are necessary for tissue regeneration [10]. The most commonly used cell therapy used the bone-marrow-derived MSCs (BMSCs), which are capable of differentiating multiple mesodermal lineages, including bone and cartilage [23]. Guo et al. [23] investigated the bioactivity of an n-HA/PA composite implant seeded with ectogenic BMSCs and found that ectogenic BMSCs had a significant impact on bone regeneration in bone-marrow-poor locations such as mandible angle. The authors suggested that the presence of endogenic BMSCs at the implantation site was found to be a critical factor in determining the outcome of the bone regeneration process, since ectogenic BMSCs were not found to enhance bone regeneration in the rich-marrow sites such as the mandibular body, implicating different tissue engineering strategies for bone defects in marrow-rich and marrow-poor sites.

Dental pulp stem cells (DPSCs) offer certain advantages over other SCs, such as accessibility, availability and multipotency, maintain an undifferentiated state upon long-term cultivation, and are little influenced by the number of passages [146]. Gutiérrez-Quintero et al. [26] reported HA/PLGA/DPSCs scaffolds without offering improved bone regeneration due to significant differences in the mRNA levels of osteogenic markers capable of determining osteoblastic stage differentiation (Runx2, OPN, COL1, and ALP). Adipose-derived SCs (ADSCs) have certain advantages compared to BMSCs, such as easy harvesting, a huge number of cells can be obtained from fat tissue, cells that are easy to cultivate and a higher proliferation capacity [147]. Probst et al. [35] found that ADSCs seeding on ceramic/polymer scaffolds improve bone regeneration in large mandibular defects and results in significantly higher bone volume and an increased amount of osteocalcin deposition.

The combination of MSCs with BMP-2 and composite ceramic/polymer scaffolds resulted in significantly more bone regeneration than when using MSCs/scaffold and BMP-2/scaffold complexes [25,28,43,49]. Local gene therapy using BMPs transfected on MSCs and porous n-HA/PA scaffolds in the repair of mandibular defects in rabbits, as well as their response during various periods, showed good biocompatibility, more significant bone formation and earlier mineralization in the implant area. BMP7-transfected MSCs resulted in significantly higher-end elastic modulus, ultimate stress, and ultimate strain four weeks after implantation of the mandibular explant [28]. In addition, no differences were observed between the MSC-only and BMP7-transfected MSC groups at 16 weeks, impying that BMP-7 enhances bone formation in the early phases of mandibular bone regeneration [28]. However, in a study investigating the efficacy of PLGA scaffolds, alone and in combination with BMP-2 and ASCs, when healing a critical-sized segmental mandibular defect in a rat model, bone regeneration was most robust in the BMP-2-treated scaffolds [40]. In this study, bone regeneration scores were graded according to a previously described semi-quantitative scale based on micro-CT images without histological examination.

In a study that compared liposome-mediated gene transfer with MSCs and adenoviral-mediated MSC transduction with BMP-2, the authors found that adenovirus-transfected MSCs resulted in nearly complete bone healing within four weeks of the scaffold being implanted [61]. Still, the authors suggested that liposomes offer several advantages compared to other vectors, such as ease of preparation, no limitation on the DNA size, and fewer immunological and safety problems; thus, they may represent the best vector systems for trials of bone regeneration by BMP-2 gene therapy [61]. Regarding the clinical translation of the MSCs therapy in human mandibular reconstruction, Sandor et al. reported the successful reconstruction of a 10 cm anterior mandibular ameloblastoma resection defect with b-TCP granules, BMP-2, and autologous ASCs [148]. Thus, we may conclude that the preclinical evaluation of MSCs is insufficient to demonstrate the clinical efficacy in mandibular bone regeneration. Presently, the main challenges that need to be resolved before the clinical application of cell therapy for mandibular defects include the choice of optimal MSC source, route of administration, and understanding of interactions between the scaffolds, host tissue, and cells.

### 4.4. Animal Models

Different animal models have been used to investigate mandibular BTE, including rats, rabbits, mini-pigs, domestic swine, dogs, sheep, and primates. Rats are cost-effective, easy to handle, and may be genetically engineered to construct different pathological states. However, rats have a higher metabolic rate and osteogenic potential compared with humans. Furthermore, the bone mineral density of rat cortical bone differs greatly from that of humans, and the operating space of rats is limited by their small size [149]. Rabbits are the most commonly used laboratory animals, as they are easy to acquire, house, and handle, with a short developmental cycle, reaching skeletal maturity at 6 months of age [150]. Rabbits exhibit faster cortical bone remodeling and bone turnover compared with rodents or primates. Due to their faster bone remodeling and large amounts of adipose tissue in the medullary spaces of the mandible, it is difficult to extrapolate in vivo results to human trials [151]. Dog models are widely used in maxillofacial research due to similarities with humans regarding the similar bone mineral density of the mandible and periodontal tissue and comparable intracortical remodeling, similar levels of collagen, and insulin-like growth factor-1 in cortical and cancellous bone. However, the rate of trabecular bone turnover in dogs is highly variable and higher compared to humans [152,153]. Pig bone models are used due to similarities in terms of bone mineral density and bone mineral concentration and the similar bone remodeling processes. Furthermore, mature swine have a similar bone structure to humans, with a well-developed Haversian system and a similar bone regeneration rate [154]. Swine are large animals, which are difficult to handle and maintain under experimental conditions [155]. The sheep model for bone regeneration was used due to its similar bone turnover and bone modeling rates to those of humans [156]. Sheep bones are sufficiently large to compare multiple surgical procedures simultaneously. However, the bones of sheep have a different microstructure and undergo seasonal periods of bone loss [157]. Non-human primates and humans share significant genetic homology, have comparable osteonal remodeling in skeletally mature individuals, and develop similar bone diseases and age-associated bone loss. Primates are generally used in bone biomechanics and loading studies when other large animal models do not adequately represent human bone. The use of non-human primates is expensive and is associated with some cultural and ethical questions [135]. The primary rationale for nHPs is the opportunity to match the genetic background and, therefore, the biological responsiveness of the model, as closely as possible to that of humans. Nonetheless, it has been assumed that the non-human primate model will provide the most predictive model for immunological and biological response due to its genetic background, particularly in the setting of delivery of BMPs, although the variation in response between primates limits these investigations [5,158]. The follow-up duration and the critical defect size varied widely and depended strongly on the animal used. Furthermore, the critical defect size was not uniform, even within a single animal model. Establishing uniform critical-sized defects is particularly difficult with small animals. Thus, it is difficult to fuse the results of the studies into unique conclusions to extrapolate to clinical conditions. Future studies on mandibular bone regeneration should maintain standardized animal models, possibly with larger animals (sheep, swine, and dogs), with standardized defects and follow-up periods.

### 4.5. Study Outcomes

Another important issue was the heterogeneity in the approaches used to evaluate in vivo bone regeneration, which, in many cases, enabled a direct comparison of outcomes between different treatment groups. Standard diagnostic approaches to the evaluation of bone regeneration in vivo comprise radiological, histological, and mechanical testing [2]. The majority of studies used a histological analysis of the explanted mandibular defect to measure the quantity and quality of bone regeneration. Micro-CT and plain radiography were commonly used to quantitatively assess new bone formation. Micro-CT offers certain advantages for new bone formation, and several objective variables could be extracted: bone mineral density, trabecular thickness, and the percentage of newly formed bone [2]. Cone-beam computed tomography (CBCT) may be an interesting alternative because it is available, economical, and less expensive than CT or micro-CT [36]. CBCT can calculate the amount of new bone from grey-scale changes; however, the results are unpredictable, and more objective means of bone characterization are still not possible [36]. Immunohistochemistry was used along with histology and radiologic examinations to evaluate the maturity and formation rate of new bone [2]. Noting that the mandible, during the function of mastication, has to withstand significant muscle forces, the biomechanical characteristics of newly formed bone are extremely substantial. Still, only 12.5% of studies performed a biomechanical testing of mandibular bone defects.

This research has several limitations. The significant variations among the included studies, which made any reasonable comparison complex, were as follows: differences in animal models, various scaffold types, various means of producing scaffolds, differences in cell source, and inconsistent evaluation methods. In addition, several studies did not have control groups. Due to variations in animal models, there were significant differences in the concentrations of growth factors used, and only a few studies determined the dose–response curve. This review included studies with various animal models with substantial differences regarding the follow-up duration and the critical defect size, even within a single animal model. Due to a lack of consistency in the defect size, it is difficult to compare the outcomes between the studies. Similarly, there is no standard animal model for mandibular bone regeneration. There was considerable heterogeneity in the evaluation of in vivo bone regeneration, which enables the direct comparison of outcomes between treatment groups. Future studies should provide standardized measurements of bone regeneration, including histological analysis, imaging results (micro-CT), and biomechanical testing of the newly formed bone for a reliable comparison of the results.

## 5. Conclusions

Mandibular BTE can be considered a highly promising treatment for the reconstruction of critical-sized bone defects. It could become an alternative to microvascular bone grafts, which are considered a gold-standard treatment. In vivo trials are critical for translating from experimental to randomized clinical trials. The review aimed to systematically review in vivo studies and analyze this concept's effectiveness in treating mandibular critical-sized defects.

Currently, there are significant discrepancies between the studies due to various study methodologies, review periods, outcome measures, and different control groups, with significant differences occurring even within a single animal model. The standardization of the animal models, operative techniques, and definition of critical-sized defects for each model is needed, as well as the duration of follow-up and the evaluation of study outcomes. The results of this review support the use of biocompatible scaffolds, especially composite polymer/ceramic scaffolds, for bone regeneration, as they obtain significant results compared to blank controls. In addition, the success of mandibular bone engineering is significantly enhanced by the use of scaffolds with bioactive molecules and/or progenitor cells. However, the clinical application of biomolecules and progenitor cells is limited by its high costs, side effects, and unpredictable responses in humans. Therefore, further research is required to understand the biological fundamentals of the interplay between scaffolds, regulatory molecules, and progenitor cells to translate these experimental findings into clinical practice.

**Supplementary Materials:** The following supporting information can be downloaded at: https://www.mdpi.com/article/10.3390/app13084668/s1, Table S1: An overview of included trials.

**Author Contributions:** Conceptualization, J.D. and G.R.; writing—original draft preparation, J.D., S.V., D.S., I.O., B.J. and M.S.; writing—review and editing, J.D., S.V. and G.R.; supervision, M.S. and G.R. All authors have read and agreed to the published version of the manuscript.

**Funding:** This research received no external funding.

**Institutional Review Board Statement:** Not applicable.

**Informed Consent Statement:** Not applicable.

**Data Availability Statement:** The data presented in this study are available on request from the corresponding author.

**Acknowledgments:** This work was supported by Internal Project $N^0$ 15/21 of Faculty of Medical Sciences, University of Kragujevac, Serbia (01-773/1, 21 January 2022).

**Conflicts of Interest:** The authors declare no conflict of interest.

## References

1. Vujovic, S.; Desnica, J.; Stanisic, D.; Ognjanovic, I.; Stevanovic, M.; Rosic, G. Applications of Biodegradable Magnesium-Based Materials in Reconstructive Oral and Maxillofacial Surgery: A Review. *Molecules* **2022**, *27*, 5529. [CrossRef]
2. Basyuni, S.; Ferro, A.; Santhanam, V.; Birch, M.; McCaskie, A. Systematic scoping review of mandibular bone tissue engineering. *Br. J. Oral Maxillofac. Surg.* **2020**, *58*, 632–642. [CrossRef]
3. Liu, L.; Shi, G.; Cui, Y.; Li, H.; Li, Z.; Zeng, Q.; Guo, Y. Individual construction of freeform-fabricated polycaprolactone scaffolds for osteogenesis. *Biomed. Tech.* **2017**, *62*, 467–479. [CrossRef]
4. Amini, A.R.; Laurencin, C.T.; Nukavarapu, S.P. Bone tissue engineering: Recent advances and challenges. *Crit. Rev. Biomed. Eng.* **2012**, *40*, 363–408. [CrossRef]
5. Oryan, A.; Alidadi, S.; Moshiri, A. Current concerns regarding healing of bone defects. *Hard Tissue* **2013**, *2*, 13. [CrossRef]
6. Jamari, J.; Ammarullah, M.I.; Saad, A.P.M.; Syahrom, A.; Uddin, M.; van der Heide, E.; Basri, H. The Effect of Bottom Profile Dimples on the Femoral Head on Wear in Metal-on-Metal Total Hip Arthroplasty. *J. Funct. Biomater.* **2021**, *12*, 38. [CrossRef]
7. Kretlow, J.D.; Young, S.; Klouda, L.; Wong, M.; Mikos, A.G. Injectable biomaterials for regenerating complex craniofacial tissues. *Adv. Mater.* **2009**, *21*, 3368–3393. [CrossRef]
8. Azevedo, H.S.; Pashkuleva, I. Biomimetic supramolecular designs for the controlled release of growth factors in bone regeneration. *Adv. Drug Deliv. Rev.* **2015**, *94*, 63–76. [CrossRef]
9. Oryan, A.; Kamali, A.; Moshiri, A.; Baghaban Eslaminejad, M. Role of Mesenchymal Stem Cells in Bone Regenerative Medicine: What Is the Evidence? *Cells Tissues Organs* **2017**, *204*, 59–83. [CrossRef]
10. Thrivikraman, G.; Athirasala, A.; Twohig, C.; Boda, S.K.; Bertassoni, L.E. Biomaterials for Craniofacial Bone Regeneration. *Dent. Clin. N. Am.* **2017**, *61*, 835–856. [CrossRef]
11. Putra, R.U.; Basri, H.; Prakoso, A.T.; Chandra, H.; Ammarullah, M.I.; Akbar, I.; Syahrom, A.; Kamarul, T. Level of Activity Changes Increases the Fatigue Life of the Porous Magnesium Scaffold, as Observed in Dynamic Immersion Tests, over Time. *Sustainability* **2023**, *15*, 823. [CrossRef]
12. Stevanovic, M.; Vujovic, S.; Stanisic, D.; Desnica, J.; Ognjanovic, I. The Use of Newly Synthesized Composite Scaffolds for Bone Regeneration—A Review of Literature. *Exp. Appl. Biomed. Res. EABR* **2022**. [CrossRef]
13. Venkataiah, V.S.; Yahata, Y.; Kitagawa, A.; Inagaki, M.; Kakiuchi, Y.; Nakano, M.; Suzuki, S.; Handa, K.; Saito, M. Clinical Applications of Cell-Scaffold Constructs for Bone Regeneration Therapy. *Cells* **2021**, *10*, 2687. [CrossRef]
14. Valdoz, J.C.; Johnson, B.C.; Jacobs, D.J.; Franks, N.A.; Dodson, E.L.; Sanders, C.; Cribbs, C.G.; Van Ry, P.M. The ECM: To Scaffold, or Not to Scaffold, That Is the Question. *Int. J. Mol. Sci.* **2021**, *22*, 12690. [CrossRef]
15. Velasco, M.A.; Narváez-Tovar, C.A.; Garzón-Alvarado, D.A. Design, materials, and mechanobiology of biodegradable scaffolds for bone tissue engineering. *BioMed Res. Int.* **2015**, *2015*, 729076. [CrossRef]
16. Liu, J.; Kerns, D.G. Mechanisms of guided bone regeneration: A review. *Open Dent. J.* **2014**, *8*, 56–65. [CrossRef]
17. Nandi, S.K.; Roy, S.; Mukherjee, P.; Kundu, B.; De, D.K.; Basu, D. Orthopaedic applications of bone graft & graft substitutes: A review. *Indian J. Med. Res.* **2010**, *132*, 15–30.
18. Alam, S.; Ueki, K.; Marukawa, K.; Ohara, T.; Hase, T.; Takazakura, D.; Nakagawa, K. Expression of bone morphogenetic protein 2 and fibroblast growth factor 2 during bone regeneration using different implant materials as an onlay bone graft in rabbit mandibles. *Oral Surg. Oral Med. Oral Pathol. Oral Radiol. Endodontology* **2007**, *103*, 16–26. [CrossRef]
19. Sheikh, Z.; Hamdan, N.; Ikeda, Y.; Grynpas, M.; Ganss, B.; Glogauer, M. Natural graft tissues and synthetic biomaterials for periodontal and alveolar bone reconstructive applications: A review. *Biomater. Res.* **2017**, *21*, 9. [CrossRef]
20. Elgali, I.; Omar, O.; Dahlin, C.; Thomsen, P. Guided bone regeneration: Materials and biological mechanisms revisited. *Eur. J. Oral Sci.* **2017**, *125*, 315–337. [CrossRef]

21. Boyce, T.; Edwards, J.; Scarborough, N. ALLOGRAFT BONE: The influence of processing on safety and performance. *Orthop. Clin. N. Am.* **1999**, *30*, 571–581. [CrossRef]
22. Zhang, L.; Mu, W.; Chen, S.; Yang, D.; Xu, F.; Wu, Y. The enhancement of osteogenic capacity in a synthetic BMP-2 derived peptide coated mineralized collagen composite in the treatment of the mandibular defects. *Biomed. Mater. Eng.* **2016**, *27*, 495–505. [CrossRef]
23. Guo, J.; Meng, Z.; Chen, G.; Xie, D.; Chen, Y.; Wang, H.; Tang, W.; Liu, L.; Jing, W.; Long, J.; et al. Restoration of critical-size defects in the rabbit mandible using porous nanohydroxyapatite-polyamide scaffolds. *Tissue Eng. Part A* **2012**, *18*, 1239–1252. [CrossRef] [PubMed]
24. Liu, Y.; Liu, S.; Fu, Y.; Chang, D.T.; Zhou, Y.H. Mineralised Collagen Scaffolds Loaded with Stromal Cell-derived Factor-1 Improve Mandibular Bone Regeneration. *Chin. J. Dent. Res.* **2014**, *17*, 23–29. [PubMed]
25. Su, J.; Xu, H.; Sun, J.; Gong, X.; Zhao, H. Dual delivery of BMP-2 and bFGF from a new nano-composite scaffold, loaded with vascular stents for large-size mandibular defect regeneration. *Int. J. Mol. Sci.* **2013**, *14*, 12714–12728. [CrossRef] [PubMed]
26. Gutiérrez-Quintero, J.G.; Durán Riveros, J.Y.; Martínez Valbuena, C.A.; Pedraza Alonso, S.; Munévar, J.C.; Viafara-García, S.M. Critical-sized mandibular defect reconstruction using human dental pulp stem cells in a xenograft model-clinical, radiological, and histological evaluation. *Oral Maxillofac. Surg.* **2020**, *24*, 485–493. [CrossRef]
27. Liu, X.; Zhao, K.; Gong, T.; Song, J.; Bao, C.; Luo, E.; Weng, J.; Zhou, S. Delivery of growth factors using a smart porous nanocomposite scaffold to repair a mandibular bone defect. *Biomacromolecules* **2014**, *15*, 1019–1030. [CrossRef]
28. Li, J.; Li, Y.; Ma, S.; Gao, Y.; Zuo, Y.; Hu, J. Enhancement of bone formation by BMP-7 transduced MSCs on biomimetic nano-hydroxyapatite/polyamide composite scaffolds in repair of mandibular defects. *J. Biomed. Mater. Res. A* **2010**, *95*, 973–981. [CrossRef]
29. Jiang, X.; Gittens, S.A.; Chang, Q.; Zhang, X.; Chen, C.; Zhang, Z. The use of tissue-engineered bone with human bone morphogenetic protein-4-modified bone-marrow stromal cells in repairing mandibular defects in rabbits. *Int. J. Oral Maxillofac. Surg.* **2006**, *35*, 1133–1139. [CrossRef]
30. Zhao, J.; Hu, J.; Wang, S.; Sun, X.; Xia, L.; Zhang, X.; Zhang, Z.; Jiang, X. Combination of beta-TCP and BMP-2 gene-modified bMSCs to heal critical size mandibular defects in rats. *Oral Dis.* **2010**, *16*, 46–54. [CrossRef]
31. Wu, W.; Chen, X.; Mao, T.; Chen, F.; Feng, X. Bone marrow-derived osteoblasts seeded into porous beta-tricalcium phosphate to repair segmental defect in canine's mandibula. *Ulus Travma Acil Cerrahi Derg* **2006**, *12*, 268–276. [PubMed]
32. Liu, X.; Liu, H.Y.; Lian, X.; Shi, X.L.; Wang, W.; Cui, F.Z.; Zhang, Y. Osteogenesis of mineralized collagen bone graft modified by PLA and calcium sulfate hemihydrate: In vivo study. *J. Biomater. Appl.* **2013**, *28*, 12–19. [CrossRef] [PubMed]
33. Wang, X.; Wu, X.; Xing, H.; Zhang, G.; Shi, Q.; E, L.; Liu, N.; Yang, T.; Wang, D.; Qi, F.; et al. Porous Nanohydroxyapatite/Collagen Scaffolds Loading Insulin PLGA Particles for Restoration of Critical Size Bone Defect. *ACS Appl. Bio. Mater.* **2017**, *9*, 11380–11391. [CrossRef] [PubMed]
34. Cui, Y.; Lu, C.; Chen, B.; Han, J.; Zhao, Y.; Xiao, Z.; Han, S.; Pan, J.; Dai, J. Restoration of mandibular bone defects with demineralized bone matrix combined with three-dimensional cultured bone marrow-derived mesenchymal stem cells in minipig models. *J. Mater. Sci. Mater. Med.* **2018**, *29*, 147. [CrossRef]
35. Probst, F.A.; Fliefel, R.; Burian, E.; Probst, M.; Eddicks, M.; Cornelsen, M.; Riedl, C.; Seitz, H.; Aszódi, A.; Schieker, M.; et al. Bone regeneration of minipig mandibular defect by adipose derived mesenchymal stem cells seeded tri-calcium phosphate-poly(D,L-lactide-co-glycolide) scaffolds. *Sci. Rep.* **2020**, *10*, 2062. [CrossRef]
36. Stevanovic, M.; Selakovic, D.; Vasovic, M.; Ljujic, B.; Zivanovic, S.; Papic, M.; Zivanovic, M.; Milivojevic, N.; Mijovic, M.; Tabakovic, S.Z.; et al. Comparison of Hydroxyapatite/Poly(lactide-co-glycolide) and Hydroxyapatite/Polyethyleneimine Composite Scaffolds in Bone Regeneration of pigs Mandibular Critical Size Defects: In Vivo Study. *Molecules* **2022**, *27*, 1694. [CrossRef]
37. He, Y.; Zhang, Z.Y.; Zhu, H.G.; Qiu, W.; Jiang, X.; Guo, W. Experimental study on reconstruction of segmental mandible defects using tissue engineered bone combined bone marrow stromal cells with three-dimensional tricalcium phosphate. *J. Craniofac Surg.* **2007**, *18*, 800–805. [CrossRef]
38. Yuan, J.; Cui, L.; Zhang, W.J.; Liu, W.; Cao, Y. Repair of canine mandibular bone defects with bone marrow stromal cells and porous beta-tricalcium phosphate. *Biomaterials* **2007**, *28*, 1005–1013. [CrossRef]
39. Tateno, A.; Asano, M.; Akita, D.; Toriumi, T.; Tsurumachi-Iwasaki, N.; Kazama, T.; Arai, Y.; Matsumoto, T.; Kano, K.; Honda, M. Transplantation of dedifferentiated fat cells combined with a biodegradable type I collagen-recombinant peptide scaffold for critical-size bone defects in rats. *J. Oral Sci.* **2019**, *61*, 534–538. [CrossRef]
40. Lee, M.K.; DeConde, A.S.; Lee, M.; Walthers, C.M.; Sepahdari, A.R.; Elashoff, D.; Grogan, T.; Bezouglaia, O.; Tetradis, S.; St John, M.; et al. Biomimetic scaffolds facilitate healing of critical-sized segmental mandibular defects. *Am. J. Otolaryngol.* **2015**, *36*, 1–6. [CrossRef]
41. Fan, J.; Guo, M.; Im, C.S.; Pi-Anfruns, J.; Cui, Z.K.; Kim, S.; Wu, B.M.; Aghaloo, T.L.; Lee, M. Enhanced Mandibular Bone Repair by Combined Treatment of Bone Morphogenetic Protein 2 and Small-Molecule Phenamil. *Tissue Eng. Part A.* **2017**, *23*, 195–207. [CrossRef] [PubMed]
42. Mankani, M.H.; Kuznetsov, S.A.; Wolfe, R.M.; Marshall, G.W.; Robey, P.G. In vivo bone formation by human bone marrow stromal cells: Reconstruction of the mouse calvarium and mandible. *Stem. Cells* **2006**, *24*, 2140–2149. [CrossRef] [PubMed]

43. Tee, B.C.; Desai, K.G.; Kennedy, K.S.; Sonnichsen, B.; Kim, D.G.; Fields, H.W.; Mallery, S.R.; Schwendeman, S.P.; Sun, Z. Reconstructing jaw defects with MSCs and PLGA-encapsulated growth factors. *Am. J. Transl. Res.* **2016**, *8*, 2693–2704.
44. Lopez, C.D.; Diaz-Siso, J.R.; Witek, L.; Bekisz, J.M.; Cronstein, B.N.; Torroni, A.; Flores, R.L.; Rodriguez, E.D.; Coelho, P.G. Three dimensionally printed bioactive ceramic scaffold osseoconduction across critical-sized mandibular defects. *J. Surg. Res.* **2018**, *223*, 115–122. [CrossRef]
45. Herford, A.S.; Lu, M.; Buxton, A.N.; Kim, J.; Henkin, J.; Boyne, P.J.; Caruso, J.M.; Rungcharassaeng, K.; Hong, J. Recombinant human bone morphogenetic protein 2 combined with an osteoconductive bulking agent for mandibular continuity defects in nonhuman primates. *J. Oral Maxillofac. Surg.* **2012**, *70*, 703–716. [CrossRef]
46. Toriumi, D.M.; O'Grady, K.; Horlbeck, D.M.; Desai, D.; Turek, T.J.; Wozney, J. Mandibular reconstruction using bone morphogenetic protein 2: Long-term follow-up in a canine model. *Laryngoscope* **1999**, *109*, 1481–1489. [CrossRef]
47. Witek, L.; Tian, H.; Tovar, N.; Torroni, A.; Neiva, R.; Gil, L.F.; Coelho, P.G. The effect of platelet-rich fibrin exudate addition to porous poly(lactic-co-glycolic acid) scaffold in bone healing: An in vivo study. *J. Biomed. Mater. Res. B Appl. Biomater.* **2020**, *108*, 1304–1310. [CrossRef]
48. Konopnicki, S.; Sharaf, B.; Resnick, C.; Patenaude, A.; Pogal-Sussman, T.; Hwang, K.G.; Abukawa, H.; Troulis, M.J. Tissue-engineered bone with 3-dimensionally printed β-tricalcium phosphate and polycaprolactone scaffolds and early implantation: An in vivo pilot study in a porcine mandible model. *J. Oral Maxillofac. Surg.* **2015**, *73*, 1016.e1–1016.e11. [CrossRef]
49. Fan, J.; Park, H.; Lee, M.K.; Bezouglaia, O.; Fartash, A.; Kim, J.; Aghaloo, T.; Lee, M. Adipose-derived stem cells and BMP-2 delivery in chitosan-based 3D constructs to enhance bone regeneration in a rat mandibular defect model. *Tissue Eng. Part A* **2014**, *20*, 2169–2179. [CrossRef]
50. Das, A.; Fishero, B.A.; Christophel, J.J.; Li, C.J.; Kohli, N.; Lin, Y.; Dighe, A.S.; Cui, Q. Poly(lactic-co-glycolide) polymer constructs cross-linked with human BMP-6 and VEGF protein significantly enhance rat mandible defect repair. *Cell Tissue Res.* **2016**, *364*, 125–135. [CrossRef]
51. DeConde, A.S.; Sidell, D.; Lee, M.; Bezouglaia, O.; Low, K.; Elashoff, D.; Grogan, T.; Tetradis, S.; Aghaloo, T.; St John, M. Bone morphogenetic protein-2-impregnated biomimetic scaffolds successfully induce bone healing in a marginal mandibular defect. *Laryngoscope* **2013**, *123*, 1149–1155. [CrossRef]
52. Arosarena, O.; Collins, W. Comparison of BMP-2 and -4 for rat mandibular bone regeneration at various doses. *Orthod. Craniofac. Res.* **2005**, *8*, 267–276. [CrossRef] [PubMed]
53. Arosarena, O.A.; Collins, W.L. Bone regeneration in the rat mandible with bone morphogenetic protein-2: A comparison of two carriers. *Otolaryngol. Head Neck Surg.* **2005**, *132*, 592–597. [CrossRef]
54. Arosarena, O.A.; Falk, A.; Malmgren, L.; Bookman, L.; Allen, M.J.; Schoonmaker, J.; Tatum, S.; Kellman, R. Defect repair in the rat mandible with bone morphogenic proteins and marrow cells. *Arch. Facial Plast. Surg.* **2003**, *5*, 103–108. [CrossRef]
55. Boyne, P.J.; Salina, S.; Nakamura, A.; Audia, F.; Shabahang, S. Bone regeneration using rhBMP-2 induction in hemimandibulectomy type defects of elderly sub-human primates. *Cell Tissue Bank.* **2006**, *7*, 1–10. [CrossRef]
56. Lohse, N.; Moser, N.; Backhaus, S.; Annen, T.; Epple, M.; Schliephake, H. Continuous delivery of rhBMP2 and rhVEGF165 at a certain ratio enhances bone formation in mandibular defects over the delivery of rhBMP2 alone–An experimental study in rats. *J. Control. Release* **2015**, *220*, 201–209. [CrossRef]
57. Moser, N.; Lohse, N.; Golstein, J.; Kauffmann, P.; Sven, B.; Epple, M.; Schliephake, H. Do we need retarded delivery of bone growth factors in facial bone repair? An experimental study in rats. *Eur. Cells Mater.* **2017**, *34*, 162–179. [CrossRef]
58. Springer, I.N.; Niehoff, P.; Açil, Y.; Marget, M.; Lange, A.; Warnke, P.H.; Pielenz, H.; Roldán, J.C.; Wiltfang, J. BMP-2 and bFGF in an irradiated bone model. *J. Craniomaxillofac. Surg.* **2008**, *36*, 210–217. [CrossRef]
59. Yahia, S.; Khalil, I.A.; El-Sherbiny, I.M. Sandwich-Like Nanofibrous Scaffolds for Bone Tissue Regeneration. *ACS Appl. Mater. Interfaces* **2019**, *11*, 28610–28620. [CrossRef]
60. Schliephake, H.; Weich, H.A.; Dullin, C.; Gruber, R.; Frahse, S. Mandibular bone repair by implantation of rhBMP-2 in a slow release carrier of polylactic acid–an experimental study in rats. *Biomaterials* **2008**, *29*, 103–110. [CrossRef]
61. Park, J.; Ries, J.; Gelse, K.; Kloss, F.; von der Mark, K.; Wiltfang, J.; Neukam, F.W.; Schneider, H. Bone regeneration in critical size defects by cell-mediated BMP-2 gene transfer: A comparison of adenoviral vectors and liposomes. *Gene Ther.* **2003**, *10*, 1089–1098. [CrossRef] [PubMed]
62. Streckbein, P.; Jäckel, S.; Malik, C.Y.; Obert, M.; Kähling, C.; Wilbrand, J.F.; Zahner, D.; Heidinger, K.; Kampschulte, M.; Pons-Kühnemann, J.; et al. Reconstruction of critical-size mandibular defects in immunoincompetent rats with human adipose-derived stromal cells. *J. Craniomaxillofac. Surg.* **2013**, *41*, 496–503. [CrossRef] [PubMed]
63. Wang, H.; Springer, I.N.; Schildberg, H.; Acil, Y.; Ludwig, K.; Rueger, D.R.; Terheyden, H. Carboxymethylcellulose-stabilized collagenous rhOP-1 device-a novel carrier biomaterial for the repair of mandibular continuity defects. *J. Biomed. Mater. Res. Part A* **2004**, *68*, 219–226. [CrossRef] [PubMed]
64. Schliephake, H.; Knebel, J.W.; Aufderheide, M.; Tauscher, M. Use of cultivated osteoprogenitor cells to increase bone formation in segmental mandibular defects: An experimental pilot study in sheep. *Int. J. Oral Maxillofac. Surg.* **2001**, *30*, 531–537. [CrossRef]
65. Ozaki, M.; Takayama, T.; Yamamoto, T.; Ozawa, Y.; Nagao, M.; Tanabe, N.; Nakajima, A.; Suzuki, N.; Maeno, M.; Yamano, S.; et al. A collagen membrane containing osteogenic protein-1 facilitates bone regeneration in a rat mandibular bone defect. *Arch. Oral Biol.* **2017**, *84*, 19–28. [CrossRef]

66. Marukawa, E.; Asahina, I.; Oda, M.; Seto, I.; Alam, M.; Enomoto, S. Functional reconstruction of the non-human primate mandible using recombinant human bone morphogenetic protein-2. *Int. J. Oral Maxillofac. Surg.* **2002**, *31*, 287–295. [CrossRef]
67. Yamada, Y.; Ueda, M.; Naiki, T.; Takahashi, M.; Hata, K.; Nagasaka, T. Autogenous injectable bone for regeneration with mesenchymal stem cells and platelet-rich plasma: Tissue-engineered bone regeneration. *Tissue Eng.* **2004**, *10*, 955–964. [CrossRef]
68. Seto, I.; Marukawa, E.; Asahina, I. Mandibular reconstruction using a combination graft of rhBMP-2 with bone marrow cells expanded in vitro. *Plast. Reconstr. Surg.* **2006**, *117*, 902–908. [CrossRef]
69. Lopez, C.D.; Diaz-Siso, J.R.; Witek, L.; Bekisz, J.M.; Gil, L.F.; Cronstein, B.N.; Flores, R.L.; Torroni, A.; Rodriguez, E.D.; Coelho, P.G. Dipyridamole Augments Three-Dimensionally Printed Bioactive Ceramic Scaffolds to Regenerate Craniofacial Bone. *Plast. Reconstr. Surg.* **2019**, *143*, 1408–1419. [CrossRef]
70. Seto, I.; Asahina, I.; Oda, M.; Enomoto, S. Reconstruction of the primate mandible with a combination graft of recombinant human bone morphogenetic protein-2 and bone marrow. *J. Oral Maxillofac. Surg.* **2001**, *59*, 53–63. [CrossRef]
71. Alfotawei, R.; Naudi, K.B.; Lappin, D.; Barbenel, J.; Di Silvio, L.; Hunter, K.; McMahon, J.; Ayoub, A. The use of TriCalcium Phosphate (TCP) and stem cells for the regeneration of osteoperiosteal critical-size mandibular bony defects, an in vitro and preclinical study. *J. Craniomaxillofac. Surg.* **2014**, *42*, 863–869. [CrossRef]
72. Abu-Serriah, M.M.; Odell, E.; Lock, C.; Gillar, A.; Ayoub, A.F.; Fleming, R.H. Histological assessment of bioengineered new bone in repairing osteoperiosteal mandibular defects in sheep using recombinant human bone morphogenetic protein-7. *Br. J. Oral Maxillofac. Surg.* **2004**, *42*, 410–418. [CrossRef] [PubMed]
73. Abu-Serriah, M.; Kontaxis, A.; Ayoub, A.; Harrison, J.; Odell, E.; Barbenel, J. Mechanical evaluation of mandibular defects reconstructed using osteogenic protein-1 (rhOP-1) in a sheep model: A critical analysis. *Int. J. Oral Maxillofac. Surg.* **2005**, *34*, 287–293. [CrossRef] [PubMed]
74. Kontaxis, A.; Abu-Serriah, M.; Ayoub, A.F.; Barbenel, J.C. Mechanical testing of recombinant human bone morphogenetic protein-7 regenerated bone in sheep mandibles. *Proc. Inst. Mech. Eng. H* **2004**, *218*, 381–388. [CrossRef] [PubMed]
75. Busuttil Naudi, K.; Ayoub, A.; McMahon, J.; Di Silvio, L.; Lappin, D.; Hunter, K.D.; Barbenel, J. Mandibular reconstruction in the rabbit using beta-tricalcium phosphate (β-TCP) scaffolding and recombinant bone morphogenetic protein 7 (rhBMP-7)—Histological, radiographic and mechanical evaluations. *J. Craniomaxillofac. Surg.* **2012**, *40*, e461–e469. [CrossRef]
76. Deng, N.; Sun, J.; Li, Y.; Chen, L.; Chen, C.; Wu, Y.; Wang, Z.; Li, L. Experimental study of rhBMP-2 chitosan nano-sustained release carrier-loaded PLGA/nHA scaffolds to construct mandibular tissue-engineered bone. *Arch. Oral Biol.* **2019**, *102*, 16–25. [CrossRef]
77. Jin, I.G.; Kim, J.H.; Wu, H.G.; Kim, S.K.; Park, Y.; Hwang, S.J. Effect of bone marrow-derived stem cells and bone morphogenetic protein-2 on treatment of osteoradionecrosis in a rat model. *J. Craniomaxillofac. Surg.* **2015**, *43*, 1478–1486. [CrossRef]
78. Yun, P.Y.; Kim, Y.K.; Jeong, K.I.; Park, J.C.; Choi, Y.J. Influence of bone morphogenetic protein and proportion of hydroxyapatite on new bone formation in biphasic calcium phosphate graft: Two pilot studies in animal bony defect model. *J. Craniomaxillofac. Surg.* **2014**, *42*, 1909–1917. [CrossRef]
79. Kim, J.; Yang, H.J.; Cho, T.H.; Lee, S.E.; Park, Y.D.; Kim, H.M.; Kim, I.S.; Seo, Y.K.; Hwang, S.J.; Kim, S.J. Enhanced regeneration of rabbit mandibular defects through a combined treatment of electrical stimulation and rhBMP-2 application. *Med. Biol. Eng. Comput.* **2013**, *51*, 1339–1348. [CrossRef]
80. Poudel, S.B.; Bhattarai, G.; Kim, J.H.; Kook, S.H.; Seo, Y.K.; Jeon, Y.M.; Lee, J.C. Local delivery of recombinant human FGF7 enhances bone formation in rat mandible defects. *J. Bone Miner. Metab.* **2017**, *35*, 485–496. [CrossRef]
81. Behnia, A.; Haghighat, A.; Talebi, A.; Nourbakhsh, N.; Heidari, F. Transplantation of stem cells from human exfoliated deciduous teeth for bone regeneration in the dog mandibular defect. *World J. Stem. Cells* **2014**, *6*, 505–510. [CrossRef] [PubMed]
82. Khojasteh, A.; Behnia, H.; Hosseini, F.S.; Dehghan, M.M.; Abbasnia, P.; Abbas, F.M. The effect of PCL-TCP scaffold loaded with mesenchymal stem cells on vertical bone augmentation in dog mandible: A preliminary report. *J. Biomed. Mater. Res. B Appl. Biomater.* **2013**, *101*, 848–854. [CrossRef]
83. Gallego, L.; Junquera, L.; García, E.; García, V.; Alvarez-Viejo, M.; Costilla, S.; Fresno, M.F.; Meana, A. Repair of rat mandibular bone defects by alveolar osteoblasts in a novel plasma-derived albumin scaffold. *Tissue Eng. Part A* **2010**, *16*, 1179–1187. [CrossRef]
84. Gallego, L.; Pérez-Basterrechea, M.; García-Consuegra, L.; Álvarez-Viejo, M.; Megías, J.; Novoa, A.; Costilla, S.; Meana, Á.; Junquera, L. Repair of segmental mandibular bone defects in sheep using bone marrow stromal cells and autologous serum scaffold: A pilot study. *J. Clin. Periodontol.* **2015**, *42*, 1143–1151. [CrossRef]
85. Park, J.H.; Jung, S.Y.; Lee, C.K.; Ban, M.J.; Lee, S.J.; Kim, H.Y.; Oh, H.J.; Kim, B.K.; Park, H.S.; Jang, S.H.; et al. A 3D-printed polycaprolactone/β-tricalcium phosphate mandibular prosthesis: A pilot animal study. *Laryngoscope* **2020**, *130*, 358–366. [CrossRef]
86. Li, X.; Song, T.; Chen, X.; Wang, M.; Yang, X.; Xiao, Y.; Zhang, X. Osteoinductivity of Porous Biphasic Calcium Phosphate Ceramic Spheres with Nanocrystalline and Their Efficacy in Guiding Bone Regeneration. *ACS Appl. Mater. Interfaces* **2019**, *11*, 3722–3736. [CrossRef]
87. Issa, J.P.; do Nascimento, C.; Bentley, M.V.; Del Bel, E.A.; Iyomasa, M.M.; Sebald, W.; de Albuquerque, R.F., Jr. Bone repair in rat mandible by rhBMP-2 associated with two carriers. *Micron* **2008**, *39*, 373–379. [CrossRef] [PubMed]
88. Hussein, K.A.; Zakhary, I.E.; Elawady, A.R.; Emam, H.A.; Sharawy, M.; Baban, B.; Akeel, S.; Al-Shabrawey, M.; Elsalanty, M.E. Difference in soft tissue response between immediate and delayed delivery suggests a new mechanism for recombinant human bone morphogenetic protein 2 action in large segmental bone defects. *Tissue Eng. Part A* **2012**, *18*, 665–675. [CrossRef] [PubMed]

89. Ekholm, M.; Hietanen, J.; Tulamo, R.M.; Muhonen, J.; Lindqvist, C.; Kellomäki, M.; Suuronen, R. The copolymer of epsilon-caprolactone-lactide and tricalcium phosphate does not enhance bone growth in mandibular defect of sheep. *J. Mater. Sci. Mater. Med.* **2006**, *17*, 139–145. [CrossRef]
90. Jégoux, F.; Goyenvalle, E.; Cognet, R.; Malard, O.; Moreau, F.; Daculsi, G.; Aguado, E. Mandibular segmental defect regenerated with macroporous biphasic calcium phosphate, collagen membrane, and bone marrow graft in dogs. *Arch. Otolaryngol. Head Neck Surg.* **2010**, *136*, 971–978. [CrossRef]
91. Srouji, S.; Rachmiel, A.; Blumenfeld, I.; Livne, E. Mandibular defect repair by TGF-beta and IGF-1 released from a biodegradable osteoconductive hydrogel. *J. Craniomaxillofac. Surg.* **2005**, *33*, 79–84. [CrossRef] [PubMed]
92. Çakır-Özkan, N.; Eğri, S.; Bekar, E.; Altunkaynak, B.Z.; Kabak, Y.B.; Kıvrak, E.G. The Use of Sequential VEGF- and BMP2-Releasing Biodegradable Scaffolds in Rabbit Mandibular Defects. *J. Oral Maxillofac. Surg.* **2017**, *75*, 221.e1–221.e14. [CrossRef] [PubMed]
93. Carlisle, P.; Guda, T.; Silliman, D.T.; Burdette, A.J.; Talley, A.D.; Alvarez, R.; Tucker, D.; Hale, R.G.; Guelcher, S.A.; BrownBaer, P.R. Localized low-dose rhBMP-2 is effective at promoting bone regeneration in mandibular segmental defects. *J. Biomed. Mater. Res. B Appl. Biomater.* **2019**, *107*, 1491–1503. [CrossRef] [PubMed]
94. Stigler, R.G.; Schimke, M.M.; Bigus, S.; Steinmüller-Nethl, D.; Tillmann, K.; Lepperdinger, G. Pervasion of beta-tricalcium phosphate with nanodiamond particles yields efficient and safe bone replacement material amenable for biofunctionalization and application in large-size osseous defect healing. *Nanomed. Nanotechnol. Biol. Med.* **2019**, *16*, 250–257. [CrossRef]
95. Wang, Y.; Cai, X.; Huang, J.; Zhou, Y.; Jiang, T.; Wang, Y. Bone regeneration in critically sized rat mandible defects through the endochondral pathway using hydroxyapatite-coated 3D-printed Ti6Al4V scaffolds. *RSC Adv.* **2018**, *8*, 31745–31754. [CrossRef]
96. Helal, M.H.; Hendawy, H.D.; Gaber, R.A.; Helal, N.R.; Aboushelib, M.N. Osteogenesis ability of CAD-CAM biodegradable polylactic acid scaffolds for reconstruction of jaw defects. *J. Prosthet. Dent.* **2019**, *121*, 118–123. [CrossRef]
97. Khojasteh, A.; Hosseinpour, S.; Dehghan, M.M.; Mashhadiabbas, F.; Rezai Rad, M.; Ansari, S.; Farzad Mohajeri, S.; Zadeh, H.H. Antibody-Mediated Osseous Regeneration for Bone Tissue Engineering in Canine Segmental Defects. *BioMed Res. Int.* **2018**, *2018*, 9508721. [CrossRef]
98. Nuntanaranont, T.; Promboot, T.; Sutapreyasri, S. Effect of expanded bone marrow-derived osteoprogenitor cells seeded into polycaprolactone/tricalcium phosphate scaffolds in new bone regeneration of rabbit mandibular defects. *J. Mater. Sci. Mater. Med.* **2018**, *29*, 24. [CrossRef]
99. Maglione, M.; Spano, S.; Ruaro, M.E.; Salvador, E.; Zanconati, F.; Tromba, G.; Turco, G. In vivo evaluation of chitosan-glycerol gel scaffolds seeded with stem cells for full-thickness mandibular bone regeneration. *J. Oral Sci.* **2017**, *59*, 225–232. [CrossRef]
100. Song, W.Y.; Liu, G.M.; Li, J.; Luo, Y.G. Bone morphogenetic protein-2 sustained delivery by hydrogels with microspheres repairs rabbit mandibular defects. *Tissue Eng. Regen. Med.* **2016**, *13*, 750–761. [CrossRef]
101. Mao, Y.; Hu, M.; Chen, L.; Chen, X.; Liu, M.; Zhang, M.; Nie, M.; Liu, X. CGF-HLC-I repaired the bone defect repair of the rabbits mandible through tight junction pathway. *Front. Bioeng. Biotechnol.* **2022**, *10*, 976499. [CrossRef] [PubMed]
102. Zhu, Y.; Cao, N.; Zhang, Y.; Cao, G.; Hao, C.; Liu, K.; Li, X.; Wang, W. The Ability and Mechanism of nHAC/CGF in Promoting Osteogenesis and Repairing Mandibular Defects. *Nanomaterials* **2022**, *12*, 212. [CrossRef] [PubMed]
103. Cao, S.S.; Li, S.Y.; Geng, Y.M.; Kapat, K.; Liu, S.B.; Perera, F.H.; Li, Q.; Terheyden, H.; Wu, G.; Che, Y.J.; et al. Prefabricated 3D-Printed Tissue-Engineered Bone for Mandibular Reconstruction: A Preclinical Translational Study in Primate. *ACS Biomater. Sci. Eng.* **2021**, *7*, 5727–5738. [CrossRef]
104. Barrientos-Lezcano, F.J.; Redondo-González, L.M.; Alberca-Zeballos, M.; Sánchez-García, A.M.; García-Sancho, J. Mandibular bone regeneration with autologous adipose-derived mesenchymal stem cells and coralline hydroxyapatite: Experimental study in rats. *Br. J. Oral Maxillofac. Surg.* **2021**, *59*, 1192–1199. [CrossRef] [PubMed]
105. Xu, H.Z.; Su, J.S. Restoration of critical defects in the rabbit mandible using osteoblasts and vascular endothelial cells co-cultured with vascular stent-loaded nano-composite scaffolds. *J. Mech. Behav. Biomed. Mater.* **2021**, *124*, 104831. [CrossRef] [PubMed]
106. Lee, J.S.; Park, T.H.; Ryu, J.Y.; Kim, D.K.; Oh, E.J.; Kim, H.M.; Shim, J.H.; Yun, W.S.; Huh, J.B.; Moon, S.H.; et al. Osteogenesis of 3D-Printed PCL/TCP/bdECM Scaffold Using Adipose-Derived Stem Cells Aggregates; An Experimental Study in the Canine Mandible. *Int. J. Mol. Sci.* **2021**, *22*, 5409. [CrossRef]
107. Park, S.A.; Lee, H.J.; Kim, S.Y.; Kim, K.S.; Jo, D.W.; Park, S.Y. Three-dimensionally printed polycaprolactone/beta-tricalcium phosphate scaffold was more effective as an rhBMP-2 carrier for new bone formation than polycaprolactone alone. *J. Biomed. Mater. Res. A* **2021**, *109*, 840–848. [CrossRef]
108. Zhang, P.; Hong, Z.; Yu, T.; Chen, X.; Jing, X. In vivo mineralization and osteogenesis of nanocomposite scaffold of poly(lactide-co-glycolide) and hydroxyapatite surface-grafted with poly(L-lactide). *Biomaterials* **2009**, *30*, 58–70. [CrossRef]
109. Terheyden, H.; Warnke, P.; Dunsche, A.; Jepsen, S.; Brenner, W.; Palmie, S.; Toth, C.; Rueger, D.R. Mandibular reconstruction with prefabricated vascularized bone grafts using recombinant human osteogenic protein-1: An experimental study in miniature pigs. Part II: Transplantation. *Int. J. Oral Maxillofac. Surg.* **2001**, *30*, 469–478. [CrossRef]
110. Lynn, A.K.; Yannas, I.V.; Bonfield, W. Antigenicity and immunogenicity of collagen. *J. Biomed. Mater. Res. B Appl. Biomater.* **2004**, *71*, 343–354. [CrossRef]
111. Kim, M.H.; Kim, B.S.; Park, H.; Lee, J.; Park, W.H. Injectable methylcellulose hydrogel containing calcium phosphate nanoparticles for bone regeneration. *Int. J. Biol. Macromol.* **2018**, *109*, 57–64. [CrossRef] [PubMed]

112. Townsend, J.M.; Andrews, B.T.; Feng, Y.; Wang, J.; Nudo, R.J.; Van Kampen, E.; Gehrke, S.H.; Berkland, C.J.; Detamore, M.S. Superior calvarial bone regeneration using pentenoate-functionalized hyaluronic acid hydrogels with devitalized tendon particles. *Acta Biomater.* **2018**, *71*, 148–155. [CrossRef] [PubMed]
113. Zhai, P.; Peng, X. Li, B. Liu, Y.; Sun, H.; Li, X. The application of hyaluronic acid in bone regeneration. *Int. J. Biol. Macromol.* **2020**, *151*, 1224–1239. [CrossRef] [PubMed]
114. Micic, M.; Antonijevic, D.; Milutinovic-Smiljanic, S.; Trisic, D.; Colovic, B.; Kosanovic, D.; Prokic, B.; Vasic, J.; Zivkovic, S.; Milasin, J.; et al. Developing a novel resorptive hydroxyapatite-based bone substitute for over-critical size defect reconstruction: Physicochemical and biological characterization and proof of concept in segmental rabbit's ulna reconstruction. Biomedizinische Technik. *Biomed. Eng.* **2020**, *65*, 491–505. [CrossRef] [PubMed]
115. Zhao, D.; Zhu, T.; Li, J.; Cui, L.; Zhang, Z.; Zhuang, X.; Ding, J. Poly(lactic-co-glycolic acid)-based composite bone-substitute materials. *Bioact. Mater.* **2020**, *6*, 346–360. [CrossRef] [PubMed]
116. Liu, C.G.; Zeng, Y.T.; Kankala, R.K.; Zhang, S.S.; Chen, A.Z.; Wang, S.B. Characterization and Preliminary Biological Evaluation of 3D-Printed Porous Scaffolds for Engineering Bone Tissues. *Materials* **2018**, *11*, 1832. [CrossRef]
117. Dong, X.P.; Zhang, Y.W.; Pei, Y.J.; Wang, Z.; Zhang, X.X.; Yu, X.L.; Ai, Z.Z.; Mei, Y.X.; Li, J.N. Three-dimensional printing for the accurate orthopedics: Clinical cases analysis. *Bio-Des. Manuf.* **2022**, *3*, 122–132. [CrossRef]
118. Liang, X.; Qi, Y.; Pan, Z.; He, Y.; Liu, X.; Cui, S.; Ding, J. Design and preparation of quasi-spherical salt particles as water-soluble porogens to fabricate hydrophobic porous scaffolds for tissue engineering and tissue regeneration. *Mater. Chem. Front.* **2018**, *8*, 1539–1553. [CrossRef]
119. Lee, H.; Yoo, J.J.; Kang, H.W.; Cho, D.W. Investigation of thermal degradation with extrusion-based dispensing modules for 3D bioprinting technology. *Biofabrication* **2016**, *8*, 015011. [CrossRef]
120. Yu, Y.; Sun, B.; Yi, C.; Mo, X. Stem cell homing-based tissue engineering using bioactive materials. *Front. Mater. Sci.* **2017**, *11*, 93–105. [CrossRef]
121. Batool, F.; Strub, M.; Petit, C.; Bugueno, I.M.; Bornert, F.; Clauss, F.; Huck, O.; Kuchler-Bopp, S.; Benkirane-Jessel, N. Periodontal Tissues, Maxillary Jaw Bone, and Tooth Regeneration Approaches: From Animal Models Analyses to Clinical Applications. *Nanomaterials* **2018**, *8*, 337. [CrossRef] [PubMed]
122. Liu, J.; Ye, X.; Wang, H.; Zhu, M.; Wang, B.; Yan, H. The influence of pH and temperature on the morphology of hydroxyapatite synthesized by hydrothermal method. *Ceram. Int.* **2003**, *29*, 629–633. [CrossRef]
123. Rodríguez-Lugo, V.; Hernández, J.S.; Arellano-Jimenez, M.J.; Hernández-Tejeda, P.H.; Recillas-Gispert, S. Characterization of hydroxyapatite by electron microscopy. *Microsc. Microanal.* **2005**, *11*, 516–523. [CrossRef] [PubMed]
124. Jokanovic, V.; Jokanovic, B.; Markovic, D.; Zivojinovic, V.; Pasalic, S.; Izvonar, D.; Plavsic, M. Kinetics and sintering mechanisms of hydro-thermally obtained hydroxyapatite. *Mater. Chem. Phys.* **2008**, *111*, 180–185. [CrossRef]
125. Ungureanu, D.N.; Angelescu, N.; Bacinschi, Z.; Stoian, E.V.; Rizescu, C.Z. Thermal stability of chemically precipitated hydroxyapatite nanopowders. *Int. J. Biol. Biomed. Eng.* **2011**, *5*, 57–64.
126. Bodhak, S.; Bose, S.; Bandyopadhyay, A. Electrically polarized HAp-coated Ti: In vitro bone cell-material interactions. *Acta Biomater.* **2010**, *6*, 641–651. [CrossRef]
127. Zhang, B.G.; Myers, D.E.; Wallace, G.G.; Brandt, M.; Choong, P.F. Bioactive coatings for orthopaedic implants-recent trends in development of implant coatings. *Int. J. Mol. Sci.* **2014**, *15*, 11878–11921. [CrossRef]
128. Fitzpatrick, V.; Martín-Moldes, Z.; Deck, A.; Torres-Sanchez, R.; Valat, A.; Cairns, D.; Li, C.; Kaplan, D.L. Functionalized 3D-printed silk-hydroxyapatite scaffolds for enhanced bone regeneration with innervation and vascularization. *Biomaterial.* **2021**, *276*, 120995. [CrossRef]
129. Jokanović, V.; Čolović, B.; Marković, D.; Petrović, M.; Jokanović, M.; Milosavljević, P.; Sopta, J. In Vivo investigation of ALBO-OS scaffold based on hydroxyapatite and PLGA. *J. Nanomater.* **2016**, *2016*, 3948768. [CrossRef]
130. Furtos, G.; Rivero, G.; Rapuntean, S.; Abraham, G.A. Amoxicillin-loaded electrospun nanocomposite membranes for dental applications. *J. Biomed. Mater. Res. B Appl. Biomater.* **2017**, *105*, 966–976. [CrossRef]
131. Xia, D.; Yang, F.; Zheng, Y.; Liu, Y.; Zhou, Y. Research status of biodegradable metals designed for oral and maxillofacial applications: A review. *Bioact. Mater.* **2021**, *6*, 4186–4208. [CrossRef] [PubMed]
132. Hang, R.; Wang, C.; Yu, Z.; Li, Z.; Xiao, Y. Biodegradable metallic wires in dental and orthopedic applications: A review. *Materials* **2018**, *8*, 212. [CrossRef]
133. Rider, P.; Kačarević, Ž.P.; Elad, A.; Rothamel, D.; Sauer, G.; Bornert, F.; Windisch, P.; Hangyási, D.; Molnar, B.; Hesse, B.; et al. Biodegradation of a Magnesium Alloy Fixation Screw Used in a Guided Bone Regeneration Model in Beagle Dogs. *Materials* **2022**, *15*, 4111. [CrossRef] [PubMed]
134. Muschler, G.F.; Raut, V.P.; Patterson, T.E.; Wenke, J.C.; Hollinger, J.O. The design and use of animal models for translational research in bone tissue engineering and regenerative medicine. *Tissue Eng. Part B Rev.* **2010**, *16*, 123–145. [CrossRef]
135. Boden, S.D.; Grob, D.; Damien, C. Ne-Osteo bone growth factor for posterolateral lumbar spine fusion: Results from a nonhuman primate study and a prospective human clinical pilot study. *Spine* **2004**, *29*, 504–514. [CrossRef]
136. Chanchareonsook, N.; Junker, R.; Jongpaiboonkit, L.; Jansen, J.A. Tissue-engineered mandibular bone reconstruction for continuity defects: A systematic approach to the literature. *Tissue Eng. Part B Rev.* **2014**, *20*, 147–162. [CrossRef] [PubMed]

137. Kim, I.S.; Lee, E.N.; Cho, T.H.; Song, Y.M.; Hwang, S.J.; Oh, J.H.; Park, E.K.; Koo, T.Y.; Seo, Y.K. Promising efficacy of Escherichia coli recombinant human bone morphogenetic protein-2 in collagen sponge for ectopic and orthotopic bone formation and comparison with mammalian cell recombinant human bone morphogenetic protein-2. *Tissue Eng. Part A* **2011**, *17*, 337–348. [CrossRef]
138. Moghadam, H.G.; Urist, M.R.; Sandor, G.K.; Clokie, C.M. Successful mandibular reconstruction using a BMP bioimplant. *J. Craniofacial Surg.* **2001**, *12*, 119–128. [CrossRef]
139. Warnke, P.H.; Springer, I.N.; Wiltfang, J.; Acil, Y.; Eufinger, H.; Wehmöller, M.; Russo, P.A.; Bolte, H.; Sherry, E.; Behrens, E.; et al. Growth and transplantation of a custom vascularised bone graft in a man. *Lancet* **2004**, *364*, 766–770. [CrossRef]
140. Heliotis, M.; Lavery, K.M.; Ripamonti, U.; Tsiridis, E.; di Silvio, L. Transformation of a prefabricated hydroxyapatite/osteogenic protein-1 implant into a vascularised pedicled bone flap in the human chest. *Int. J. Oral Maxillofac. Surg.* **2006**, *35*, 265–269. [CrossRef]
141. Herford, A.S.; Boyne, P.J. Reconstruction of mandibular continuity defects with bone morphogenetic protein-2 (rhBMP-2). *J. Oral Maxillofac. Surg.* **2008**, *66*, 616–624. [CrossRef] [PubMed]
142. Chao, M.; Donovan, T.; Sotelo, C.; Carstens, M.H. In situ osteogenesis of hemimandible with rhBMP-2 in a 9-year-old boy: Osteoinduction via stem cell concentration. *J. Craniofac. Surg.* **2006**, *17*, 405–412. [CrossRef] [PubMed]
143. Clokie, C.M.; Sándor, G.K. Reconstruction of 10 major mandibular defects using bioimplants containing BMP-7. *J. Can. Dent. Assoc.* **2008**, *74*, 67–72.
144. Glied, A.N.; Kraut, R.A. Off-label use of rhBMP-2 for reconstruction of critical-sized mandibular defects. *N. Y. State Dent. J.* **2010**, *76*, 32–35.
145. Herford, A.S.; Cicciù, M. Recombinant human bone morphogenetic protein type 2 jaw reconstruction in patients affected by giant cell tumor. *J. Craniofac. Surg.* **2010**, *21*, 1970–1975. [CrossRef]
146. Scadden, D.T. The stem-cell niche as an entity of action. *Nature* **2006**, *441*, 1075–1079. [CrossRef]
147. Monaco, E.; Bionaz, M.; Hollister, S.J.; Wheeler, M.B. Strategies for regeneration of the bone using porcine adult adipose-derived mesenchymal stem cells. *Theriogenology* **2011**, *75*, 1381–1399. [CrossRef] [PubMed]
148. Sándor, G.K.; Tuovinen, V.J.; Wolff, J.; Patrikoski, M.; Jokinen, J.; Nieminen, E.; Mannerström, B.; Lappalainen, O.P.; Seppänen, R.; Miettinen, S. Adipose stem cell tissue-engineered construct used to treat large anterior mandibular defect: A case report and review of the clinical application of good manufacturing practice-level adipose stem cells for bone regeneration. *J. Oral Maxillofac. Surg.* **2013**, *71*, 938–950. [CrossRef]
149. Aerssens, J.; Boonen, S.; Lowet, G.; Dequeker, J. Interspecies differences in bone composition, density, and quality: Potential implications for in vivo bone research. *Endocrinology* **1998**, *139*, 663–670. [CrossRef]
150. Gilsanz, V.; Roe, T.F.; Gibbens, D.T.; Schulz, E.E.; Carlson, M.E.; Gonzalez, O.; Boechat, M.I. Effect of sex steroids on peak bone density of growing rabbits. *Am. J. Physiol.* **1988**, *255*, E416–E421. [CrossRef]
151. Castañeda, S.; Largo, R.; Calvo, E.; Rodríguez-Salvanés, F.; Marcos, M.E.; Díaz-Curiel, M.; Herrero-Beaumont, G. Bone mineral measurements of subchondral and trabecular bone in healthy and osteoporotic rabbits. *Skelet. Radiol.* **2006**, *35*, 34–41. [CrossRef] [PubMed]
152. Wancket, L.M. Animal Models for Evaluation of Bone Implants and Devices: Comparative Bone Structure and Common Model Uses. *Vet. Pathol.* **2015**, *52*, 842–850. [CrossRef] [PubMed]
153. Reitan, K.; Kvam, E. Comparative behavior of human and animal tissue during experimental tooth movement. *Angle Orthod.* **1971**, *41*, 1–14. [CrossRef]
154. Harper, R.A.; Pfeiffer, F.M.; Choma, T.J. The minipig as a potential model for pedicle screw fixation: Morphometry and mechanics. *J. Orthop. Surg. Res.* **2019**, *14*, 246. [CrossRef] [PubMed]
155. Schorn, L.; Sproll, C.; Ommerborn, M.; Naujoks, C.; Kübler, N.R.; Depprich, R. Vertical bone regeneration using rhBMP-2 and VEGF. *Head Face Med.* **2017**, *13*, 11. [CrossRef] [PubMed]
156. Jinno, Y.; Jimbo, R.; Lindström, M.; Sawase, T.; Lilin, T.; Becktor, J.P. Vertical Bone Augmentation Using Ring Technique with Three Different Materials in the Sheep Mandible Bone. *Int. J. Oral Maxillofac. Implants* **2018**, *33*, 1057–1063. [CrossRef] [PubMed]
157. Carrel, J.P.; Wiskott, A.; Moussa, M.; Rieder, P.; Scherrer, S.; Durual, S. A 3D printed TCP/HA structure as a new osteoconductive scaffold for vertical bone augmentation. *Clin. Oral Implants. Res.* **2016**, *27*, 55–62. [CrossRef]
158. Triplett, R.G.; Nevins, M.; Marx, R.E.; Spagnoli, D.B.; Oates, T.W.; Moy, P.K.; Boyne, P.J. Pivotal, randomized, parallel evaluation of recombinant human bone morphogenetic protein-2/absorbable collagen sponge and autogenous bone graft for maxillary sinus floor augmentation. *J. Oral Maxillofac. Surg.* **2009**, *67*, 1947–1960. [CrossRef]

*applied sciences*

MDPI

*Review*

# The Appliance of A-PRF and CGF in the Treatment of Impacted Mandibular Third Molar Extraction Sockets—Narrative Review

**Daniel Selahi [1,†], Maciej Spiegel [2,*,†], Jakub Hadzik [1,*], Artur Pitułaj [1], Filip Michalak [1], Paweł Kubasiewicz-Ross [1] and Marzena Dominiak [1]**

1 Department of Dental Surgery, Faculty of Dentistry, Wroclaw Medical University, Krakowska 26, 50-425 Wroclaw, Poland
2 Department of Pharmacognosy and Herbal Medicines, Faculty of Pharmacy, Wroclaw Medical University, Borowska 211A, 50-556 Wroclaw, Poland
* Correspondence: maciej.spiegel@student.umw.edu.pl (M.S.); jakub.hadzik@umw.edu.pl (J.H.)
† These authors contributed equally to this work.

**Abstract:** Tooth extractions, especially of impacted lower third molars, are among the most common procedures performed in dental practices. The continuity of the patient's oral mucosa, which is interrupted during them, can manifest itself in general discomfort, pain, swelling, and even trismus. In the age of cosmetic dentistry, when lost teeth are restored through implant, prosthetic, and orthodontic treatment, each tooth extraction actually reduces the amount of available alveolar bone. This has prompted researchers to develop extraction sockets treatment procedures that reduce the negative consequences of surgical intervention while also enhancing the rate of alveolar bone and soft tissue regeneration using minimally invasive approaches. This is expected to enable or significantly facilitate further stages of treatment. The aim of this paper is to review the literature on the use of autologous blood preparations, which are considered to aid regenerative processes when applied to extraction sockets.

**Keywords:** advanced platelet-rich plasma; concentrated growth factors; post-extraction sockets; A-PRF; CGF; regeneration; autologous blood products; dentistry

**Citation:** Selahi, D.; Spiegel, M.; Hadzik, J.; Pitułaj, A.; Michalak, F.; Kubasiewicz-Ross, P.; Dominiak, M. The Appliance of A-PRF and CGF in the Treatment of Impacted Mandibular Third Molar Extraction Sockets—Narrative Review. *Appl. Sci.* **2023**, *13*, 165. https://doi.org/10.3390/app13010165

Academic Editor: Vittorio Checchi

Received: 15 November 2022
Revised: 16 December 2022
Accepted: 19 December 2022
Published: 23 December 2022



## 1. Introduction

During the extraction, the periodontal ligaments are torn, and the tooth is luxated and removed, resulting in the tissues disruption. In the case of an impacted tooth, the surgical intervention is usually more invasive than a simple tooth extraction—procedures such as cutting, detaching the flap and often removing the bone around the tooth are required. The level of difficulty, and therefore the length of the extraction, has an impact on healing. It is influenced by factors such as the position of the tooth in the bone or its size and shape. A statistically significant correlation between the gonial angle and the position of lower third molars was shown by Barone S et al. in 2021, who confirmed that a higher incidence of impacted lower third molars was associated with a lower value of the gonial angle, which may facilitate the decision to extract germs of the lower wisdom teeth at an early stage of development [1]. The difficulty of extraction of impacted lower wisdom teeth in relation to various factors was examined by Park et al. They confirmed that older age, male sex, depth of impaction, position of the retained tooth, large or/and bulbous roots, ankylosis and blurred root image on panoramic radiographs are factors that increase the difficulty of extraction [2]. Unfortunately, tooth extractions, like all surgical procedures, are associated with postoperative complications. Cho et al., in their review article, showed that the use of painkillers such as paracetamol and ibuprofen reduce pain, and trismus and swelling could be reduced by using corticosteroids, while antibiotics administered immediately before extraction can reduce the risk of infection and alveolar osteitis (but postoperative use does not seem to make sense), and gels and mouthwash with chlorhexidine reduce the incidence of alveolar osteitis [3].

Previously, the only way to heal the alveoli of extracted teeth was a natural dressing made of a blood clot. The recovery period was associated with swelling, discomfort and a dry socket, and there was a risk of hemorrhage and nerve damage during the procedure [4]. This prompted critics to seek alternative treatments such as dressings that modulate inflammatory responses and accelerate healing [5].

Human plasma derivatives, also known as tissue fibrin adhesives, were the first of their kind to be introduced in Europe in the late 1970s. The general mechanism of action relies on the formation of a fibrin clot, which is the end product of the blood clotting process. They are used to seal wound edges and provide a homeostatic surface, as well as a bonding substance for biomaterial particles in bone augmentation surgery. The commercial preparation was made from cryoprecipitated donor plasma and contained two lyophilized components: fibrinogen/fibronectin/factor–XIII dissolved in an antifibrinolytic solution (e.g., aprotinin), and thrombin concentrate dissolved in a dilute calcium chloride solution. Activated factor XIII catalyzes crosslinking between fibrin molecules in the presence of calcium cations, resulting in a water-insoluble fibrin matrix that serves as a clot scaffold.

However, the use of such treatment puts patients at risk of infection with pathogens such as hepatitis (HBV, HCV). This led researchers to seek procedures based on the use of autologous preparations derived from patients' serum. Combining whole plasma from patients with bovine thrombin produced fibrin glues. Unfortunately, their manufacture was characterized by very low physical reproducibility (in terms of viscosity and elasticity, for example) [6].

## 2. Materials and Methods

There are few studies and review articles in the scientific literature on modern techniques for the treatment of post-extraction sockets. Nonetheless, knowledge of this topic is essential for refining practice and advancing this field of dental surgery. With that in mind, the aim of this review is to present the current state of knowledge on the management of post-extraction sockets in the form of a narrative summary. Current treatment practices and research in the field of regenerative dentistry are discussed.

Papers on PRF and CGF were searched in the Pubmed, Medline, and Scopus databases. Following the extraction of third molars, particular emphasis was placed on facts about their appliance. The articles were compiled in April 2021 and included most of the latest news from the previous 20 years.

D.S. and M.S. briefly assessed the abstracts of the resulting publications for inclusion in this review. If the article was relevant and presented unique findings, databases were also searched for the keywords included, allowing us to expand our review to include relevant but rarely published materials. This is due to the novelty of the recommended approach to the treatment of third molar sockets. The final list of items considered was selected after much deliberation. It resulted in a total of 58 articles.

This review is divided into two parts: A-PRF and CGF. The topic of their mechanisms of action, applications, and a discussion of their claimed results are presented.

## 3. Results

In 1998, Marx et al. [7]. developed platelet-rich plasma (PRP) as a breakthrough in the use of platelet preparations derived from blood with higher angiogenic or osteogenic potential than the clot found in the socket after extraction. He obtained it by centrifuging 400 to 450 mL of a patient's whole blood at 5600 RPM (revolutions per minute) with the addition of citrate phosphate dextrose (an anticoagulant). The previous procedure resulted in three layers of preparation, starting from the lowest: red blood cells, PRP (platelet-rich plasma, also called "buffy coat"), and PPP (platelet-poor plasma). After the PPP layer was collected, the remaining blood was centrifuged at 2400 RPM to properly separate the PRP from the red blood cells. To start the coagulation process, PRP must be mixed with 10%

calcium chloride and bovine thrombin. Individual 10 mL syringes were used for mixing, with 6 mL of PRP, 1 mL of calcium chloride + thrombin and 1 mL of air collected as a mixing element. A proper PRP preparation with a gel consistency is formed after mixing in the syringe for 6 to 10 s.

After extensive research, Jo et al. [8]. presented a modification to the PRP technique in 2013. According to the original concept, citrate phosphate dextrose is used as an anticoagulant, and calcium gluconate + bovine thrombin is used as a coagulant. After a 5-min centrifugation of 9 mL of the patient's blood at 900 RPM, three fractions are visible: red blood cells, buffy coat, and platelets with white blood cells. The top two fractions were collected and centrifuged again (1500 RPM, 15 min), after which this top layer of PPP is collected, leaving only 2 mL of PRP in the tube. When PRP is treated with 0.2 mL of 10% calcium gluconate, it forms a gel with 4.2 times the platelet concentration of peripheral blood. Both centrifuges use plastic tubes.

Anitua et al. [9,10] proposed another concept of an autologous blood derivative from the PRP family that accelerates the healing process, calling their product PRGF (Plasma Rich In Growth Factors). After a single 8-min centrifugation at 1850 RPM using 5 mL plastic tubes containing the anticoagulant sodium citrate, a fibrin clot was produced from the patient's blood. The centrifugation results in the three visible layers, starting from the bottom: a layer of red blood cells, a middle transitional layer called a buffy coat, and an upper layer of cell-free plasma, which includes two empirically defined layers: upper plasma with low-growth factors (PPGF), and lower plasma rich in growth factors (PRGF), which is collected from all centrifuged tubes and transferred to a pooled one, to which calcium chloride is added to induce clotting, and after 15 to 20 min PRGF gel is obtained. It is noteworthy that the authors do not use bovine thrombin (except from the previously mentioned modifications) for clot formation, and one of its salient features is the absence of both erythrocytes and leukocytes. According to the authors' findings, the absence of polynuclear neutrophils within the damaged tissues, which are the body's first line of defense against pathogens, may have a beneficial effect on healing. This is because they produce matrix metalloproteinases MMP-8 and MMP-9, which can impede tissue repair, as well as free radicals (active forms of oxygen and nitrogen), which can damage cells in surrounding tissues in addition to bacteria.

The aforementioned family of PRP preparations is the first generation of platelet concentrates. Their main disadvantage is the need for coagulants and anticoagulants in the manufacturing process, which usually involves repeated centrifugation. In addition, the use of bovine thrombin can cause coagulopathies by stimulating the formation of antibodies against blood clotting components V and XI, as well as thrombin [11]. Therefore, researchers conducted additional studies to develop an autologous biomaterial that would not require the use of chemicals in the manufacturing process.

Choukroun's breakthrough was classified as the second generation of platelet concentrates, called L-PRF (Platelet-Rich Fibrin) concentrates, which he produced and presented in 2001 [12,13]. Unlike previous concepts, the protocol for obtaining PRF does not require any additives; only the patient's blood, a glass tube and a centrifuge are needed to obtain a clot, and the process is physiological, using the autogenous thrombin present in the collected blood [14]. The original procedure used 10 mL plastic tubes with a glass cover on the inside, and the collected blood was centrifuged for 10 min at 3000 RPM. When the blood contacts the inside surface of the glass tube, the clotting cascade is activated; fibrinogen accumulated during the centrifugation process in the upper part of the tube, as a result of the action of thrombin, is transformed into a fibrin clot occupying the central part of the tube, inside which platelets, white blood cells and growth factors are trapped; the upper layer is platelet-poor plasma and the lower layer is red blood cells [5].

PRFM, T-PRF, liquid i-PRF, Vivostat PRF and A-PRF, A-PRF+, CGF are among the second generation formulations and are described below:

- PRFM (Platelet-Rich Fibrin Matrix), is a method of producing platelet-rich fibrin without the use of additional bovine thrombin. In the first stage (low speed centrifugation), red blood cells are separated from platelets and plasma proteins in a 9 mL tube containing sodium citrate. In the second centrifugation, fibrinogen is converted to cross-linked fibrin containing platelets in the presence of $CaCl_2$ [15].

- T-PRF (Titanium-prepared Platelet-Rich Fibrin): the patient's blood is collected into 10 mL titanium tubes and centrifuged without anticoagulants at 3500 RPM for 15 min [16].
- i-PRF (injectable Platelet-Rich Fibrin): from 10 mL of a patient's blood drawn into a plastic tube, centrifugation at 700 RPM for 3 min produces a liquid form of fibrin without the use of anticoagulants [17].
- A Vivostat PRF-120 mL of whole blood is collected and processed in the Vivostat Processor Unit using the "platelet" program. After 26 min. of centrifugation, 6 mL of preparation is obtained (without the use of thrombin) [18].
- L-PRF (Leukocyte and Platelet-Rich Fibrin) was invented by Joseph Choukroun in 2001, and the clot was obtained by centrifuging the blood at 3000 RPM in 10 mL plastic tubes for 10 min [13].
- A-PRF (Advanced Platelet-Rich Fibrin), A-PRF+ (Advanced Platelet-Rich Fibrin +) and CGF (concentrated growth factors) will be described below.

In 2014, Ghanaati and Choukroun et al. [19] presented a modification of the original system for producing platelet-rich fibrin, called the new A-PRF (advanced platelet-rich fibrin) procedure. Blood was collected from patients and immediately centrifuged in sterile 10 mL vacuum glass tubes for 14 min at 1500 RPM. When the centrifugation speed was reduced while the process was prolonged, the researchers discovered an increase in the presence of neutrophils captured between fibrin fibers. Products of neutrophil degranulation influence the conversion and differentiation of monocytes into macrophages. In turn, growth factors secreted from macrophage granules can influence bone and soft tissue regeneration.

In collaboration with Choukroun, Fujioka-Kobayashi et al. [20] proposed a variation of the aforementioned procedure in 2017, naming the produced product A-PRF+. Patient blood was collected into a 10 mL glass vacuum tube and centrifuged at 1300 RPM for 8 min to obtain A-PRF+. In vitro, the researchers found that the A-PRF and A-PRF+ regimens released more growth factors (e.g., PDGF-Platelet-derived growth factor, TGF-1-Transforming growth factor beta 1, EGF-Epidermal growth factor, IGF-1-Insulin-like growth factor 1) from fibrin than the original L-PRF regimen. Furthermore, A-PRF+, a platelet rich fibrin, released more growth factors than A-PRF fibrin.

In 2006, another researcher, Sacco, named his unique method of generating fibrin clots by centrifugation with varying centrifugation settings "CGF". Unfortunately, until the publication of Rodella et al. in 2011 [21], there were no studies confirming the biological efficacy and histological aspect of this novel technique. Vacuum blood collection tubes are made out of PET plastic, and the centrifugation strategy for CGF is as follows:

- 30 s of acceleration,
- 2 min of centrifugation at 2700 RPM,
- 4 min at 2400 RPM,
- 4 min at 2700 RPM,
- 3 min at 3000 RPM,
- 36 s deacceleration till it fully stops

Platelets and growth factors TGF-1, PDGF-BB, and VEGF were found in equal amounts in CGF and A-PRF+ fibrin clots, with a slight predominance of the aforementioned numbers in A-PRF+ [22].

## 4. APRF

### 4.1. General Mechanism

A-PRF, a biomaterial used in current tissue engineering procedures, has been developed to accelerate healing processes at the application site. During the centrifugation process, no additives are used to activate coagulation, resulting in a tube with three distinct layers, starting from the bottom: a layer of red blood cells, a PRF fibrin clot with a layer tangential to the red blood cells called the buffy coat (the highest concentration of white blood cells and platelets), and a top layer of cell-free plasma [5].

The fibrin clot formed during the production of traditional PRF or its modification, A-PRF, is a three-dimensional scaffold that replaces the extracellular matrix in cell regeneration and newly formed vessels. Platelets trapped between fibrin fibers, B and T lymphocytes, monocytes, stem cells and neutrophils, as well as secreted growth factors such as TGF-1, PDGF, and VEGF, play a role in healing. As previously reported, neutrophils influence monocyte differentiation and conversion to macrophages by releasing the contents of their granules, which contain growth factors that can positively influence soft tissue and bone regeneration [19,23].

As a result, A-PRF, like other second generation preparations, is highly regarded by clinicians worldwide and is used in the treatment of musculoskeletal trauma [24], drug-induced bone necrosis in the form of a membrane applied to exposed jawbone to reduce bacterial contamination and risk of reinfection [25], in periodontal reconstructive procedures [26], in implants, and maxillary sinus floor lifts [27], and as a local hemostatic agent, specifically recommended after multiple extractions in patients taking antiplatelet drugs [28].

The extraction of molars is one of the most common surgical procedures performed in dental clinics worldwide. As with any medical procedure, it carries the risk of intra- or postoperative complications. The most common of these are dry socket, post-operative socket infection and damage to the inferior alveolar nerve, which may be reversible or irreversible. In addition, postoperative discomfort, swelling of the surrounding tissues, trismus and, in rare cases, hemorrhage, are associated with the extraction process [29]. As a result, clinicians are looking for better, more effective techniques for dealing with extraction sockets that are also cheap and simple to use to reduce the negative consequences of the procedure. One of these has been fibrin clots taken from the patient's own blood before surgery, such as L-PRF, A-PRF, and CGF.

### 4.2. Regeneration of Soft Tissues and Bones

When extracting an impacted tooth, it is often necessary to remove a significant amount of surrounding bone. Improper management of the post-extraction socket can lead to a significant loss of alveolar height after extraction, resulting in recession on the second molar in the distal/buccal region of the tooth. Therefore, in order to preserve the height of the ridge, the alveolus needs to be adequately protected, which is achieved with bone substitute materials, fibrin preparations derived from the patient's blood, or a combination of both.

Three months after extraction, Talal M Zahid et al. [30] found no significant differences between the test side (with A-PRF augmentation) and the control side (without A-PRF augmentation). CAL (clinical attachment level) and GR (gingival recession) measurements yielded similar results. In conclusion, the authors of the aforementioned study did not discover any additional benefit of A-PRF over natural healing in terms of pocket shallowing, reconstruction of the connective tissue attachment and minimization of the recessions formed; a slight advantage in healing with A-PRF could be seen by analyzing data from different measurement points around the tooth at different times after extraction. Unfortunately, this benefit did not include improved bone healing.

Gupta et al. [31] discovered a significant difference between alveolar healing using postoperative A-PRF and bone healing as gauged by measures of bone density using extraoral RVG imaging (performed on controls after 1, 3, and 6 months). The researchers found comparable improvements in soft tissue healing after A-PRF.

The findings of the above in vivo studies do not seem to confirm the results of in vitro studies comparing L-PRF (low-speed centrifugation) and A-PRF+ (high-speed centrifugation) and L-PRF, A-PRF, and A-PRF+ in terms of content, including growth factors, which have been shown to have higher concentrations in A-PRF+ compared to L-PRF [20,32].

In 2019, Masahiro To et al. [33] confirmed the osteogenic effect of A-PRF+ in sockets after extraction. In a study on Beagle dogs with removed premolars, the researchers observed significantly faster bone recovery in A-PRF-dressed sockets compared to control sockets (without A-PRF), including post mortem histology and immunofluorescence of healing tissues after 14 and 30 days.

Animal studies were also carried out in 2012 by Dominiak et al. in the group of 36 New Zealand White (NZW) rabbits, in which a bone defect 5 mm in diameter and 10 mm deep was made in the femur under general anesthesia. Subsequently, in 12 rabbits (group I), the defect was filled with bone substitute material (xenograft Bio-Oss Collagen®) and covered with a collagen membrane (Bio-Gide Perio®); in 12 rabbits from group 2, a layer of platelet rich plasma (PRP) was placed to the defect after application of the biomaterial. Group 3 (also 12 rabbits) was the control group that was treated without the regenerative techniques. After the animals were sacrificed, a histological examination of the dissection preparations was performed, which showed the most intense osteogenesis 1 month after treatment in group 2 (with PRP application). At subsequent stages of healing (after 3, 6 and 12 months), more intense osteogenesis was shown in group 1 (xenogenic material and resorbable collagen membrane). The worst results were obtained in the control group, while the use of two regenerative methods influenced the speed, quality and overall healing of intraosseous defects [34].

### 4.3. *Analgesic and Antiedemic Effect*

Tooth extraction, as with any surgical procedure, causes tissue disruption and a subsequent inflammatory response by the body during the healing phase.

Under normal conditions, the extraction socket fills with blood, which forms a clot within a few to several minutes. The clot is quickly replaced by richly vascularized granulation tissue (day 3), which is replaced by connective tissue (day 21) which fills 2/3 of the socket and gives rise to bone formation (osteoid). After 6 weeks, the socket is filled with immature bone.

In a 2018 study by Talal M Zahid and Mohammed Nadershah [30], which was the first randomized study of alveolar healing using A-PRF, augmentation of the post-extraction socket with A-PRF clot significantly reduced postoperative pain and swelling within 7 days of surgery according to the authors. Gupta et al. [31] also observed a reduction in post-extraction discomfort when A-PRF was used (compared to a control group without augmentation). On day 1, there was no difference in post-extraction swelling or trismus between the groups, but on day 3 in the A-PRF group, both pain and the potential for a broad opening of the mouth were significantly reduced, and patients showed significantly greater potential for a broad opening of the mouth.

Caymaz et al. [35] conducted a study in 2018 comparing the healing process using a primary PRF (L-PRF) and A-PRF regimen. Patients with bilaterally retained third molars underwent surgical extraction (twice, with at least 21 days between procedures), with L-PRF inserted into one of the extraction sockets (group 2) and A-PRF inserted into the other (group 1). Discomfort on days 1, 2, and 3 days after extraction was significantly greater in group 2 (L-PRF) than in group 1 (A-PRF). On day 7, there was no discernible difference in discomfort between group 1 and group 2. The aforementioned relationship can also be seen in the amount of analgesics used; patients with the L-PRF dressing took significantly more pain medication on days 2 and 3 after surgery. There were no differences in the amount of painkillers consumed by the groups on days 1 and 7. There were no differences in swelling and trismus between the groups on the first, second, third and seventh postoperative days.

The above study shows that the use of A-PRF instead of L-PRF after extraction of the lower third molar has a significant effect on reducing postoperative pain, while no association favoring one of the above techniques in reducing swelling and trismus was found.

Torul et al. [36] obtained additional findings by evaluating the effects of A-PRF and CGF on the incidence of swelling, trismus, and postoperative discomfort after lower third molar extraction. The researchers found that the CGF group had greater trismus and horizontal postoperative swelling, as well as greater vertical swelling, than the A-PRF group in a study of 75 patients (25 in each group). Although not statistically significant, the above results can be attributed to the higher concentration of white blood cells and growth factors in the A-PRF and CGF fibrin clots compared to classic PRF, which may result in an increased inflammatory response in the early postoperative period. In addition, the researchers found no reduction in pain symptoms with the administration of A-PRF and CGF compared to the control group.

## 5. CGF

Concentrated Growth Factors (CGF) are derivatives of PRF and were developed by Sacco in 2006 [14,37]. CGF is a fibrin-rich organic matrix obtained by centrifuging of the patient's venous blood, and is considered a third generation platelet enrichment that does not require any additional reagents to induce platelet activation as well as fibrin polymerization [38]. It contains growth factors, platelets, fibronectin, immune cells and CD34+ stem cells that play a vital role in regeneration processes, immunomodulatory responses, as well as having the ability to induce angiogenesis, chemotaxis and tissue remodeling, while being a matrix for cell migration [39–42].

Due to the use of a different centrifugation speed, CGF contains a denser matrix that has more growth factors than both PRP and PRF, making it also more efficient at releasing them into the surrounding space, which can be especially useful in dentistry [43]. Among the numerous growth factors identified within CGF are platelet-derived growth factor (PDGF), transforming growth factor β-1 and 2 (TGF-β1 and TGF-β2), fibroblast growth factor (FGF), bone morphogenetic protein 2 (BMP-2), vascular endothelial growth factor (VEGF), brain derived growth factor (BDGF), and insulin-like growth factor (IGF). They stimulate cell proliferation, matrix remodeling, and promote angiogenesis [5,12,21,44]. It is noteworthy that CGF is associated with a sustained release of growth factors over 7–10 days, which can be used in aesthetic facial rejuvenation procedures, such as the treatment of wrinkles [45]. The ability to promote angiogenesis has applications in the regeneration of immature necrotic teeth in endodontics as an effective alternative to apexification [46]. It has been confirmed that CGF fibrous membrane is able to promote periodontal tissue regeneration involving hUCMSCs, which is achieved by upregulating the expression of TAZ and osteogenic differentiation-related genes [47]. The use of CGF together with a coronally advanced flap (CAF) leads to an increase in the amount of keratinized gingiva 6 months after maxillary recession coverage compared to a simple CAF procedure [48].

On the other hand, according to Akcan and Ünsal, CTG is superior to CGF in covering recessions, with CGF having a more positive effect on postoperative pain [49]. The biological properties of CGF, together with its viscosity and mechanical properties, allow it to improve the handling of other graft materials, promote wound healing, bone growth and maturation, as well as to stabilize bone grafts when used simultaneously [50]. Because of these properties, CGF has been widely used in jawbone regeneration procedures. Numerous studies have shown positive results with CGF as a biomaterial used in sinus lift procedures, which induces rapid and reliable bone formation [51–53].

CGF also induces osteoblastic differentiation promoting the early osseointegration of dental implants, leading to an increase in bone density around them [54]. There are some limitations to the use of CGF. First of all, platelet counts are affected by blood pH; changes in blood pH can interfere with cell proliferation. Furthermore, the time of CGF preparation and the volume of blood can affect the results [43,45] (See Table 1).

**Table 1.** Summary of the purpose and results of individual authors' research on A-PRF/CGF; + positive outcome, − negative outcome, +/− non-conclusive outcome.

| | Material | Aim of the Research | Results | Effect | Authors/Year | Ref. |
|---|---|---|---|---|---|---|
| 1 | A-PRF | histochemical study of the clot and its composition | A-PRF might influence bone and soft tissue regeneration, especially through the presence of monocytes/macrophages and their growth factors. The relevance and feasibility of this tissue-engineering concept have to be proven through in vivo studies. | + (in vitro) | Ghanaati et al., 2014 | [19] |
| 2 | A-PRF | To evaluate the potential of advanced platelet-rich fibrin (A-PRF) as a regenerative biomaterial for bone regeneration and postoperative sequlae after impacted third molar extractions. | Placement of A-PRF clot in the extraction socket could lessen postoperative pain and increase patient comfort after third molar extraction | + (in vivo) | Zahid et al., 2019 | [30] |
| 3 | A-PRF | To evaluate the efficacy and healing potential of modified formulation of PRF, commonly known as advanced PRF (A-PRF) in impacted mandibular third molar extraction sockets. | A-PRF has enhanced the healing potential of soft tissue as well as bone in extraction socket. Using A-PRF as well relief of immediate postoperative symptoms like pain, swelling and trismus. | + (in vivo) | Gupta et al., 2020 | [31] |
| 4 | A-PRF | To evaluate the potential of advanced platelet-rich fibrin (A-PRF) on bone formation after extraction of beagle dogs premolars. | A-PRF application may result in enhanced new bone formation and may aid in accelerating bone formation. | + (in vivo) | Masahiro et al., 2019 | [33] |
| 5 | A-PRF | To investigate and compare the postoperative effects of leukocyte- and platelet-rich fibrin (L-PRF) and advanced platelet-rich fibrin (A-PRF) in terms of pain, swelling, and trismus after mandibular third molar surgery. | Using of A-PRF after mandibular third molar extraction significantly reduces postoperative pain compared to the L-PRF group. However, there was no significant difference between groups in terms of swelling and trismus. | +/− (in vivo) | Caymaz et al., 2018 | [35] |
| 6 | A-PRF, CGF | To investigate the effects of concentrated growth factors (CGF) and advanced platelet-rich fibrin (A-PRF) on edema, pain, and trismus after mandibular third molar surgery. | A-PRF and CGF seem to have no positive effects on pain, edema, and trismus after third molar surgery. | − (in vivo) | Torul et al., 2020 | [36] |
| 7 | CGF | To investigate the biological effects of concentrated growth factor on human dental pulp stem cells. | Concentrated growth factor (CGF) promoted cell proliferation, migration, and the dental pulp stem cell–mediated dentinogenesis and angiogenesis process. | + (in vitro) | Jin et al., 2018 | [42] |
| 8 | A-PRF, CGF | to evaluate the effect of platelet-rich plasma (PRP), platelet-rich fibrin (PRF), and concentrated growth factor (CGF) on bone healing | The addition of PRP, PRF, and CGF had significantly increased bone formation at the 6th week. The effect of PRP, PRF, and CGF was similar. | + (in vivo) | Kim et al., 2014 | [50] |

## 6. Study Limitations

The paper itself is narrative in nature. The efficacy of narrative reviews is irreplaceable in tracking the development of a scientific principle or a clinical concept. This ability to conduct a wider exploration could be lost in the restrictive framework of a systematic review.

Author bias may be present in this type of review topic. When reading and evaluating a narrative review, keep in mind that the author's bias may or may not be present. Furthermore, due to the scarcity of literature on the use of platelet concentrates in the treatment of post-extraction teeth, especially lower third molars, it is impossible to perform a meaningful systematic review.

## 7. Conclusions and Perspectives

Autologous platelet concentrates were thought to revolutionize both bones and soft tissue regeneration, thus indirectly affecting the quality of life of patients throughout the postoperative recovery period. Therefore, they have found their application in many medical fields, including dentistry [55]. Many authors of clinical studies involving the aforementioned tissue-engineering technologies confirm their efficacy in reducing post-extraction pain and emphasize the anti-inflammatory component of their action, which manifests itself, among other things, in the reduction of trismus and postoperative swelling.

A number of studies have been conducted to determine the efficacy of A-PRF and CGF in the treatment of edema, pain, and trismus. The therapeutic effect is clearly evident in some publications, but appears to have no significant impact on the recovery process in others. Instead, some studies highlight the lack of benefit associated with the use of the aforementioned approaches, casting doubt on their use.

In line with the above, the vast majority of publications treating the topic of blood concentrates either state their beneficial effect on the healing of post-extraction wounds or extraction sockets, or indicate that there is no perceived benefit from their use. However, it should be remembered that autologous platelet concentrates are not the panacea of bone healing. PRP, PRGF, A-PRF and CGF, depending on their generation, show differences in the quantitative composition of platelets, leukocytes, growth factors (including TGF-$\beta$1, PDGF-BB, VEGF) and pro-inflammatory cytokines (including IL-1$\beta$, IL-6) [22]. The amount of the latter increases in the blood of people who have an ongoing inflammatory process or who suffer from systemic diseases such as diabetes. This may result in a prolongation of the inflammatory phase of post-extraction wound healing by increasing the production of local pro-inflammatory cytokines [56]. They result in an imbalance between polarized pro-inflammatory M1 macrophages and inflammation-silencing M2 macrophages in favor of the former. Activated M1 macrophages continuously produce pro-inflammatory cytokines, causing bone resorption through increased osteoclast activity and the inhibition of bone formation by osteoblasts, resulting in impaired and prolonged soft and hard tissue healing [57,58].

Unfortunately, there is a lack of studies in the current literature comparing the amount of pro-inflammatory cytokines in a patient's peripheral blood with their levels after centrifugation in blood concentrates. Undoubtedly, more studies are needed to clarify the correlation between pro-inflammatory cytokine levels and alveolar healing after extraction and to assess the risk of treatment with blood concentrates in patients with systemic diseases causing chronic inflammation.

The tissue-engineering technologies discussed in the article above are relatively new and are constantly being refined by a large number of researchers, necessitating additional clinical trials on large groups of patients to collect more data.

**Author Contributions:** Conceptualization, M.D.; methodology, M.S. and D.S.; validation, D.S., M.S. and M.D.; formal analysis. P.K.-R. and M.D.; investigation, D.S. and M.S.; writing—original draft preparation, D.S., M.S. and A.P.; writing—review and editing, D.S., M.S., F.M., J.H. and M.D.; supervision, M.D. and J.H.; project administration, M.S. and M.D.; funding acquisition, D.S. and M.D. All authors have read and agreed to the published version of the manuscript.

**Funding:** The APC was funded by Wroclaw Medical University, grant SIMPLE: STM.B040.20.075.

**Institutional Review Board Statement:** Not applicable.

**Informed Consent Statement:** Not applicable.

**Data Availability Statement:** Available on request.

**Conflicts of Interest:** The authors declare that they have no conflict of interest.

## References

1. Barone, S.; Antonelli, A.; Averta, F.; Diodati, F.; Muraca, D.; Bennardo, F.; Giudice, A. Does Mandibular Gonial Angle Influence the Eruption Pattern of the Lower Third Molar? A Three-Dimensional Study. *J. Clin. Med.* **2021**, *10*, 4057. [CrossRef] [PubMed]
2. Park, K.-L. Which factors are associated with difficult surgical extraction of impacted lower third molars? *J. Korean Assoc. Oral Maxillofac. Surg.* **2016**, *42*, 251–258. [CrossRef] [PubMed]
3. Cho, H.; Lynham, A.J.; Hsu, E. Postoperative interventions to reduce inflammatory complications after third molar surgery: Review of the current evidence. *Aust. Dent. J.* **2017**, *62*, 412–419. [CrossRef] [PubMed]
4. Caruana, A.; Savina, D.; Macedo, J.P.; Soares, S.C. From Platelet-Rich Plasma to Advanced Platelet-Rich Fibrin: Biological Achievements and Clinical Advances in Modern Surgery. *Eur. J. Dent.* **2019**, *13*, 280–286. [CrossRef]
5. Dohan, D.M.; Choukroun, J.; Diss, A.; Dohan, S.L.; Dohan, A.J.; Mouhyi, J.; Gogly, B. Platelet-rich fibrin (PRF): A second-generation platelet concentrate. Part I: Technological concepts and evolution. *Oral Surg. Oral Med. Oral Pathol. Oral Radiol. Endodontol.* **2006**, *101*, e37–e44. [CrossRef]
6. Soffer, E.; Ouhayoun, J.P.; Anagnostou, F. Fibrin sealants and platelet preparations in bone and periodontal healing. *Oral Surg. Oral Med. Oral Pathol. Oral Radiol. Endodontol.* **2003**, *95*, 521–528. [CrossRef]
7. Marx, R.E.; Carlson, E.R.; Eichstaedt, R.M.; Schimmele, S.R.; Strauss, J.E.; Georgeff, K.R. Platelet-rich plasma: Growth factor enhancement for bone grafts. *Oral Surg. Oral Med. Oral Pathol. Oral Radiol. Endodontol.* **1998**, *85*, 638–646. [CrossRef]
8. Jo, C.H.; Roh, Y.H.; Kim, J.E.; Shin, S.; Yoon, K.S. Optimizing Platelet-Rich Plasma Gel Formation by Varying Time and Gravitational Forces During Centrifugation. *J. Oral Implant.* **2013**, *39*, 525–532. [CrossRef]
9. Anitua, E.; Prado, R.; Sánchez, M.; Orive, G. Platelet-Rich Plasma: Preparation and Formulation. *Oper. Tech. Orthop.* **2012**, *22*, 25–32. [CrossRef]
10. Anitua, E.; Sánchez, M.; Prado, R.; Orive, G. Plasma rich in growth factors: The pioneering autologous technology for tissue regeneration. *J. Biomed. Mater. Res. Part A* **2011**, *97A*, 536. [CrossRef] [PubMed]
11. Raja, V.S.; Naidu, E.M. Platelet-rich fibrin: Evolution of a second-generation platelet concentrate. *Indian J. Dent. Res.* **2008**, *19*, 42. [CrossRef] [PubMed]
12. Choukroun, J.; Adda, F.; Schoeffler, C.; Vervelle, A. Une opportunity en paro-implantologie: Le PRF. *Implantodontie* **2001**, *42*, 55–62.
13. Miron, R.; Choukroun, J.; Ghanaati, S. Controversies related to scientific report describing g-forces from studies on platelet-rich fibrin: Necessity for standardization of relative centrifugal force values. *Int. J. Growth Factors Stem Cells Dent.* **2018**, *1*, 80. [CrossRef]
14. Dohan, D.M.; Choukroun, J.; Diss, A.; Dohan, S.L.; Dohan, A.J.; Mouhyi, J.; Gogly, B. Platelet-rich fibrin (PRF): A second-generation platelet concentrate. Part II: Platelet-related biologic features. *Oral Surg. Oral Med. Oral Pathol. Oral Radiol. Endodontol.* **2006**, *101*, e45–e50. [CrossRef] [PubMed]
15. Simon, B.; Zatcoff, A.; Kong, J.J.; O'Connell, S. Clinical and Histological Comparison of Extraction Socket Healing Following the Use of Autologous Platelet-Rich Fibrin Matrix (PRFM) to Ridge Preservation Procedures Employing Demineralized Freeze Dried Bone Allograft Material and Membrane. *Open Dent. J.* **2009**, *3*, 92–99. [CrossRef]
16. Tunalı, M.; Özdemir, H.; Küçükodacı, Z.; Akman, S.; Fıratlı, E. In vivo evaluation of titanium-prepared platelet-rich fibrin (T-PRF): A new platelet concentrate. *Br. J. Oral Maxillofac. Surg.* **2013**, *51*, 438–443. [CrossRef] [PubMed]
17. Miron, R.J.; Fujioka-Kobayashi, M.; Hernandez, M.; Kandalam, U.; Zhang, Y.; Ghanaati, S.; Choukroun, J. Injectable platelet rich fibrin (i-PRF): Opportunities in regenerative dentistry? *Clin. Oral Investig.* **2017**, *21*, 2619–2627. [CrossRef]
18. Leitner, G.C.; Gruber, R.; Neumuller, J.; Wagner, A.; Kloimstein, P.; Hocker, P.; Kormoczi, G.F.; Buchta, C. Platelet content and growth factor release in platelet-rich plasma: A comparison of four different systems. *Vox Sang.* **2006**, *91*, 135–139. [CrossRef]
19. Ghanaati, S.; Booms, P.; Orlowska, A.; Kubesch, A.; Lorenz, J.; Rutkowski, J.; Landes, C.; Sader, R.; Kirkpatrick, C.; Choukroun, J. Advanced Platelet-Rich Fibrin: A New Concept for Cell-Based Tissue Engineering by Means of Inflammatory Cells. *J. Oral Implant.* **2014**, *40*, 679–689. [CrossRef]

20. Fujioka-Kobayashi, M.; Miron, R.J.; Hernandez, M.; Kandalam, U.; Zhang, Y.; Choukroun, J. Optimized Platelet-Rich Fibrin With the Low-Speed Concept: Growth Factor Release, Biocompatibility, and Cellular Response. *J. Periodontol.* **2017**, *88*, 112–121. [CrossRef]
21. Rodella, L.F.; Favero, G.; Boninsegna, R.; Buffoli, B.; Labanca, M.; Scarì, G.; Sacco, L.; Batani, T.; Rezzani, R. Growth factors, CD34 positive cells, and fibrin network analysis in concentrated growth factors fraction. *Microsc. Res. Tech.* **2011**, *74*, 772–777. [CrossRef] [PubMed]
22. Masuki, H.; Okudera, T.; Watanebe, T.; Suzuki, M.; Nishiyama, K.; Okudera, H.; Nakata, K.; Uematsu, K.; Su, C.-Y.; Kawase, T. Growth factor and pro-inflammatory cytokine contents in platelet-rich plasma (PRP), plasma rich in growth factors (PRGF), advanced platelet-rich fibrin (A-PRF), and concentrated growth factors (CGF). *Int. J. Implant Dent.* **2016**, *2*, 19. [CrossRef]
23. Dohan Ehrenfest, D.M.; Pinto, N.R.; Pereda, A.; Jiménez, P.; Del Corso, M.; Kang, B.-S.; Nally, M.; Lanata, N.; Wang, H.-L.; Quirynen, M. The impact of the centrifuge characteristics and centrifugation protocols on the cells, growth factors, and fibrin architecture of a leukocyte- and platelet-rich fibrin (L-PRF) clot and membrane. *Platelets* **2018**, *29*, 171–184. [CrossRef] [PubMed]
24. Masoudi, E.A.; Ribas, J.; Kaushik, G.; Leijten, J.; Khademhosseini, A. Platelet-Rich Blood Derivatives for Stem Cell-Based Tissue Engineering and Regeneration. *Curr. Stem Cell Rep.* **2016**, *2*, 33–42. [CrossRef] [PubMed]
25. Maluf, G.; Caldas, R.J.; Silva Santos, P.S. Use of Leukocyte- and Platelet-Rich Fibrin in the Treatment of Medication-Related Osteonecrosis of the Jaws. *J. Oral Maxillofac. Surg.* **2018**, *76*, 88–96. [CrossRef]
26. Rock, L. Potential of platelet rich fibrin in regenerative periodontal therapy: Literature review. *Can. J. Dent. Hyg.* **2013**, *47*, 33–37.
27. Del Corso, M.; Mazor, Z.; Rutkowski, J.L.; Ehrenfest, D.M.D. The Use of Leukocyte- and Platelet-Rich Fibrin During Immediate Postextractive Implantation and Loading for the Esthetic Replacement of a Fractured Maxillary Central Incisor. *J. Oral Implantol.* **2012**, *38*, 181–187. [CrossRef]
28. Brancaccio, Y.; Antonelli, A.; Barone, S.; Bennardo, F.; Fortunato, L.; Giudice, A. Evaluation of local hemostatic efficacy after dental extractions in patients taking antiplatelet drugs: A randomized clinical trial. *Clin. Oral Investig.* **2020**, *25*, 1159–1167. [CrossRef]
29. Blondeau, F.; Nach, D.G. Extraction of Impacted Mandibular Third Molars: Postoperative Complications and Their Risk Factors. *J. Can. Dent. Assoc.* **2007**, *73*, 325.
30. Zahid, T.M.; Nadershah, M. Effect of Advanced Platelet-rich Fibrin on Wound Healing after Third Molar Extraction: A Split-mouth Randomized Double-blind Study. *J. Contemp. Dent. Pract.* **2019**, *20*, 1164–1170. [CrossRef]
31. Gupta, N.; Agarwal, S. Advanced–PRF: Clinical evaluation in impacted mandibular third molar sockets. *J. Stomatol. Oral Maxillofac. Surg.* **2021**, *122*, 43–49. [CrossRef] [PubMed]
32. Miron, R.J.; Xu, H.; Chai, J.; Wang, J.; Zheng, S.; Feng, M.; Zhang, X.; Wei, Y.; Chen, Y.; de Almeida Barros Mourão, C.F.; et al. Comparison of platelet-rich fibrin (PRF) produced using 3 commercially available centrifuges at both high (~700 g) and low (~200 g) relative centrifugation forces. *Clin. Oral Investig.* **2020**, *24*, 1171–1182. [CrossRef] [PubMed]
33. To, M.; Su, C.; Hidaka, K.; Okudera, T.; Matsuo, M. Effect of advanced platelet-rich fibrin on accelerating alveolar bone formation in dogs: A histological and immunofluorescence evaluation. *Anat. Sci. Int.* **2019**, *94*, 238–244. [CrossRef] [PubMed]
34. Dominiak, M.; Łysiak-Drwal, K.; Solski, L.; Żywicka, B.; Rybak, Z.; Gedrange, T. Evaluation of healing processes of intraosseous defects with and without guided bone regeneration and platelet rich plasma. An animal study. *Ann. Anat.-Anat. Anz.* **2012**, *194*, 549–555. [CrossRef] [PubMed]
35. Caymaz, M.; Uyanik, L. Comparison of the effect of advanced platelet-rich fibrin and leukocyte- and platelet-rich fibrin on outcomes after removal of impacted mandibular third molar: A randomized split-mouth study. *Niger. J. Clin. Pr.* **2019**, *22*, 546–552. [CrossRef]
36. Torul, D.; Omezli, M.M.; Kahveci, K. Evaluation of the effects of concentrated growth factors or advanced platelet rich-fibrin on postoperative pain, edema, and trismus following lower third molar removal: A randomized controlled clinical trial. *J. Stomatol. Oral Maxillofac. Surg.* **2020**, *121*, 646–651. [CrossRef]
37. Kshirsagar, J.T.; Rubine, S. Innovation in regeneration–Concentrated growth factor. *Int. J. Appl. Dent. Sci.* **2017**, *3*, 206–208.
38. Yılmaz, O.; Özmeriç, A.; Alemdaroğlu, K.B.; Celepli, P.; Hücümenoğlu, S.; Şahin, Ö. Effects of concentrated growth factors (CGF) on the quality of the induced membrane in Masquelet's technique—An experimental study in rabbits. *Injury* **2018**, *49*, 1497–1503. [CrossRef]
39. Bernardi, S.; Mummolo, S.; Tecco, S.; Continenza, M.A.; Marzo, G. Histological Characterization of Sacco's Concentrated Growth Factors Membrane. *Int. J. Morphol.* **2017**, *35*, 114–119. [CrossRef]
40. Qiao, J.; An, N. Effect of concentrated growth factors on function and Wnt3a expression of human periodontal ligament cells in vitro. *Platelets* **2016**, *28*, 281–286. [CrossRef]
41. Nityasri, A.S.; Pradeep, K.Y. Role of CGF (Concentrated Growth Factor) in periodontal regeneration. *J. Dent. Health Oral Disord. Ther.* **2018**, *9*, 350–352.
42. Jin, R.; Song, G.; Chai, J.; Gou, X.; Yuan, G.; Chen, Z. Effects of concentrated growth factor on proliferation, migration, and differentiation of human dental pulp stem cells in vitro. *J. Tissue Eng.* **2018**, *9*, 204173141881750. [CrossRef] [PubMed]
43. Sohn, D.-S.; Heo, J.-U.; Kwak, D.-H.; Kim, D.-E.; Kim, J.-M.; Moon, J.-W.; Lee, J.-H.; Park, I.-S. Bone Regeneration in the Maxillary Sinus Using an Autologous Fibrin-Rich Block With Concentrated Growth Factors Alone. *Implant. Dent.* **2011**, *20*, 389–395. [CrossRef] [PubMed]
44. Yu, B.; Wang, Z. Effect of concentrated growth factors on beagle periodontal ligament stem cells in vitro. *Mol. Med. Rep.* **2013**, *9*, 235–242. [CrossRef]

45. Mijiritsky, E.; Assaf, H.; Peleg, O.; Shacham, M.; Cerroni, L.; Mangani, L. Use of PRP, PRF and CGF in Periodontal Regeneration and Facial Rejuvenation—A Narrative Review. *Biology* **2021**, *10*, 317. [CrossRef]
46. Cheng, J.; Yang, F.; Li, J.; Hua, F.; He, M.; Song, G. Treatment Outcomes of Regenerative Endodontic Procedures in Traumatized Immature Permanent Necrotic Teeth: A Retrospective Study. *J. Endod.* **2022**, *48*, 1129–1136. [CrossRef]
47. Li, W.; Wang, F.; Dong, F.; Zhang, Z.; Song, P.; Chen, H.; Wang, J. CGF Membrane Promotes Periodontal Tissue Regeneration Mediated by hUCMSCs through Upregulating TAZ and Osteogenic Differentiation Genes. *Stem Cells Int.* **2021**, *2021*, 14. [CrossRef]
48. Doğan, Ş.B.; Dede, F.; Ballı, U.; Atalay, E.N.; Durmuşlar, M.C. Concentrated growth factor in the treatment of adjacent multiple gingival recessions: A split-mouth randomized clinical trial. *J. Clin. Periodontol.* **2015**, *42*, 868–875. [CrossRef]
49. Akcan, S.K.; Ünsal, B. Gingival recession treatment with concentrated growth factor membrane: A comparative clinical trial. *J. Appl. Oral Sci.* **2020**, *28*, e20190236. [CrossRef]
50. Kim, T.-H.; Kim, S.-H.; Sándor, G.K.; Kim, Y.-D. Comparison of platelet-rich plasma (PRP), platelet-rich fibrin (PRF), and concentrated growth factor (CGF) in rabbit-skull defect healing. *Arch. Oral Biol.* **2014**, *59*, 550–558. [CrossRef]
51. Kim, J.-M.; Sohn, D.-S.; Bae, M.-S.; Moon, J.-W.; Lee, J.-H.; Park, I.-S. Flapless Transcrestal Sinus Augmentation Using Hydrodynamic Piezoelectric Internal Sinus Elevation With Autologous Concentrated Growth Factors Alone. *Implant. Dent.* **2014**, *23*, 168–174. [CrossRef] [PubMed]
52. Chen, Y.; Cai, Z.; Zheng, D.; Lin, P.; Cai, Y.; Hong, S.; Lai, Y.; Wu, W.D. Inlay osteotome sinus floor elevation with concentrated growth factor application and simultaneous short implant placement in severely atrophic maxilla. *Sci. Rep.* **2016**, *6*, 27348. [CrossRef] [PubMed]
53. Sohn, D.S.; Moon, J.W.; Moon, Y.S.; Park, J.S.; Jung, H.S. The use of concentrated growth factor (CGF) for sinus augmentation. *J. Oral Implant.* **2009**, *38*, 25–38.
54. Gupta, D.; Lokwani, B.V.; Agrawal, R.S.; Mehta, S.; Nirmal, N.J. The use of concentrated growth factor in dental implantology: A systematic review. *J. Indian Prosthodont. Soc.* **2020**, *20*, 3–10. [CrossRef] [PubMed]
55. Pietruszka, P.; Chruścicka, I.; Duś-Ilnicka, I.; Paradowska-Stolarz, A. PRP and PRF—Subgroups and Divisions When Used in Dentistry. *J. Pers. Med.* **2021**, *11*, 944. [CrossRef] [PubMed]
56. Ko, K.I.; Sculean, A.; Graves, D.T. Diabetic wound healing in soft and hard oral tissues. *Transl. Res.* **2021**, *236*, 72–86. [CrossRef]
57. Pajarinen, J.; Lin, T.; Gibon, E.; Kohno, Y.; Maruyama, M.; Nathan, K.; Lu, L.; Yao, Z.; Goodman, S.B. Mesenchymal stem cell-macrophage crosstalk and bone healing. *Biomaterials* **2019**, *196*, 80–89. [CrossRef]
58. Shin, R.L.-Y.; Lee, C.-W.; Shen, O.Y.-J.; Xu, H.; Lee, O.K.-S. The Crosstalk between Mesenchymal Stem Cells and Macrophages in Bone Regeneration: A Systematic Review. *Stem Cells Int.* **2021**, *2021*, 8835156. [CrossRef]

*applied sciences*

MDPI

*Perspective*

# Prediction of Mandibular Third Molar Impaction Using Linear and Angular Measurements in Young Adult Orthopantomograms

**Stefano Mummolo [1], Gianni Gallusi [1], Enrico M. Strappa [2], Filippo Grilli [1], Antronella Mattei [1], Fabiana Fiasca [1], Fabrizio Bambini [3] and Lucia Memè [3,*]**

[1] Department of Life, Health and Environmental Sciences, Università degli Studi dell'Aquila, 67100 L'Aquila, Italy; stefano.mummolo@univaq.it (S.M.); gianni.gallusi@gmail.com (G.G.); filippo.grilli@gmail.com (F.G.); antonella.mattei@univaq.it (A.M.); fabiana.fiasca@univaq.it (F.F.)

[2] Department of Health Technologies, IRCCS Ospedale Galeazzi-Sant'Ambrogio, University of Milan, 20157 Milan, Italy; estrappa@yahoo.it

[3] Department of Clinical Sciences, Polytechnic University of Marche, 60126 Ancona, Italy; f.bambini@staff.univpm.it

* Correspondence: l.meme@staff.univpm.it

**Abstract:** This retrospective study aimed to evaluate a possible correlation between the characteristics of the mandibular ramus and lower third molar impaction by comparing a group of subjects with an impacted lower third molar and a second group with normal eruption for an early prediction of this pathology. This comparison was made using linear and angular measurements, which were taken on digital panoramic radiographs. **Materials and methods:** A total of 726 orthopantomographs (OPT) were examined, and 81 were considered suitable for the present study. The results were divided into two groups: a control group and an experimental group. The control group comprised 38 cases in which patients had at least one lower third molar that had erupted, and the experimental group comprised 43 cases in which patients had at least one lower third molar that was impacted or partially impacted. In total, 16 variables (11 linear, 4 angular, and 1 ratio) were determined and measured by an experienced observer. **Results:** The control group had a larger retromolar space, a larger impaction angle and a higher ratio of retromolar area to the third molar, compared to the experimental group. In contrast, the experimental group showed a deeper sigmoid notch depth than the control group did. In the control group, moderate positive correlations were found between both the length of the coronoid and the width of the third molar, and the retromolar space. Furthermore, in the experimental group, moderate positive correlations were found between both the angular condyle–coronoid process and the inclination of the lower posterior teeth, and the retromolar space. **Conclusion:** this study showed that the angle of a lower third molar, in relation to mandibular pain, can be an index for predicting tooth inclusion.

**Keywords:** third molar impaction; mandibular ramus dimensions; molar inclusion

**Citation:** Mummolo, S.; Gallusi, G.; Strappa, E.M.; Grilli, F.; Mattei, A.; Fiasca, F.; Bambini, F.; Memè, L. Prediction of Mandibular Third Molar Impaction Using Linear and Angular Measurements in Young Adult Orthopantomograms. *Appl. Sci.* **2023**, *13*, 4637. https://doi.org/10.3390/app13074637

Academic Editors: Gabriele Cervino and Vittorio Checchi

Received: 14 February 2023
Revised: 28 March 2023
Accepted: 30 March 2023
Published: 6 April 2023



## 1. Introduction

The inclusion of lower third molars has always represented a complex situation in dentistry. This occurs in about 73% of young adults in Europe [1–5].

However, the eruption of third molars can vary based on race and other factors such as diet, genetics, and the degree of tooth usage [6].

In fact, these are the teeth that most often undergo bone inclusion [1–9] and this can lead to complications in surgical treatment—given the possible risks of such a procedure [10]—and in the stability of possible orthodontic treatment.

The physiological eruption of the third molar occurs between the ages of 17 and 24 years [11]. Third molar retention can manifest itself with different clinical conditions: complete bone impaction, osteomucosal impaction and mucosal impaction.

The phenomenon of bone inclusion can be the cause of suppurative pericoronaritis or can be totally asymptomatic. Impacted third molars can lead to the development of cysts and tumors, which can cause significant damage to the jawbone and surrounding teeth. A study published in 2014 by Steed MB et al. found that impacted wisdom teeth were associated with cysts and tumors, although they are relatively rare, highlighting the importance of the early detection and removal of impacted third molars [4]. The impacted lower third molars are also extracted more commonly due to dental caries involving either the impacted third molar itself or the distal surface of the second molar [5].

However, in a study that was conducted in 2020 by Ghaeminia et al. [12], it was concluded that "Insufficient evidence was found to support or refute routine prophylactic removal of asymptomatic impacted wisdom teeth in adults. A single trial comparing removal versus retention found no evidence of a difference on late lower incisor crowding at 5 years; however, no other relevant outcomes were measured. Watchful monitoring of asymptomatic third molar teeth may be a more prudent strategy".

Furthermore, a major revision was previously published by G. Mettes [13] in The Cochrane Library, 2012. This manuscript was concluded by stating that "insufficient evidence was found to support or refute routine prophylactic removal of asymptomatic impacted wisdom teeth in adults. A single trial comparing removal versus retention found no evidence of a difference on late lower incisor crowding at 5 years; however, no other relevant outcomes were measured. Watchful monitoring of asymptomatic third molar teeth may be a more prudent strategy".

The extraction of the lower third molar can be the cause of different complications. For example, in 2016, a study was published by Jessica Yolanda Jeevitha [14] and revealed that it is possible to observe fractures on the mandible either intraoperatively or in four weeks, postoperatively. This was also highlighted by Bodner et al. [15] in 2011.

In 2022, Boffano P. et al. [16] published a manuscript in which they concluded that the "inadequate management of surgical instruments, the application of excessive force, incorrect surgical technique, underestimating the difficulty of the extraction, not performing the correct odontosection of the lower third molar and performing extensive ostectomies may be some of the causes of iatrogenic fractures".

An important complication that can arise from the extraction of a lower third molar when it is impacted on the seventh tooth is the secondary presence of an empty space close to the distal root of the seventh tooth. This empty space leaves the distal root of the seventh tooth completely or partially exposed. An in vitro study was published in 2022 by Bambini F. [17], which investigated how to support bone regeneration in this area. In their study, they tested the dentin—which could be used as a filler in the postextraction alveolus of the tooth for the preservation of the dental socket that was derived from the trituration of the dentin of an extracted eighth tooth. Another approach for preserving the alveolus was published by both Rossi et al. [18,19] and by Grassi et al. [20], in 2022. In these studies, they investigated alveolar preservation using bovine cortical lamina and fibrin glue.

The etiology of third molar inclusion is still under discussion; however, craniofacial development is certainly an important aspect of third molar inclusion [21], as inclusion is often associated with poor growth in the length of the mandible [4–7]; therefore, it is associated with a type II skeletal class [22]. Consequently, it is also important to consider the decrease in the space between the lower second molar and the mandibular ramus.

These factors occur due to a change in craniofacial growth during the developmental process, as a result of a decrease in the masticatory activity of the maxillary bones, which thus causes a decrease in their development. Another demographic factor that has been implicated in the etiology of impacted wisdom teeth is age. A systematic review and meta-analysis by Chen, Y.W., et al. (2017) demonstrated that older age was a significant risk factor for impacted wisdom teeth, with the highest prevalence of impaction occurring in patients over the age of 25. The authors proposed that older age may result in increased bone density and decreased jawbone size, contributing to the development of impaction [23].

In addition to morphological and demographic factors, a significant genetic component has also been identified in the etiology of impacted wisdom teeth. In a twin study, Trakinienė G et al. (2018) reported heritability estimates ranging from 40 to 60% for the development of impacted wisdom teeth. The authors suggested that the genetic contribution may be due to the influence of genetic factors on tooth size and jaw size [24]. Lastly, poor oral hygiene can also increase the risk of impaction. Caymaz, M.G. et al. (2021) found that patients with impacted wisdom teeth were more likely to have periodontitis and gingivitis compared to patients without impacted wisdom teeth. The authors proposed that poor oral hygiene may lead to an increase in the risk of impaction by creating an environment that is conducive to bacterial growth [25].

OPTs are extensively utilized in the field of dentistry due to their ability to offer a swift, cost-effective, and low radiation dosage option, while also providing a bilateral perspective of the mandible, unlike more complex diagnostic instruments). Furthermore, it is regarded as a suitable radiographic approach for evaluating the space occupied by the lower third molar and the linear and angular dimensions of the mandible [2,26].

This retrospective radiograph study aimed to evaluate a possible correlation between the characteristics of the mandibular ramus and lower third molar inclusion by comparing a group of subjects with lower third molar inclusion to a second group with normal eruption to establish an early means of predicting this pathology. The comparison was made using linear and angular measurements taken on digital panoramic radiographs [2].

## 2. Materials and Methods

This study was carried out as a retrospective radiographic research study and was performed in a private clinic (A.G., E.M.), in compliance with the principles of the Declaration of Helsinki, on medical protocol and ethics.

Orthopanoramic radiographs taken in the period between January 2015 and December 2021 were considered.

A total of 726 OPTs were examined, but only 81 were suitable for the present study considering the following evaluation criteria: patients with included or erupted lower third molars, no history of pathology associated with third molars, no previous orthodontic treatment, complete formation of the tooth's root and good OPT quality [27].

The radiographs were all taken on the Carestream C8100 3D CBCT digital radiography machine, with an OPT function.

We analyzed both sides of the maxillary bones indiscriminately. We only considered the side that was included in the selection criteria.

OPTs with one side of the third molar impacted and the other side fully erupted were excluded.

The radiographs included patients aged between 18 and 25 years old, of both sexes (50 male and 31 female).

The results were divided into 2 groups:

Group A: control group comprising 38 cases with at least one lower third molar erupted.

Group B: experimental group comprising 43 cases with at least one lower third molar included or partially included and, therefore, not in functional occlusion.

Groups were further divided into male and female groups, male experimental group B (MB) ($n$ = 24), male control group A (MA) ($n$ = 26), female experimental group B (FB) ($n$ = 19) and female control group A (FA) ($n$ = 12), and were compared with their equivalent subgroups in the control group.

Interpretation of the digital panoramic radiographic images was performed using Carestream Dental Imaging Software.

Using the digital ruler and protractor functions, 16 variables (11 linear, 4 angular and 1 ratio) were determined and measured by an experienced observer (Figures 1 and 2) [1–9,21,28–33].

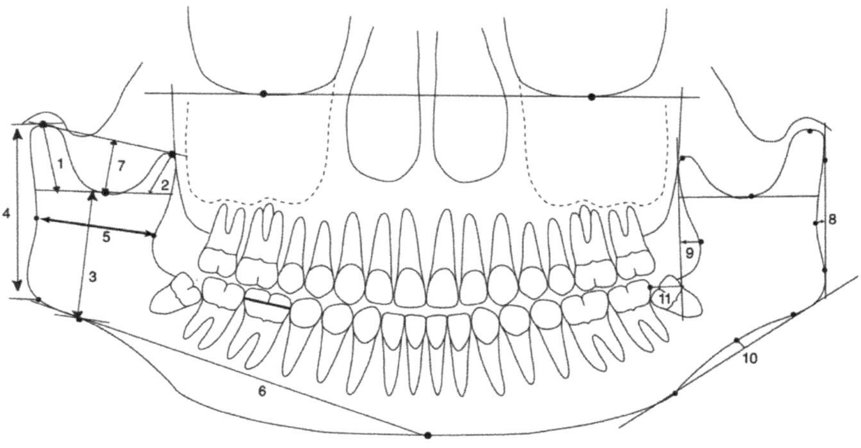


**Figure 1.** Linear measurements.

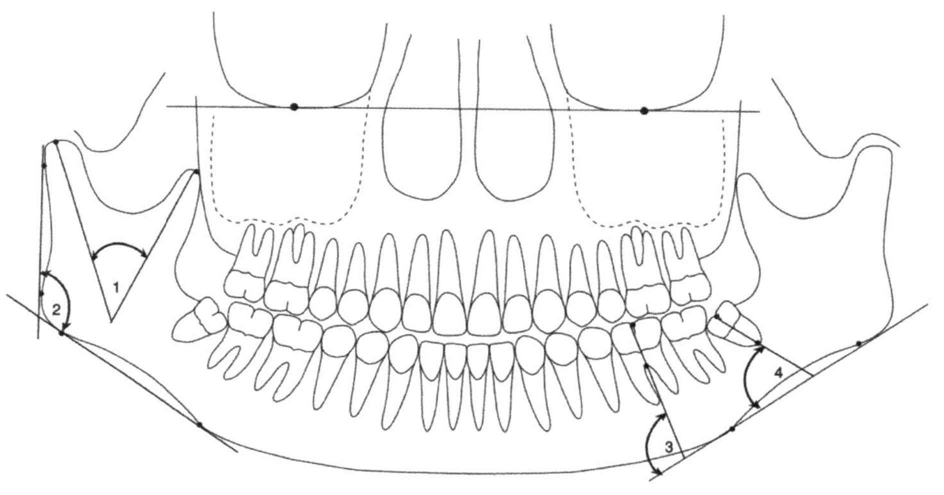


**Figure 2.** Angular measurements.

The 11 linear measurements are represented in Figure 1 and listed in Table 1 with their corresponding numbers:

1. Condyle length from the highest point of the mandibular condyle's head to lowest point of the mandibular sigmoid notch plane, along the long axis of the condylar process.
2. Coronoid length from the highest point of the mandibular coronoid process to the lowest point of the mandibular sigmoid notch plane, along the long axis of the coronoid process.
3. Ramus height from the lowest point of the mandibular sigmoid notch to the point in the antegonial notch of the mandible, the ramus and body of the mandible are joined.
4. Total ramus height from the highest point of the mandibular condyle's head to the intersection point of the ramus plane and the mandibular plane.
5. Ramal width from the deepest point of the anterior ramus notch concavity to the deepest point of the posterior ramus notch concavity.
6. Mandibular body length from the intersection point of the ramus plane and the mandibular plane to the midpoint of the mandible.

7. Sigmoid notch depth: the perpendicular line from the lowest point of the mandibular sigmoid notch to a line from the condylion and coronoid process.
8. Posterior ramus notch depth from the perpendicular line from the deepest point of the posterior ramus notch concavity to the line that connects the point where the external contour of the cranial base intersects with the dorsal contour of the condylar head to the point of maximal convexity on the posterior border of the angular process of the mandible.
9. Anterior ramus notch depth from the perpendicular line from the deepest point of the anterior ramus notch concavity to the perpendicolar line to the plane of the sigmoid notch and tangent to the descending anterior border of the ramus of the mandible.
10. Antegonial notch depth from the perpendicular line from the deepest point of the mandibular inferior border notch concavity to the mandibular plane.
11. Third molar width from the mesial aspect to distal aspect of third molar.

**Table 1.** Reference points: 13 variables (8 linear, 4 angular and 1 ratio) determined and measured.

| Variable | Control Group (A) | | Experimental Group (B) | | *p* Value * |
|---|---|---|---|---|---|
| | Mean | SD | Mean | SD | |
| 1. Condyle length (cm) | 1.77 | 0.41 | 1.84 | 0.45 | 0.463 |
| 2. Coronoid length (cm) | 1.37 | 0.46 | 1.53 | 0.36 | 0.080 |
| 3. Ramus height (cm) | 6.37 | 0.57 | 6.18 | 0.68 | 0.199 |
| 4. Total ramus height (cm) | 7.40 | 0.73 | 7.30 | 0.80 | 0.540 |
| 5. Ramal width (cm) | 3.62 | 0.52 | 3.66 | 0.39 | 0.676 |
| 6. Mandibular body length (cm) | 10.97 | 1.24 | 10.90 | 1.11 | 0.787 |
| 7. Sigmoid notch depth (cm) | 1.43 | 0.33 | 1.59 | 0.31 | **0.030** |
| 8. Posterior ramus notch depth (cm) | 0.25 | 0.14 | 0.30 | 0.14 | 0.088 |
| 9. Anterior ramus notch depth (cm) | 0.27 | 0.22 | 0.24 | 0.19 | 0.490 |
| 10. Antegonial notch depth (cm) | 0.23 | 0.24 | 0.20 | 0.15 | 0.515 |
| 11. Third molar width (cm) | 1.38 | 0.27 | 1.41 | 0.14 | 0.424 |
| Retromolar space (cm) | 1.52 | 0.63 | 1.14 | 0.60 | **0.007** |
| 1. Angle condyle—coronoid process (deg) | 30.13 | 5.35 | 29.53 | 4.81 | 0.599 |
| 2. Gonial angle (deg) | 124.84 | 6.78 | 122.63 | 68.33 | 0.195 |
| 3.Inclination of lower posterior teeth (deg) | 95.53 | 5.93 | 92.65 | 6.23 | 0.521 |
| 4. Angle of impaction (deg) | 88.61 | 16.72 | 68.53 | 34.06 | **0.002** |
| Retromolar space/3M width (ratio) | 1.09 | 0.40 | 0.81 | 0.44 | **0.004** |

* using Student's *t*-test.

The 4 angular measurements are represented in Figure 2 and listed in Table 1 with their corresponding numbers:

1. Angle condyle—coronoid process: the intersection between the highest point of the mandibular condyle's head to the highest point of the mandibular coronoid process.
2. Gonial angle: the intersection between the line that connects the point where the external contour of the cranial base intersects with the dorsal contour of the condylar head to the point of maximal convexity on the posterior border of the angular process of the mandible and the mandibular plane.
3. Inclination of lower posterior teeth: the intersection between the mandibular plane and the long axis of the first molar.

4. Angle of impaction: the intersection between the mandibular plane and the long axis of the third molar.

*Statistical Analysis*

The mandibular dimensions of the sample were compared with those of the control group. Descriptive statistics, as mean and standard deviation, were used to examine the characteristics of the sample. Data analyzed were normally distributed (through a Shapiro–Wilk test), and Student's *t*-test was used to analyze the statistical differences between the two groups.

Groups were further divided into male and female groups: male impaction group B (MB) ($n = 24$), male control group A (MA) ($n = 26$), female impaction group B (FB) ($n = 19$) and female control group A (FA) ($n = 12$). The impaction groups were also compared to their equivalent subgroups in Group A using an unpaired *t*-test.

Furthermore, Pearson's correlation and linear regression tests were used to assess the degree of relationship between the retromolar space and mandibular measurements. Statistical analyses were performed using the STATA/IC 15.1 statistical package. All tests were two-tailed, and *p*-values of $\leq 0.05$ were considered statistically significant.

## 3. Results

The results showed that the control group demonstrated a larger retromolar space ($1.52 \pm 0.63$ vs. $1.14 \pm 0.60$, $p = 0.007$), a larger impaction angle ($88.61 \pm 16.72$ vs. $68.53 \pm 34.06$, $p = 0.002$), and a higher ratio of retromolar area to the third molar ($1.09 \pm 0.40$ vs. $0.81 \pm 0.44$, $p = 0.004$), compared to the experimental group (Table 1). In contrast, the experimental group demonstrated a deeper sigmoid notch depth ($1.59 \pm 0.31$ vs. $1.43 \pm 0.33$, $p = 0.030$) than the control group.

In both groups, a moderate negative correlation was found between the depth of the anterior branch notch ($p = 0.001$ and $p = 0.002$, respectively) and the retromolar space. A strong positive correlation was found between both the retromolar area and the third molar ratio ($p < 0.001$), and the retromolar space.

In the control group, moderate positive correlations were found between both the length of the coronoid ($p = 0.029$) and the width of the third molar ($p = 0.004$). In addition, in the control group, a moderate negative correlation was found between the depth of the antegonial notch ($p = 0.019$) and the retromolar space.

Furthermore, in the experimental group, moderate positive correlations ($p = 0.008$) were found between both the angular condyle–coronoid process and the inclination of the lower posterior teeth, and the retromolar space (Table 2).

**Table 2.** Pearson's correlation and linear regression tests values.

| Variable | Control Group (A) | | | | Experimental Group (B) | | | |
|---|---|---|---|---|---|---|---|---|
| | Retromolar Space | | | | Retromolar Space | | | |
| | r | $R^2$ | $R^2$ (ADJ) | *p* Value | r | $R^2$ | $R^2$ (ADJ) | *p* Value |
| Condyle length | −0.172 | 0.029 | 0.003 | 0.303 | −0.157 | 0.025 | 0.001 | 0.314 |
| Coronoid length | 0.354 | 0.125 | 0.101 | **0.029** | 0.035 | 0.001 | −0.023 | 0.826 |
| Ramus height | 0.222 | 0.049 | 0.023 | 0.181 | 0.151 | 0.023 | −0.001 | 0.335 |
| Total ramus height | 0.197 | 0.039 | 0.012 | 0.236 | 0.194 | 0.038 | 0.014 | 0.213 |
| Ramal width | 0.307 | 0.095 | 0.069 | 0.061 | 0.025 | 0.001 | −0.024 | 0.875 |
| Mandibular body length | 0.081 | 0.007 | −0.021 | 0.629 | −0.288 | 0.083 | 0.061 | 0.061 |
| Sigmoid notch depth | 0.064 | 0.004 | −0.024 | 0.701 | −0.149 | 0.022 | −0.002 | 0.339 |
| Posterior ramus notch depth | −0.192 | 0.037 | 0.010 | 0.249 | 0.188 | 0.035 | 0.012 | 0.227 |

**Table 2.** *Cont.*

| Variable | Control Group (A) | | | | Experimental Group (B) | | | |
|---|---|---|---|---|---|---|---|---|
| | Retromolar Space | | | | Retromolar Space | | | |
| | r | $R^2$ | $R^2$ (ADJ) | *p* Value | r | $R^2$ | $R^2$ (ADJ) | *p* Value |
| Anterior ramus notch depth | −0.521 | 0.271 | 0.251 | **0.001** | −0.454 | 0.206 | 0.187 | **0.002** |
| Antegonial notch depth | −0.379 | 0.144 | 0.120 | **0.019** | 0.295 | 0.087 | 0.065 | 0.055 |
| Third molar width | 0.456 | 0.208 | 0.186 | **0.004** | 0.095 | 0.009 | −0.015 | 0.545 |
| Gonial angle | 0.312 | 0.097 | 0.072 | 0.056 | 0.182 | 0.033 | 0.010 | 0.243 |
| Angle condyle—coronoid process | 0.071 | 0.005 | −0.023 | 0.673 | 0.402 | 0.162 | 0.141 | **0.008** |
| Inclination of lower posterior teeth | 0.142 | 0.020 | −0.007 | 0.396 | 0.397 | 0.157 | 0.137 | **0.008** |
| Angle of impaction | 0.176 | 0.031 | 0.004 | 0.290 | 0.245 | 0.060 | 0.037 | 0.113 |
| Retromolar space/3M width (ratio) | 0.966 | 0.933 | 0.931 | **<0.001** | 0.971 | 0.942 | 0.941 | **<0.001** |

r = Pearson correlation coefficient; $R^2$ = squared multiple correlation coefficient; $R^2$ (ADJ) = adjusted coefficient of determination.

Considering sex, male control group MA showed larger retromolar space (1.54 ± 0.59 vs. 1.10 ± 0.58, $p = 0.010$), larger angle of impaction (90.93 ± 8.69 vs. 69.46 ± 32.66, $p = 0.002$) and higher retromolar area to the third molar ratio (1.09 ± 0.39 vs. 0.77 ± 0.39, $p = 0.006$) than male experimental group MB (Table 3).

**Table 3.** Comparison between male group A (MA) and the male group B (MB).

| Variable | Control Group (Male Group A, *n* = 26) | | Experimental Group (Male Group B, *n* = 24) | | *p* Value * |
|---|---|---|---|---|---|
| | Mean | SD | Mean | SD | |
| Condyle length (cm) | 1.76 | 0.43 | 1.86 | 0.37 | 0.365 |
| Coronoid length (cm) | 1.49 | 0.48 | 1.55 | 0.36 | 0.608 |
| Ramus height (cm) | 6.43 | 0.52 | 6.13 | 0.67 | 0.087 |
| Total ramus height (cm) | 7.48 | 0.70 | 7.25 | 0.79 | 0.294 |
| Ramal width (cm) | 3.69 | 0.55 | 3.58 | 0.33 | 0.421 |
| Mandibular body length (cm) | 10.81 | 1.11 | 10.88 | 1.18 | 0.836 |
| Sigmoid notch depth (cm) | 1.47 | 0.36 | 1.60 | 0.29 | 0.137 |
| Posterior ramus notch depth (cm) | 0.24 | 0.13 | 0.30 | 0.16 | 0.110 |
| Anterior ramus notch depth (cm) | 0.26 | 0.19 | 0.24 | 0.18 | 0.656 |
| Antegonial notch depth (cm) | 0.22 | 0.24 | 0.20 | 0.14 | 0.737 |
| Third molar width (cm) | 1.39 | 0.12 | 1.41 | 0.15 | 0.608 |
| Retromolar space (cm) | 1.54 | 0.59 | 1.10 | 0.58 | **0.010** |
| Angle condyle—coronoid process (deg) | 31.04 | 5.38 | 28.75 | 5.06 | 0.129 |
| Gonial angle (deg) | 124.81 | 7.48 | 122.33 | 8.76 | 0.287 |
| Inclination of lower posterior teeth (deg) | 91.15 | 5.70 | 92.70 | 6.65 | 0.753 |
| Angle of impaction (deg) | 90.93 | 8.69 | 69.46 | 32.66 | **0.002** |
| Retromolar space/3M width (ratio) | 1.09 | 0.39 | 0.77 | 0.39 | **0.006** |

* using Student's *t*-test.

Female experimental group FB showed higher coronoid length (1.50 ± 0.37 vs. 1.10 ± 0.28, $p = 0.004$) than female control group (FA) (Table 4).

**Table 4.** Comparison between female group A (FA) and group B (FB).

| Variable | Control Group (Female Group A, $n$ = 12) | | Experimental Group (Female Group B, $n$ = 19) | | $p$ Value * |
|---|---|---|---|---|---|
| | Mean | SD | Mean | SD | |
| Condyle length (cm) | 1.81 | 0.36 | 1.82 | 0.53 | 0.943 |
| Coronoid length (cm) | 1.10 | 0.28 | 1.50 | 0.37 | **0.004** |
| Ramus height (cm) | 6.23 | 0.67 | 6.25 | 0.70 | 0.930 |
| Total ramus height (cm) | 7.23 | 0.77 | 7.35 | 0.82 | 0.688 |
| Ramal width (cm) | 3.46 | 0.41 | 3.75 | 0.45 | 0.077 |
| Mandibular body length (cm) | 11.32 | 1.48 | 10.93 | 1.04 | 0.396 |
| Sigmoid notch depth (cm) | 1.35 | 0.23 | 1.56 | 0.33 | 0.069 |
| Posterior ramus notch depth (cm) | 0.27 | 0.17 | 0.30 | 0.13 | 0.537 |
| Anterior ramus notch depth (cm) | 0.28 | 0.26 | 0.24 | 0.20 | 0.584 |
| Antegonial notch depth (cm) | 0.25 | 0.25 | 0.20 | 0.16 | 0.505 |
| Third molar width (cm) | 1.35 | 0.46 | 1.42 | 0.13 | 0.525 |
| Retromolar space (cm) | 1.49 | 0.76 | 1.19 | 0.65 | 0.255 |
| Angle condyle—coronoid process (deg) | 28.17 | 4.95 | 30.53 | 4.41 | 0.177 |
| Gonial angle (deg) | 124.92 | 5.23 | 123.00 | 7.83 | 0.461 |
| Inclination of lower posterior teeth (deg) | 96.50 | 5.50 | 92.58 | 5.81 | 0.072 |
| Angle of impaction (deg) | 83.58 | 26.98 | 67.37 | 36.62 | 0.197 |
| Retromolar space/3M width (ratio) | 1.07 | 0.45 | 0.85 | 0.50 | 0.240 |

*: using Student's $t$-test.

## 4. Discussion

Various studies have been carried out on the predictability of the eruption of the mandibular lower third molar, based on the size of the bony structures of the mandible. These studies have been conducted using both lateral cephalometric and orthopanoramic radiographs; however, not many authors have compared the different radiographic techniques [21,26,28–33] for mandibular measurements. The few authors who have compared the different techniques have found excellent results when using both methods. Therefore, they have concluded that they are both valid tools for diagnostic investigation in this area and that the choice between them depends on the experience of the clinician. They are routinely used in dentists' normal professional practice [23] both to obtain an initial general diagnosis of a patient's oral health status and for more in-depth examinations of third molar inclusion, for which digital orthopanoramic examinations are also used.

The subjects were selected upon the consideration that an age between 18 to 25 years of age is the average age of eruption and complete formation of the mandibular third molar. Various studies have reported [29–31] that the ideal age for studying the incidence of the lower third molar is between 20 and 25 years. In total, 81 subjects were considered, and the age range was extended to between 18 and 25 years of age, on the condition that the tooth's root had been completely formed.

In our study, we found that the length of the condyle–coronoid process in the experimental group was greater than that in the control group. This result was partially in agreement with that of Capelli [5], who found an association between a greater ascending ramus size and the inclusion of the lower third molar.

In contrast, the height of the branch and its total size were larger in the control group than in the experimental group. Significant differences were found in these measurements, which differed from the result obtained by Hassan [30], who found uniformity between results.

Regarding the branch width, the experimental group showed a slightly wider measurement than the control group did. This result was in line with Hassan's study [30], although Hassan's results showed a sharper difference.

In our study, the measurements of the length of the mandibular body were uniform for both groups; therefore, there were no statistically significant differences.

This result was in agreement with the the results of the studies of Kaplan [32] and Djerkes [6], in which the values of this measurement were statistically insignificant; however, in contrast to the studies of Hassan [30] and Capelli [5], the length of the mandibular body was larger in the control group.

According to the results of our study, the sigmoid notch was deeper in the experimental group than in the control group ($p < 0.030$), and this may be related to the greater size of the bony structures of the mandible. In fact, this corresponded to the results obtained through the measurements of the length of the condyle and coronoid process, which were longer in the experimental group than in the control group.

This result contrasts with that of Yamaki's study [1], which showed higher measurements for the control group than the experimental group in relation to the depth of the sigmoid notch. This may have been due to the use of a different measurement technique or a different sampling method.

It should be noted, however, that the depth of the notch of the anterior and posterior branches in our study showed no relevant differences, as the posterior depth was greater in the experimental group, but the anterior depth was greater in the control group.

Regarding the retromolar space, our study found a significant difference between the two groups: the control group reported a mean measurement of 1.52 cm, which was significantly higher than the space in the experimental group, which was 1.14 cm, on average ($p < 0.001$). This result is in line with the results of the studies carried out by Hattab [31] in Jordan (a measurement of 1.44 cm for the control group and of 1.10 cm for the experimental group was found) and by Qamruddin [34] in Pakistan (a measurement of 1.63 cm for the control group and 1.12 cm for the experimental group was found).

According to Uthman [27], the retromolar space measurable from orthopanoramic radiographs should be more than 12 mm. This figure corresponded to the measurements in our study.

Regarding the the space-witdth ratio of the lower third molar, the results that we obtained show that the control group had a ratio of 1.09 and that the experimental group had a ratio of 0.81. These ratios were very similar to those found by the studies already mentioned by Hattab [31] and Al-Gunaid [1].

In the angular measurements, however, the gonial angle was wider in the control group than in the experimental group. This result agreed with the results of the previous studies by Ganss [8] and Richardson [22]; however, they contrasted with those of Hattab [31] and Al-Gunaid [1], who found a wider angle for the experimental group than for the control group.

Finally, Behbehani [4] stated that a smaller gonial angle may be associated with an increased risk of lower third molar inclusion [10,27,35,36]. This was in agreement with our results.

In our study, the angulation of the lower posterior teeth, specifically the first and second molars, was greater in the experimental group. The control group showed a smaller angle and a more upright position. This result aligned with previous studies that have concluded that the inclination of the posterior teeth is a possible cause of the inclusion of lower third molars.

On the other hand, it should be noted that, in our study, the inclination of the lower third molars was greater in the experimental group than it was in the control group, and this difference was highly significant ($p < 0.002$).

This result agreed with the results of previous studies by Ricketts [37], Hassan [30], Capelli [5] and Hugoson [38] and confirmed that the angle of a lower third molar, in relation to mandibular pain, can be an index for predicting tooth inclusion.

To investigate whether there are any gender differences in mandibular geometry related to third molar impaction, the sample was divided into males and females. The impaction groups (FB and MB) were compared with their respective control groups.

Most of the differences between the control groups and the experimental groups were found among males; the male control group showed a larger retromolar space and retromolar area to the third molar ratio than the male experimental group did. This result agreed with the results of previous studies by Hassan [30]

Their results also disagree with those of Kaplan [32], who found no significant sex predilection when comparing the experimental group to the control group. The variation influenced by sex gender observed in different studies appears to be linked to the variability in the timing of mandibular skeletal maturity between males and females. This could be attributed to the continued growth of the mandible in males until the age at which third molars are about to erupt.

## 5. Conclusions

By evaluating the relevant data present in the existing literature, through accurate and simple data analysis, our observational cross-sectional study has found an associative link between some of the investigated variables in the conformation of the mandible associated with the impaction of third molars, in accordance with some of the literature.

Such a study requires further investigation with experimental studies (randomized clinical trials). In this way, it will be possible to identify and confirm the predictive factors in the impaction of mandibular third molars in relation to mandibular dimensions.

**Author Contributions:** Conceptualization, L.M. and F.B.; methodology, G.G., F.G. and A.M.; software, E.M.S. and F.F.; validation, L.M., G.G. and F.B.; formal analysis, S.M., F.B. and L.M.; investigation, F.G., A.M. and F.F.; resources, L.M. and F.B.; data curation, G.G. and F.F.; writing—original draft preparation, L.M. and G.G.; writing—review and editing, E.M.S., F.B. and S.M.; visualization, L.M., G.G., S.M. and F.G.; supervision, L.M.; project administration, F.B. and S.M. All authors have read and agreed to the published version of the manuscript.

**Funding:** This research received no external funding.

**Institutional Review Board Statement:** Not applicable.

**Informed Consent Statement:** Not applicable.

**Data Availability Statement:** Not applicable.

**Conflicts of Interest:** The authors declare no conflict of interest.

## References

1. Al-Gunaid, T.H.; Bukhari, A.K.; El Khateeb, S.M.; Yamaki, M. Relationship of Mandibular Ramus Dimensions to Lower Third Molar Impaction. *Eur. J. Dent.* **2019**, *13*, 213–221. [CrossRef] [PubMed]
2. Al-Zoubi, H.; Alharbi, A.A.; Ferguson, D.J.; Zafar, M.S. Frequency of impacted teeth and categorization of impacted canines: A retrospective radiographic study using orthopantomograms. *Eur. J. Dent.* **2017**, *11*, 117–121. [CrossRef] [PubMed]
3. Andreasen, J.O. Epidemiology of third molar impaction. In *Textbook and Color Atlas of Tooth Impactions*; Andreasen, J.O., Peterson, J.K., Laskin, D.M., Eds.; Munksgaard: Copenhagen, Denmark, 1997; pp. 222–223.
4. Behbehani, F.; Årtun, J.; Thalib, L. Prediction of mandibular third-molar impaction in adolescent orthodontic patients. *Am. J. Orthod. Dentofac. Orthop.* **2006**, *130*, 47–55. [CrossRef] [PubMed]
5. Capelli, J., Jr. Mandibular growth and third molar impaction in extraction cases. *Angle Orthod.* **1991**, *61*, 223–229. [PubMed]
6. Dierkes, D.D. An investigation of the mandibular third molars in orthodontic cases. *Angle Orthod.* **1975**, *45*, 207–212.
7. Forsberg, C.M.; Vingren, B.; Wesslén, U. Mandibular third molar eruption in relation to available space as assessed on lateral cephalograms. *Swed. Dent. J.* **1989**, *13*, 23–31.
8. Ganss, C.; Hochban, W.; Kielbassa, A.M.; Umstadt, H.E. Prognosis of third molar eruption. *Oral Surg. Oral Med. Oral Pathol.* **1993**, *76*, 688–693. [CrossRef]
9. Gonca, M.; Gunacar, D.N.; Kose, T.E.; Karamehmetoglu, I. Evaluation of mandibular morphologic measurements and trabecular structure among subgroups of impacted mandibular third molars. *Oral Radiol.* **2021**, *38*, 63–71. [CrossRef]
10. Vaibhav, N.; Vivek, G.; Shetty, A.; Mohammad, I.; Ahmed, N.; Umeshappa, H. Efficacy of various routes of dexamethasone administration in reducing postoperative sequelae following impacted third molar surgery. *Ann. Maxillofac. Surg.* **2020**, *10*, 61–65. [CrossRef]

11. Garcia, R.I.; Chauncey, H.H. The eruption of third molarsin adults: A 10-year longitudinal study. *Oral Surg. Oral Med. Oral Pathol.* **1989**, *68*, 9–13. [CrossRef]
12. Ghaeminia, H.; Nienhuijs, M.E.; Toedtling, V.; Perry, J.; Tummers, M.; Hoppenreijs, T.J.; Van der Sanden, W.J.; Mettes, T.G. Interventions for treating trouble-free impacted wisdom teeth in adults. *Cochrane Database Syst Rev.* **2020**, *5*, CD003879. [CrossRef]
13. Mettes, T.D.; Ghaeminia, H.; Nienhuijs, M.E.; Perry, J.; van der Sanden, W.J.; Plasschaert, A. Surgical removal versus retention for the management of asymptomatic impacted wisdom teeth. *Cochrane Database Syst Rev.* **2012**, *13*, CD003879. [CrossRef]
14. Jeevitha, J.Y.; Thiagarajan, A.; Sivalingam, B. Influence and Impact of Mandibular Ramal Dimensions on the Incidence of Lower Third Molar Impaction: A Prospective Study. *J. Pharm. Bioallied Sci.* **2022**, *14* (Suppl. 1), S364–S368. [CrossRef]
15. Bodner, L.; Brennan, P.A.; McLeod, N.M. Characteristics of iatrogenic mandibular fractures associated with tooth removal: Review and analysis of 189 cases. *Br. J. Oral Maxillofac. Surg.* **2011**, *49*, 567–572. [CrossRef]
16. Boffano, P.; Roccia, F.; Gallesio, C.; Berrone, S. Pathological mandibular fractures: A review of the literature of the last two decades. *Dent. Traumatol.* **2013**, *29*, 185–196. [CrossRef]
17. Memè, L.; Strappa, E.M.; Monterubbianesi, R.; Bambini, F.; Mummolo, S. SEM and FT-MIR Analysis of Human Demineralized Dentin Matrix: An In Vitro Study. *Appl. Sci.* **2022**, *12*, 1480. [CrossRef]
18. Rossi, R.; Modoni, M.; Monterubbianesi, R.; Dallari, G.; Memè, L. The 'Guided Tissue Regeneration (GTR) Effect' of Guided Bone Regeneration (GBR) with the Use of Bone Lamina: A Report of Three Cases with More than 36 Months of Follow-Up. *Appl. Sci.* **2022**, *12*, 11247. [CrossRef]
19. Rossi, R.; Memè, L.; Strappa, E.M.; Bambini, F. Restoration of Severe Bone and Soft Tissue Atrophy by Means of a Xenogenic Bone Sheet (Flex Cortical Sheet): A Case Report. *Appl. Sci.* **2023**, *13*, 692. [CrossRef]
20. Grassi, A.; Memè, L.; Strappa, E.M.; Martini, E.; Bambini, F. Modified Periosteal Inhibition (MPI) Technique for Extraction Sockets: A Case Series Report. *Appl. Sci.* **2022**, *12*, 12292. [CrossRef]
21. Khalil, H. Skeletal tracing of impacted and erupted mandibular third molar areas using panoramic radiographs. *Biosci. Biotechnol. Res. Asia* **2016**, *7*, 1–6.
22. Richardson, M.E. The etiology and prediction of mandibular third molar impaction. *Angle Orthod.* **1977**, *47*, 165–172. [PubMed]
23. Chen, Y.W.; Lee, C.T.; Hum, L.; Chuang, S.K. Effect of flap design on periodontal healing after impacted third molar extraction: A systematic review and meta-analysis. *Int. J. Oral. Maxillofac. Surg.* **2017**, *46*, 363–372. [CrossRef] [PubMed]
24. Trakiniene, G.; Šidlauskas, A.; Švalkauskienė, V.; Smailienė, D.; Urbonė, J. The magnification in the lower third and second molar region in the digital panoramic radiographs. *J. Forensic. Dent. Sci.* **2017**, *9*, 91–95. [CrossRef]
25. Caymaz, M.G.; Buhara, O. Association of Oral Hygiene and Periodontal Health with Third Molar Pericoronitis: A Cross-Sectional Study. *Biomed. Res. Int.* **2021**, *2021*, 6664434. [CrossRef]
26. Ongkosuwito, E.M.; Dieleman, M.M.; Kuijpers-Jagtman, A.M.; Mulder, P.G.; van Neck, J.W. Linear mandibular measurements: Comparison between orthopantomograms and lateral cephalograms. *Cleft Palate Craniofac. J.* **2009**, *46*, 147–153. [CrossRef]
27. Uthman, A.T. Retromolar space analysis in relation to selected linear and angular measurements for an Iraqi sample. *Oral Surg. Oral Med. Oral Pathol. Oral Radiol. Endodontol.* **2007**, *104*, e76–e82. [CrossRef]
28. Gupta, S.; Jain, S. Orthopantomographic Analysis for Assessment of Mandibular Asymmetry. *J. Indian Orthod. Soc.* **2012**, *46*, 33–37. [CrossRef]
29. Haralabakis, H. Observations on the time of eruption, congenital absence and impaction of the third molar teeth. *Trans. Eur. Orthod. Soc.* **1957**, *33*, 308–309.
30. Hassan, A.H. Mandibular cephalometric characteristic of a Saudi sample of patients having impacted third molars. *Saudi Dent. J.* **2011**, *23*, 73–80. [CrossRef]
31. Hattab, F.N.; Alhaija, E.S. Radiographic evaluation of mandibular third molar eruption space. *Oral Surg. Oral Med. Oral Pathol. Oral Radiol. Endod.* **1999**, *88*, 285–291. [CrossRef]
32. Kaplan, R.G. Some factors related to mandibular third molar impaction. *Angle Orthod.* **1975**, *45*, 153–158. [PubMed]
33. Niedzielska, I.A.; Drugacz, J.; Kus', N.; Kręska, J. Panoramic radiographic predictors of mandibular third molar eruption. *Oral Surg. Oral Med. Oral Pathol. Oral Radiol. Endodontol.* **2006**, *102*, 154–158. [CrossRef]
34. Qamruddin, I.; Qayyum, W.; Haider, S.M.; Siddiqui, S.W.; Rehan, F. Differences in various measurements on panoramic radiograph among erupted and impacted lower third molar groups. *J. Pak. Med. Assoc.* **2012**, *62*, 883–887.
35. Shiller, W.R. Positional changes in mesio-angular impacted mandibular third molars during a year. *J. Am. Dent. Assoc.* **1979**, *99*, 460–464. [CrossRef]
36. Ventä, I.; Murtomaa, H.; Turtola, L.; Meurman, J.; Ylipaavalniemi, P. Clinical follow-up study of third molar eruption from ages 20 to 26 years. *Oral Surg. Oral Med. Oral Pathol.* **1991**, *72*, 150–153. [CrossRef]
37. Ricketts, R.M. A principle of arcial growth of the mandible. *Angle Orthod.* **1972**, *42*, 368–386.
38. Hugoson, A.; Kugelberg, C.F. The prevalence of third molars in a Swedish population. An epidemiological study. *Community Dent. Health* **1988**, *5*, 121–138.

applied sciences

MDPI

*Review*

# A Molecular View on Biomaterials and Dental Stem Cells Interactions: Literature Review

**Fernando J. Aguilar-Ayala [1,†], Fernando J. Aguilar-Pérez [1,†], Geovanny I. Nic-Can [2], Rafael Rojas-Herrera [3], Gabriela Chuc-Gamboa [1], David Aguilar-Pérez [1] and Beatriz A. Rodas-Junco [2,*]**

1 Facultad de Odontología, Universidad Autónoma de Yucatán, Mérida 97000, Mexico; faguilar@correo.uady.mx (F.J.A.-A.); fernando.aguilar@correo.uady.mx (F.J.A.-P.); martha.chuc@correo.uady.mx (G.C.-G.); david.aguilar@correo.uady.mx (D.A.-P.)
2 CONACYT—Facultad de Ingeniería Química, Universidad Autónoma de Yucatán, Mérida 97000, Mexico; geovanny.nic@correo.uady.mx
3 Facultad de Ingeniería Química, Universidad Autónoma de Yucatán, Mérida 97000, Mexico; rafael.rojas@correo.uady.mx
* Correspondence: beatriz.rodas@correo.uady.mx or barodasju@conacyt.mx
† These authors contributed equally to this work.

**Abstract:** Biomaterials and stem cells are essential components in the field of regenerative medicine. Various biomaterials have been designed that have appropriate biochemical and biophysical characteristics to mimic the microenvironment of an extracellular matrix. Dental stem cells (DT-MSCs) represent a novel source for the development of autologous therapies due to their easy availability. Although research on biomaterials and DT-MSCs has progressed, there are still challenges in the characteristics of biomaterials and the molecular mechanisms involved in regulating the behavior of DT-MSCs. In this review, the characteristics of biomaterials are summarized, and their classification according to their source, bioactivity, and different biological effects on the expansion and differentiation of DT-MSCs is summarized. Finally, advances in research on the interaction of biomaterials and the molecular components involved (mechanosensors and mechanotransduction) in DT-MSCs during their proliferation and differentiation are analyzed. Understanding the molecular dynamics of DT-MSCs and biomaterials can contribute to research in regenerative medicine and the development of autologous stem cell therapies.

**Keywords:** biomaterials; dental stem cells; differentiation; dental tissue; regenerative medicine

**Citation:** Aguilar-Ayala, F.J.; Aguilar-Pérez, F.J.; Nic-Can, G.I.; Rojas-Herrera, R.; Chuc-Gamboa, G.; Aguilar-Pérez, D.; Rodas-Junco, B.A. A Molecular View on Biomaterials and Dental Stem Cells Interactions: Literature Review. *Appl. Sci.* **2022**, *12*, 5815. https://doi.org/10.3390/app12125815

Academic Editor: Vittorio Checchi

Received: 11 May 2022
Accepted: 31 May 2022
Published: 8 June 2022



## 1. Introduction

The oral cavity has aroused particular interest as a source for obtaining mesenchymal stem cells (MSCs) because there are different oral tissues from which MSCs can be isolated. Dental tissue-derived mesenchymal stem cells (DT-MSCs) are easy to culture, as they can be obtained from a wide range of primary and permanent teeth without ethical controversy. This makes them a valuable and accessible source of autologous stem cells [1]. Most DT-MSCs are derived from the neural crest and can differentiate into multiple cell types, including epithelial cells, odontoblasts, osteoblasts, chondroblasts, adipocytes, neuronal cells, glial cells, and muscle cells. Thus, they are currently considered a promising resource for their therapeutic application in regenerative medicine. However, as in other types of stem cells, for its application to be successful, its proliferation and differentiation must be controlled in an environment that mimics in vivo conditions. Therefore, an artificial niche, such as biomaterials, is a fundamental strategy to exploit the therapeutic potential of DT-MSCs. Currently, in the design of biomaterials, characteristics, such as the physical chemistry of the material, its biological interaction, mechanical properties, specific biological functionalities, and shape or geometry at different scales, such as on the macro, micro, and nano levels, are considered during their cell–biomaterial interactions [2]. However, the biomaterial's chemical composition (natural or synthetic) also plays an important role in improving stem cells' in vitro biological response. In this sense, natural biomaterials offer the advantage of being biocompatible and biodegradable, while synthetic ones also allow the possibility of improving their chemical and physical properties for a specific application. In summary, research on biomaterials and DT-MSCs has progressed; however, challenges remain regarding the ideal characteristics of biomaterials and the molecular mechanisms involved in regulating behavior in DT-MSCs. Therefore, the aim of this literature review is to provide a molecular view of biomaterial–cell interaction to understand how signals from biomaterials act as potent regulators of the microenvironment in DT-MSCs. In the first part, the background on DT-MSCs is presented, with a specific focus on their biological characteristics. Next, the state of the art is analyzed with respect to the different chemical and physical characteristics of biomaterials and the molecular mechanisms involved during their interaction with DT-MSCs. In this sense, various in vitro and in vivo experimental studies are considered that report valuable information to understand the behavior and differentiation of these cells in biomaterials.

## 2. Dental Stem Cells

Mesenchymal stem cells (MSCs) are a group of cells capable of self-renewal and function as a repair system for damaged tissues. When a stem cell divides, each cell has the potential to remain a stem cell or to become another type of cell with a more specialized function. Thus, stem cells have two characteristics: the ability to self-renew and differentiate in any cell lineage (e.g., osteogenic, chondrogenic, adipogenic, myogenic, and neurogenic) comparable to those established for bone marrow-derived MSCs. They can be classified according to their origin in embryonic stem cells, adult stem cells (tissue-specific), and induced pluripotent cells (iPS) [3]. All of them are attractive for their use in the regeneration of damaged tissues; however, their clinical application is still limited due to the transplanted cells' low survival and differentiation potential. For a thorough understanding of the origin and biology of different stem cells, the reader is referred to excellent reviews on this subject [4,5].

Oral cavity tissues are rich sources of adult stem cells. These cells are called dental tissue-derived mesenchymal stem cells (DT-MSCs), and the method of obtaining them is relatively easy in dental tissues and, even better, they are a source of autologous stem cells [1,6]. Likewise, they present a high proliferation, ability to differentiate into multiple cell types, and the expression of positive and embryonic markers of MSCs (i.e., OCT4, Nanog, SOX2, and KLF4), which makes them more attractive for their application in regenerative medicine [1,7–9]. Different types of DT-MSCs have been identified, such as dental pulp stem cells (DPSCs), exfoliated deciduous tooth stem cells (SHEDs), periodontal ligament stem cells (PDLSCs), dental follicle stem cells (DFSCs), and stem cells from the apical papilla (SCAP) (Figure 1) [1]. Although these types of cells have been shown to have stem, clonogenicity, and self-renewal characteristics, their differentiation capacity varies according to the origin of the cells. Some authors have pointed out that this behavior could be due to: (1) the heterogeneity of DT-MSCs and (2) the microenvironment of stem cells in dental tissues, for example, teeth in pre-eruptive formation (dental follicle and apical papilla) versus erupted teeth (dental pulp or periodontal ligament) [3,10,11]. Thus, one of the challenges for the clinical application of DT-MSCs is to mimic the appropriate microenvironment so that cells can proliferate or differentiate properly [3]; to achieve this, cells need extracellular matrix (ECM) components (Figure 1). Numerous studies have focused on developing artificial ECM microenvironments that are favorable for DT-MSC regeneration activities. The combination of DT-MSCs with biomaterials is one of the key procedures for developing autologous therapeutics in the regeneration of dental and nondental tissues. Next, the relevant aspects of biomaterials will be reviewed, as well as the most important cellular and molecular mechanisms involved in the regenerative process of stem cells of dental origin.

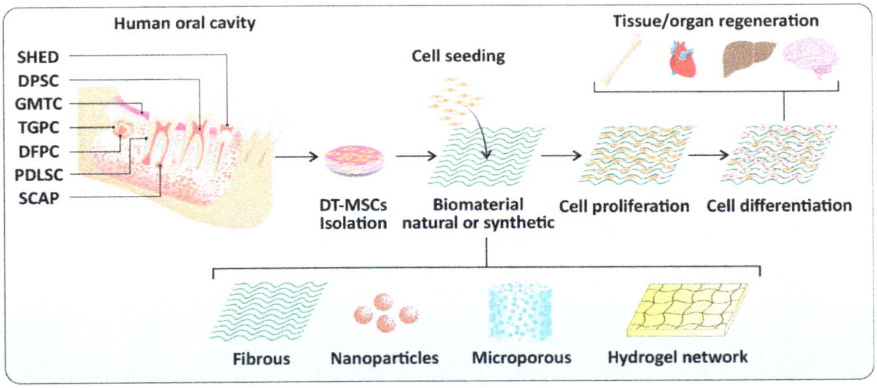


**Figure 1.** Human dental stem cells can be harvested from different tissues, including stem cells from human exfoliated deciduous teeth (SHEDs), dental pulp stem cells (DPSCs), gingival-derived mesenchymal stem cells (GMSCs), tooth germ progenitor cells (TGPCs), dental follicle progenitor cells (DFPCs), periodontal ligament stem cells (PDLSCs), stem cells from the apical papilla (SCAPs). Seeding dental stem cells on different biomaterials, differentiation, and potential clinical application for the regeneration of different tissues.

## 3. Biomaterials

Biomaterials are natural, synthetic, or semisynthetic substances designed to be implanted into biological environments [12]. In regenerative medicine, biomaterials are a vehicle for cells, as they provide a structure for their proliferation and secretion activities [13]. Several authors point out specific characteristics that a biomaterial must have for its application in regenerative medicine (Figure 2). Among them are nontoxicity, biocompatibility (ability to interact with the tissues of living beings), and chemical composition (it must mimic the components of the extracellular matrix) to promote a suitable environment for cell growth and differentiation [13–16].

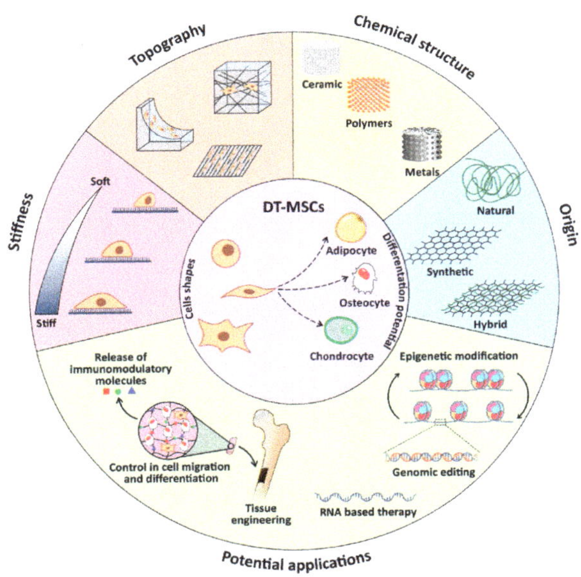


**Figure 2.** Schematic diagram of important features of a biomaterial to guide the fate of dental stem cells.

The interaction between stem cells and the chemical composition of biomaterials are critical factors that influence cell behavior. Biomaterials must be a bioactive matrix that provides the cells with sites of adhesion, growth, and three-dimensional spatial organization [17,18]. There is a great variety of biomaterials reported in the literature, among which are natural or synthetic polymers, extracellular matrix, self-assembly systems, hydrogels, and bioceramics that have been used with DT-MSCs (Table 1) [15,18].

**Table 1.** Relevant experimental findings of the interaction of different biomaterials and DT-MSC.

| Biomaterial | Cells Type | Findings | Reference |
|---|---|---|---|
| 3D-printed hydroxyapatite scaffolds containing peptide hydrogels | DPSCs | (Mice) blood vessel ingrowth, pulp-like tissue formation, and osteodentin deposition, suggesting osteogenic/odontogenic differentiation of hDPSCs | Lambrichts et al. (2017) [19] |
| Chitosan scaffolds with or without arginine-glycine-aspartic acid or fibronectin | DPSCs | Fibronectin-immobilized chitosan scaffolds may serve as suitable three-dimensional substrates for dental pulp stem cell attachment and proliferation | Asghari Sana et al. (2017) [20] |
| Silk fibroin-based 2D films and 3D scaffolds | DPSCs | Good in vitro biocompatibility of silk fibroin-based biomaterials, mainly when 3D scaffolds rather than 2D films are used. | Pecci-Lloret et al. (2017) [21] |
| Collagen and titanium | DPSCs | Compared with human sarcoma osteogenic cell line, DPPSC showed higher initial adhesion levels and similar osteogenic differentiation. These results promote the use of DPPSC as a new pluripotent-like cell model to evaluate the biocompatibility and the differentiation capacity of biomaterials used in bone regeneration | Núñez-Toldrà et al. (2017) [22] |
| Crosslinked type I and type II collagen hydrogels | DPSCs | Cells can potentially migrate from the hydrogels and migrate into the nucleus pulposus tissue | Yao and Flynn (2018) [23] |
| Polycaprolactone cone in an odontoblastic differentiation medium | DPSCs | Cells isolated from both carious and healthy mature teeth were able to colonize and proliferate and could be differentiated into functional odontoblast-like cells. | Louvrier et al. (2018) [24] |
| Commercial dental composite resins | GMSCs | Inflamed GMSCs retain their stem cell properties and could be used as a valuable cell line for testing dental biomaterials | Soancă et al. (2018) [25] |
| Calcium enriched mixture (CEM) cement, Biodentine, mineral trioxide aggregate (MTA), octacalcium phosphate (OCP), and Atlantik | SCAPs | Tested biomaterials could induce odontogenic/osteogenic differentiation in SCAPs. MTA had a more significant potential for induction of differentiation of SCAPs to odontoblast-like cells, while OCP had a higher potential to induce differentiation of SCAPs to osteoblast-like cells | Saberi et al. (2019) [26] |
| gelatin methacrylate (GelMA) hydrogel | BMSC, DPSCs, and SCAP | Among stem cells from different craniofacial regions, BMSCs appear more suitable for engineering mature vascularized networks than DPSCs or SCAPs | Parthiban et al. (2020) [27] |
| Three-dimensional (3D) graphene oxide (GO)/sodium alginate (GOSA) and reduced GOSA (RGOSA) scaffolds | DPSCs | The cytotoxicity of GO-based scaffolds showed that DPSCs could be seeded in serum-free media without cytotoxic effects. This is critical for human translation as cellular transplants are typically serum-free. | Mansouri et al. (2021) [28] |
| NeoMTA Plus, ProRoot MTA and Biodentine | DPSCs | Materials are not cytotoxic and do not induce apoptosis | Birant et al. (2021) [29] |
| Calcium phosphate cement | DPSCs | CPC is promising for dental pulp-capping, base, and liner applications to promote dentin regeneration | Gu et al. (2021) [30] |
| Chitosan/gelatin/ nanohydroxyapatite scaffolds | DPSCs | Scaffolds support the viability and proliferation of DPSCs, and provide a biomimetic microenvironment favoring odontogenic differentiation and in vitro biomineralization without the addition of any inductive factors | Vagropoulou et al. (2021) [31] |
| Granular hydroxyapatite scaffold | SHED and DPSCs | gHA scaffold is an optimal scaffold as it induced osteogenesis in vitro.<br>SHED had the highest osteogenic potential | Hagar et al. (2021) [32] |
| Polylactic acid and hydroxyapatite 3D-printed composite | DPSCs | Bone forming ability of composite in Winstar rats' bone defects. Additionally, inflammatory reaction during biodegradation. | Gendviliene et al. (2021) [33] |

**Table 1.** *Cont.*

| Biomaterial | Cells Type | Findings | Reference |
| --- | --- | --- | --- |
| Nanohydroxyapatite/ collagen/poly(l-lactide) | SCAPs | These cells are alternative sources for alveolar bone engineering in regenerative medicine (mice). | Ling-Ling et al. (2021) [34] |
| Core/shell poly (methyl methacrylate) (PMMA)/ silk fibroin (SF) fibers | DPSCs | Composite mats composed of core/shell PMMA/SF fibers could be considered a promising candidate for tissue engineering applications and drug delivery strategies | Atila et al. (2022) [35] |
| Chitosan and covalent tetra-armed poly (ethylene glycol) composite encapsulating acetylsalicylic acid (ASA) | PLSCs | The capacity of PDLSCs and ASA-laden CG to enhance new bone regeneration in situ using a mouse calvarial bone defect model. | Zhang et al. (2022) [36] |

Table 1. Relevant findings of the biomaterial/oral cavity SCs interaction reported in the literature.

### 3.1. Natural Biomaterials

Research carried out in the field of biomaterials using cells of dental origin has increased in recent years. Most studies have focused on explaining the cellular mechanisms that lead to the formation of dental structures (for example, dentin, the periodontal ligament, dental pulp, or enamel), which has contributed to this knowledge, leading to the design of novel biomaterials destined to stimulate regeneration in dental and nondental tissues.

Natural biomaterials are constituents of the ECM or represent macromolecular properties that are similar to the ECM. These can be classified into two main categories, protein-based and natural biomaterials based on polysaccharides. Collagen, fibrin, and elastin are the most explored natural protein-based biomaterials [13,37]. Polysaccharide-based biomaterials are natural polymers consisting of sugar monomers. Chitosan, alginate, glycosaminoglycans (GAGs), and hyaluronic acid are examples [38]. Most natural biomaterials present favorable biocompatibility and immunogenicity and low cost [39], making them attractive for their application in tissue engineering in the field of endodontics. One of the most widely studied biomaterials in the dental field is collagen due to its role in ECM in dental pulp and dentin, its function as a natural hemostatic agent [40], its hydrophilicity, biocompatibility, biodegradability, and its low immunogenicity and cytotoxicity [41]. In this sense, biomaterials based on type I collagen (Col-I) have been developed to generate tissues, such as dental pulp [42], dentin [43], and guided bone regeneration treatments [44]. This shows that collagen-based biomaterials are an important element in dental research; however, the difficulties encountered in regenerative endodontics of root canals indicate irregular biodegradation and the generation of connective tissue instead of dentin in vivo. Another widely investigated polysaccharide is chitosan (CHS), which is purified mainly from chitin. Chemically, CHS is a polymeric material comprised of N-acetylglucosamine and glucosamine copolymer units [45]. CHS has also been reported to be a direct pulp cap with the purpose of initiating the formation of reparative dentin to help protect the pulp, favoring the differentiation of DPSCs into odontoblast-like cells [46]. The use of CHS in conjunction with DPSCs has been studied to induce bone regeneration and for the treatment of chronic periodontitis. [47]. For example, Kamal and Khalil (2018) [48] used CHS with DPSCs to evaluate the potential for bone formation around dental implants. They noted that this method helped bone maturation around the implant, suggesting its potential use in bone regeneration [48].

Fibrin is a fibrillar biopolymer and the main component of the blood coagulation matrix. This protein has been reported as a vehicle for the release of dental stem cells since it facilitates their union, growth, and differentiation [49,50]. Its advantages include excellent biocompatibility, bioresorbability, hemostatic properties, nontoxicity of degradation products, and the short-term generation of an ECM produced by stem cells incorporated into the biomaterial. Although there is increasing development of biomaterials with natural polymers due to their similarity with ECM, the biochemical characteristics of fibrin make it suitable as a platform for autologous cell release. For a better understanding of the composition, structure, biochemical characteristics and mechanical properties of fibrin, the reader is referred to excellent reviews about this biomaterial [51–53]. One of the interesting features of fibrin is that it can form a three-dimensional network of elastic fibers which can promote biological interactions during the regeneration of target tissues. [49]. To date, two types of fibrin-based products have been used: glue and hydrogels. The first type is obtained from human plasma (homologous or autologous) as a source of fibrinogen and functions as a bioadhesive for hemostasis in surgical procedures (i.e., allogeneic plasma commercial Tissucol/Tisseel, Beriplast, and Quixil), while hydrogels are made from allogeneic fibrinogen and purified thrombin. One advantage of hydrogels is that they can be biofunctionalized to increase the cellular response through the incorporation of cell binding sequences, such as arginine–glycine–aspartic acid (RGD), for a better function as a cell vehicle [50–54]. The use of fibrin gel as a vehicle for carrying cells in a three-dimensional scaffold has been extensively investigated for the regeneration of bone tissue. In dental tissues, numerous approaches have been developed to achieve regeneration, for example, fibrin hydrogels or modified fibrin hydrogels (polyethylene glycol, chitosan, collagen) for dental pulp regeneration [18,50,55]. However, these approaches are limited because a specific spatial geometry is not achieved for each patient, nor is there control of the union, proliferation, and migration of cells within the structure. Three-dimensional (3D) bioprinting is now the most attractive approach for its application in regenerative medicine in dental and nondental tissues. This is a manufacturing technique that allows stem cells to be precisely placed within the biomaterial that acts as a temporary ECM [56,57]. With this technology, it has been possible to design a fibrin-based bio-ink with DPSCs to form an autologous dentin-pulp complex [58] or in bone regeneration [59].

### 3.2. Synthetic Biomaterials

Biomaterials of synthetic origin are used due to the growing necessity of specific characteristics of scaffolds for regenerative medicine due to the limitations of the natural biomaterials that need to be modified, the limited mechanical strength, and the difficulty of obtaining 3D scaffolds required for tissue engineering, providing cells with the necessary environment to proliferate and differentiate into a lineage-specific manner [60]. Biomaterials of synthetic origin have been widely used for the last 100 years, considering that inert materials (i.e., metal alloys) were the first to be implanted in the human body for the reconstruction of affected tissues and/or organs [61]. Currently, a range of materials are used for regenerative medicine, primarily for their characteristics, such as biocompatibility, physicochemistry, mechanical behavior, biodegradability, and modulation of cell response, among others. A variety of engineered synthetic biomaterials that are chemically and physically designed to fulfill the cellular specific needs of these critical parameters have been reported in the literature [62]. Some synthetic biomaterials, such as metallic alloys, ceramics, polymers, and hydrogels, are reported to be promotors of stem cell differentiation [63].

Regarding synthetic metal biomaterials, inert titanium alloys are commonly used in dentistry for bone tissue engineering due to their ability to induce osteogenic differentiation of dental stem cells; as reported in the literature, composite biomaterials with a polymeric matrix of polycaprolactone diol-based segmented polyurethanes and titanium particles enhance the viability of pulp stem cells and osteoblasts, as it increases with the amount of titanium in composites [64]. According to Hanafy, mineral trioxide aggregates and nanohydroxyapatite could enhance the odontogenic differentiation of human dental pulp stem cells, as assessed by tracing genes characteristic of different stages of odontoblasts via qRT–PCR and calcific nodule formation evaluated by Alizarin red staining [65].

Ceramics, as bioactive glass, promote odontogenic differentiation of DPSCs; as reported by Ahn et al. (2020) [66] in their study, composites of mesoporous bioactive glass nanoparticles (MBNs) and graphene oxide (GO) were prepared and analyzed, and they concluded that MBN/GO promoted the proliferation and odontogenic differentiation of DPSCs [66]. In another study, composites of nano bioactive glass synthesized by the sol-gel method ($58SiO_2$:$40CaO$:$5P_2O_5$) and Biodentine (Septodont, Saint Maur des Fosses, France) were prepared and tested, and they found cell adhesion and proliferation on nBG/BD nanocomposites and increased odontogenic differentiation of DPSCs, as measured by alkaline phosphatase activity after 7 and 14 days of exposure [67].

Polymers and composites of polymeric matrices are biomaterials that have been the focus of increased interest in recent years due to their capability for being designed, modified, and reinforced according to the requirements for an extensive range of therapeutic and regenerative purposes. Polymers for regenerative medicine include polyethylene glycol (PEG), polylactic acid (PLA), poly(lactic-co-glycolic acid) (PLGA), polyvinyl alcohol (PVA), and polycaprolactone (PCL) [13]. A study by Wang concluded that poly(L-lactic acid) (PLLA), with recombinant human bone morphogenetic protein 2 (BMP-2), produced odontogenic differentiation of SCAP, leading to in vivo dentin regeneration [68]. Another study with PCL scaffolds reported attachment, growth, and proliferation of human SCAPs with calcification nodules detected [69]. Alipour et al. (2019) [70] reported that PCL-PEG-PCL/zeolite nanofibrous scaffolds produced adhesion and proliferation of DPSCs and their osteo/odontogenic differentiation and concluded that zeolite nanoparticles on PCL-PEG-PCL scaffolds could have a crucial role in osteoblastic physiology [70]. One of the essential aspects of polymers is their degradability/biodegradability, which can be modulated according to the needs of therapeutics, and even synthetic polymers can be designed to carry and deliver drugs to a specific target by their degradation process [63].

Hydrogels are derived from polymers, and they are a three-dimensional, hydrophilic polymer or copolymer network that can soak up large amounts of water or biological fluids due to their affinity to absorb water, which is attributed to the presence of hydrophilic groups; they are commonly temperature-sensitive biomaterials [62]. Luo et al. (2021) [71] reported that a methacryloyl gelatin (GelMA) hydrogel and human basic fibroblast growth factor seeded with DPSCs wrapped by a cellulose/soy protein isolate composite membrane was proven to be a promising tissue engineering approach to treat significant gap defects in peripheral nerve injuries [71]. Synthetic hydrogels appear to be promising for tissue engineering since in vivo-forming hydrogels can be prepared as a solution and can easily incorporate cells and growth factors to be injected to fill the shape of the in vivo cavity via minimally invasive procedures, as described by Jang et al. (2016) [72] who obtained an in vivo forming solution of methoxy polyethylene glycol-b-poly($\varepsilon$-caprolactone), DPSCs, and osteogenic factors. They concluded that DPSCs embedded in an in vivo-forming hydrogel may provide benefits as a noninvasive formulation for bone tissue engineering applications [72].

## 4. Dental Stem Cells and Biomaterial Interactions

Biomaterials (natural or synthetic) are essential components in the construction of scaffolds, providing an artificial three-dimensional environment to regulate the behavior of stem cells. In addition, they allow for evaluating the effect of the physical environment in the cells [73]. An important aspect to consider is the biomaterial–cell interaction since they affect the adhesion, viability, proliferation, matrix production, and differentiation of stem cells [74]. Knowledge of how the interaction between cells and biomaterials is carried out is essential for achieving effective repair in regenerative medicine. Mechanobiology is an interdisciplinary field that investigates the mechanisms by which stem cells can sense (mechanosensing) and respond (mechanotransduction) to changes in their environment [75]. A comprehensive review of the mechanobiology in stem cells in response to mechanical signals can be reviewed in Argentati et al. (2019) [76]. In this section, we describe the mechano-molecular players recruited and interconnected with each other during the biomaterial–DT-MSCs interaction and their impact on cell proliferation and differentiation.

### 4.1. Mechasensors in Dental Stem Cells

Currently, the design of biomaterials with specific characteristics is a novel approach for evaluating the effect of chemical, physical or topographic changes in stem cells during their proliferation and differentiation under in vitro conditions. The reason for this is that stem cells are very sensitive to forces and can convert mechanical stimuli into a chemical response [77]. There is much evidence that DPSCs are mechanosensitive cells and capable of recognizing physical and mechanical signals during their differentiation process. In this context, the participation of mechanosensors, such as mechanosensitive ion channels, cytoskeleton proteins, and assembly proteins, has been recognized in DPSCs.

Mechanosensitive ion channels (MICs) are receptors that convert extracellular mechanical force into intracellular biochemical information. However, how do the channels mediate these sensations and turn them into a stimulus? Does this occur through direct or indirect activation of the channel? To answer this question, Xiao et al. (2016) [78] proposed two scenarios. The first is that mechanical force is released into the channel by lipid bilayer tension, generating a hydrophobic mismatch that helps the channel open. In the second, the participation of accessory proteins (for example, those of the cytoskeleton or the components of the ECM) has been proposed, and mechanical stress transmitted by the cytoskeleton causes $Ca^{2+}$ release from the endoplasmic reticulum via the inositol trisphosphate receptor ($IP_3R$) [78]. There are reports of MICs that play an important role in the transduction of mechanical forces in the activation of signaling pathways involved in cell proliferation and differentiation in stem cells. In this context, two MICs have been recognized in DPSCs: Piezo proteins and members of the transient receptor potential (TRP) channel family.

The Piezo channel is a three-bladed helix-shaped trimeric complex that includes two subtypes: Piezo1 and Piezo2 [79]. In stem cells, these proteins play an important role in shear stress and traction signals during their proliferation [80–82]. Several researchers agree that when the Piezo protein is activated, there is an influx of $Ca^{2+}$ [65]. However, there is still controversy about whether the integrity of the cytoskeleton is affected by the activity of the channel in response to mechanical stimuli. The role of Piezo proteins in DPSCs has been studied through adjuvant therapies for the repair of dental tissues. An example of this is the use of low-intensity pulsed ultrasound (LIPUS) recognition therapy employed in dental tissue repair [64]. In cells, LIPUS acts as a mechanobiological stimulus that activates various signaling pathways that regulate cell proliferation and differentiation. For example, Jin et al. (2015) [83] investigated the presence of Piezo1 and Piezo2 in DPSCs and PDLSCs and their involvement in LIPUS-associated proliferation and MAPK signaling. The authors demonstrated that DPSC proliferation was associated with LIPUS stimulation by activating MAPK signaling, while in PLSCs, it could occur through another mechanism [83]. Another study by Mousawi et al. (2020) [84] examined the role of Piezo1 in ATP release in DPSCs migration in vitro. The authors reported that the activation of Piezo1 induces the release of ATP, modulating the activity of P2 receptors and inducing the activation of proline-rich tyrosine kinase 2 (PYK2) and MEK/ERK. Another ionic channel broadly expressed in DPSCs is the transient receptor potential (TRP) channel, including transient receptor potential melastatin types 4 and 7 (TRPM4 and TRPM7, respectively) [85–87].

TRPM controls $Ca^{2+}$ signals and is sensitive to mechanical stimuli, such as patch-clamp pipette suction and patch-clamp pipette stretching. Xiao et al. (2015) [88] reported that, in human bone marrow MSCs subjected to stretching or suction, TRPM7 activation appears to be independent of actin polymerization disruption since suction-induced TRPM7 activation was not abolished [88]. In DPSCs, research has also focused on TRPM7 and osteogenesis. For example, Cui et al. (2013) [87] reported that TRPM7 participates in the pulp-repair process through the regulation of proliferation, migration, and osteogenic differentiation of DPSCs, while TRPM4 is necessary for adipogenesis in stem cells of DFSCs in rats [87]. The authors agree that the activation of TRPM gives rise to the release of $Ca^{2+}$ mediated by $IP_3$ type 2 ($IP_3R2$) from the endoplasmic reticulum, amplifying $Ca^{2+}$ signaling and inducing osteogenesis through the activation of the transcription factor NFATc1 [88–90]. Taking these results together, the data suggest that MICs are important molecular sensors. However, studies have only focused on DPSCs and osteogenesis. It would be interesting to see if a similar regulatory pathway is conserved in other types of DT-MSCs.

Other important mechanosensors are macromolecular complexes that include cytoskeletal proteins (microtubules, f-actin microfilaments, intermediate filaments, and actin-linking proteins), nucleoskeletal-related proteins (SUN1, SUN2, lamins), adherens junctions (cadherins, α-catenin, β-catenin), focal adhesion proteins (vinculin), integrins, and ECM-related proteins (fibronectin) [57,58]. These mechanosensors turn on the rearrangement of molecular components by activating several intracellular signaling pathways that are involved in growth, cell proliferation, and the regulation of gene expression (Figure 3).

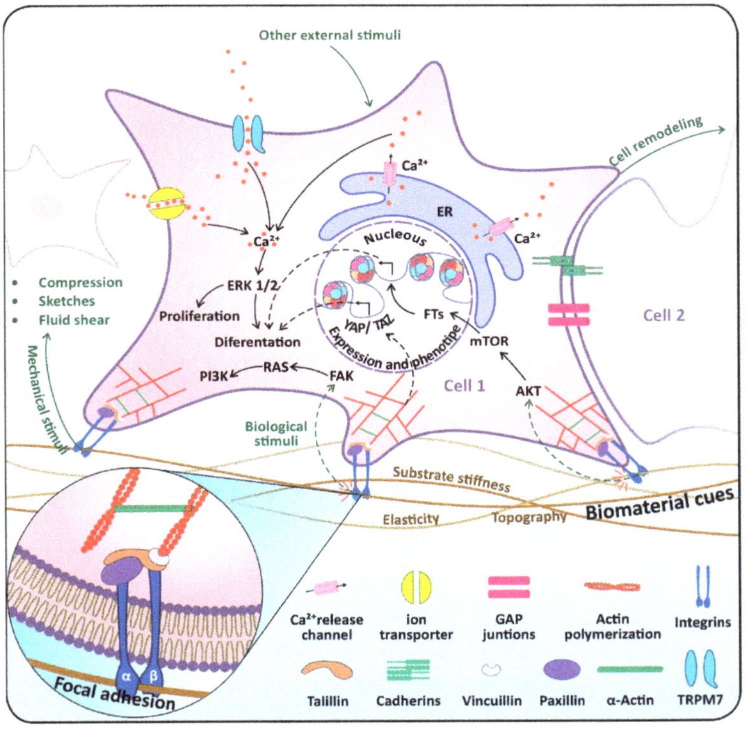


**Figure 3.** Schematic diagram for signals and signaling pathways in DT-MSCs during their interaction with biomaterials. DT-MSCs are an entity interconnected by multiple molecular components during their interaction with biomaterials. Mechanical stimulus or signals from the biomaterials are perceived in the cell membrane, which activates various proteins such as Piezo channel or TRPM, that trigger the influx or release of $Ca^{2+}$ which have strong connection with cell signaling involved in the proliferation and differentiation. Therefore, cell–cell (cadherins and gap junction) and cell–biomaterial communication is facilitated by remodeling the cytoskeleton (actin) and favoring focal adhesion sites (FAK) that activate signaling pathways (PI3K, AKT, mTOR, ERK, YAP/TAZ) that regulate the behavior of stem cells, improving their cellular response (proliferation or differentiation) in the presence of biomaterials. ER: endoplasmic reticulum; PI3K: Phosphoinositide 3-kinases, ERK: extracellular signal-regulated kinase; FAK: focal adhesion kinase; FT: transcription factor; YAP: Yes-associated protein; TAZ: Transcriptional coactivator with PDZ-binding motif; AKT: Ser/Thr protein kinase; RAS: GTPases protein.

The cytoskeleton plays important roles in cell morphology, adhesion, growth, and signaling [91]. In this context, stem cells alter their cytoskeleton in response to mechanical forces that cause cell reorganization through actin polymerization and microtubule assembly or by disassembling cytoskeletal components and their ECM junctions [75]. Topography of biomaterials is a promising approach to guide cytoskeleton behavior and differentiation in stem cells. Several works have focused on analyzing how the topographic signals (macro, micro, or nanoscale) of biomaterials affect the behavior of components of the cytoskeleton in DT-MSCs. For example, Du et al. (2019) [92] determined that the topographic signals of a poly(lactic-co-glycolic acid) bilayer (PLGA) change F-actin alignment and DPSCs morphology by modulating Yes-associated protein (YAP) signaling to control osteogenic differentiation/odontogenicity [92]. Collart-Dutilleul et al. (2014) [93] studied the influence of the micropore size of a nanostructured silicon biomaterial on DPSCs adhesion through the formation of lamellipodia (dense network of actin filaments) and filopodia. They concluded that the porosity of the biomaterial promotes the formation of filopodia and increases cell migration [93]. In another study, Conserva et al. (2018) [94] studied the growth of DPSCs by laser ablation laser-microgrooved (8-µm-sized microgrooves or microchannels) surfaces. Their results showed that DPSCs proliferated following the direction of the microgrooves, which could have significant implications for bone regeneration [94]. Additionally, Bachhuka et al. (2017) [95] reported that DPSCs proliferated faster where there was a greater density of nanotopography favoring osteogenic differentiation [95]. Marconi et al. (2021) [96] investigated the in vitro effects of titanium implants on PDLSC culture. The authors reported that the topography of the titanium implant surface enhances the release of ECM components in PDLSCs, which has an impact on the process of implant osseointegration [96]. Other authors, such as Hasturk et al. (2019) [97], proposed a novel biomaterial with 4- and 8-µm square prism micropillars on a poly(methyl methacrylate) surface as an alternative to enhance the osteogenesis of DPSCs. Their results showed that the interpillar spaces generated a high degree of tension in the cytoskeleton and induced differentiation toward the bone lineage [97]. These studies showed that the interaction between biomaterials and the cytoskeleton is important during the osteogenic differentiation response in DT-MSCs; however, there is still a long way to go to understand the mechanisms involved in biomaterial–DT-MSC interactions in other differentiation processes.

The ECM surrounding cells exerts a mechanical influence that determines phenotype, motility, and matrix production. This allows tissues to function correctly by modulating stem cell adhesion, proliferation, migration, and differentiation [73,75]. During their growth, stem cells secrete structural components of the extracellular matrix (collagen, elastin, laminin, fibronectin, hyaluronic acid, chondroitin sulfate, and syndecans) that function as mediators between the cells and the ECM. One of the strategies for the study of ECM mechanosensors in DPSCs and their physical environment is the development of scaffolds with components of the ECM. For example, Ravindran et al. (2014) [98] generated a scaffold ECM from dental pulp to induce odontogenic differentiation in DPSCs, PDLSCs, and HMSCs as a strategy for the treatment of dental caries [98]. Another example is the work of Paduado et al. (2016) [99], who demonstrated that a hydrogel scaffold derived from decellularized and demineralized bovine bone (bECM) favors the odontogenic differentiation of DPSCs and could be applied for the regeneration treatment of dentin and pulp. Currently, research groups focus on the search for alternative sources of ECM substrates of human origin, such as for human cell culture, due to the limitations represented using commercial biomaterials that are derived from animal sources or cancer lines (for example, Matrigel, which is derived from mouse sarcoma) for clinical application [99]. In this context, a novel study was reported by Heng et al. (2016) [100], who used decellularized matrix (DECM) from SHED stem cells and PLSCs as a substrate for ex vivo culture of DPSCs. Their results showed that DECM of dental cells enhanced DPSCs adhesion, which correlated with increased expression of vinculin, a key focal adhesion protein [100].

Another approach that has been addressed is the analysis of adhesion proteins, such as integrins. Integrins are heterodimeric receptors composed of alpha and beta subunits linked by noncovalent bonds. The combination of these subunits results in various receptors that exhibit preferential affinity for specific ECM molecules. For example, $\alpha 2\beta 1$ integrin recognizes the Asp-Gly-Glu-Ala amino acid sequence in collagen, while $\alpha5\beta1$ recognizes the RGD sequence in fibronectin and $\alpha v\beta3$ in vitronectin [101]. The adhesion process in animal cells is mediated by integrins, which generate supramolecular protein complexes with cytoskeletal proteins called focal contacts (FAs) (Figure 3). FAs are networks of proteins that provide structural integrity to cells and constitute a dynamic bridge between the ECM and actin of the cytoskeleton (Figure 3). In the case of stem cells, this process is essential for tissue integration of the biomaterial. In this context, Lee et al. (2014) [102] studied the interaction between PDLSCs and a mussel-inspired polydopamine (PDA) adhesive biomaterial through the expression of integrins $\alpha5$ and $\beta1$. The authors demonstrated that integrin–PI3K linkages mediate cell adhesion and regulate osteogenic differentiation of PDLSCs [102]. Likewise, using silica-based materials, Hung and colleagues [103] investigated the role of $\alpha v$ integrin in the odontogenic differentiation of DPSCs. They reported that the silicon-containing biomaterial favored cell adhesion through increased fibronectin adsorption and integrin expression [103]. Liu et al. (2013) [104] analyzed the effect of crystal alignment (ordered/disorganized) of apatite (an enamel-like substrate) on the expression of adhesion-related genes to produce an enamel/dentin superstructure in vitro. The authors reported that the ordered alignment of apatite provided a favorable environment for DPSCs adhesion, which was linked to the upregulated expression of integrins alpha 7 and 8 (ITGA 7 and 8), integrin beta 3 and 4 (ITGB3 and 4), vitronectin receptor-integrin alpha V (ITGAV), and the key adhesion protein fibronectin 1 (FN1) [104].

### 4.2. Mechanotransduction Pathways in Dental Stem Cells

As mentioned in the previous section, the attachment of cells to biomaterial substrates is essential to establishing communication between cells and the ECM microenvironment. In this way, the activated biochemical signals can modulate specific signaling pathways to regulate cell activity in processes, such as adhesion, proliferation, and differentiation. This section will address current studies on the signaling pathways involved in the differentiation process in biomaterials with DPSCs.

Biomaterials act as adhesion substrates that send mechanical signals to cells, influencing the differentiation of DT-MSCs. Stem cell differentiation during biomaterial interactions involves many signaling pathways (Figure 3). For example, Yun et al. (2015) [105] examined with DPSCs a scaffold of magnetite and polycaprolactone nanoparticles and the signaling pathways involved in the mechanisms of adhesion, migration, and odontogenic differentiation. Their results demonstrated that integrin (subunits $\alpha1$, $\alpha2$, $\beta1$, and $\beta3$) signaling with activation of FAK/MAPK and NF-$\kappa$B by the scaffold is involved in cellular events in DPSCs [105]. Another study by Lee et al. (2014) [102] evaluated the osteoinductive effect of a bioadhesive on PDLSCs for use as a dental implant. They reported that the biomaterial stimulated osteogenic differentiation of PDLSCs through activation of $\alpha5/\beta1$ integrin-PI3K signaling [102]. Additionally, Zhang et al. (2012) [106] investigated whether MAPK signaling pathways are a mediator in odontogenic differentiation of DPSCs cultured on five different biomaterials. Their results showed enhanced odontogenic differentiation and dentin-like tissue formation in natural biomaterials derived from mineralized tissue (dentin matrix and bovine bone ceramic) through the phosphorylation of ERK1/2 and p38 [106]. Another study by Guo et al. in 2018 [107] employed a pharmacological perturbation approach to identify which signaling pathways were involved in the differentiation and mineralization of DPSCs cultured on a fluorapatite-modified polycaprolactone nanofiber biomaterial. The authors reported that the Hedgehog, insulin, and Wnt signaling pathways are involved in biomaterial-induced DPSCs differentiation and can activate the osteogenesis process through autophagic modulation [107].

There are currently novel biomaterial designs in the literature that have been used to investigate the signaling pathways involved during DPSCs differentiation. The design of nanoarrays as therapeutic platforms has aroused particular interest because dental stem cells can recognize nanofibrous topology and respond to biochemical signals from their environment. In this context, Lim et al. (2016) [108] designed in vitro nanofiber arrays containing bioactive glass nanoparticles that release dexamethasone, a signaling molecule of odontogenesis. The authors reported that the integrin pathway ($\alpha 2$, $\alpha 5$, $\beta 1$), bone morphogenetic protein, and mTOR signaling pathways are possible mechanisms involved in the stimulation of odontogenesis. Other signaling pathways have also been reported in cell differentiation events in three-dimensional nanomaterials [108]. For example, Zhou et al. (2018) [109] designed a biomaterial containing a tetrahedral DNA nanostructure (TDN) self-assembled by four specific single-stranded DNAs (ssDNAs) by complementary base pairing. The authors reported that TDN stimulated the osteogenic differentiation of PDLSCs by activating the Wnt/β-catenin pathway, while in DPSCs, TDN increased the expression of HES1, HEY1, and NOTCH1, which are crucial factors of the Notch pathway [109]. These results indicate that although the cells have the same dental origin, their biochemical response can be different for the same biomaterial, which will be interesting to study in the future to develop methodologies for the regeneration of dental and nondental tissues.

One approach that has been addressed is to study signaling events in the epigenome, for which signals from biomaterials, such as topography, elasticity, material chemistry, and mechanical forces/stimulus, influence the state of the epigenome [110]. The term epigenetics refers to heritable changes in gene expression patterns that do not involve alterations in the DNA sequence [111]. It will be interesting to determine how biomaterial signals act by modulating epigenome mechanisms, including chromatin remodeling, DNA methylation, and posttranslational modifications at the amino-terminal tails of nucleosome histones. To date, there are few reports that have investigated how biomaterials with different physical and chemical characteristics alter the epigenome in stem cells [63,111]. However, we have not been able to find reports focused on DT-MSCs.

## 5. Conclusions

Although current results are promising, there are still many unsolved questions regarding the mechanical regulation of stem cell activities, and the study of MSCs during these processes is just beginning. In the coming years, the development and application of new techniques in live imaging, tissue culture, and real-time mechanical stimulation delivery will significantly increase our current knowledge about mechanobiology, as well as stem cell biology. If well the studies discussed here highlight the players involved in the response and processes of DT-MSCs during their interaction with biomaterials, much remains to be investigated. In this scenario, we consider it essential to tackle the following aspects:

- Design and develop of smart biomaterials that favor the proliferation and differentiation of DT-MSCs on a large scale.
- Integrate multi-omic tools would allow a global perspective of the interactions between cells and biomaterials at the genomic, proteomic, and metabolomic levels.
- Delivery into the mechanogenomic field to facilitate the design of highly functionalized biomaterials and the epigenetic manipulation that can be performed to control the fate of DT-MSCs for their application in regenerative medicine.

**Author Contributions:** Conceptualization, B.A.R.-J.; writing—original draft preparation, F.J.A.-A. and F.J.A.-P., writing—reviewed editing, B.A.R.-J., G.C.-G. and D.A.-P., technical assistance R.R.-H. and G.I.N.-C. All authors have read and agreed to the published version of the manuscript.

**Funding:** This research received no external funding.

**Institutional Review Board Statement:** Not applicable.

**Informed Consent Statement:** Not applicable.

**Data Availability Statement:** Not applicable.

**Acknowledgments:** This work was supported by Facultad de Ingeniería Química and Facultad de Odontología from Universidad Autónoma de Yucatán. The authors also acknowledge the support of the Seeding Labs program. The authors would like to thank Julio Montero del Toro for the design of the images.

**Conflicts of Interest:** The authors declare no conflict of interest.

## References

1. Rodas-Junco, B.A.; Canul-Chan, M.; Rojas-Herrera, R.A.; De-la-Peña, C.; Nic-Can, G.I. Stem cells from dental pulp: What epigenetics can do with your tooth. *Front. Physiol.* **2017**, *8*, 999. [CrossRef] [PubMed]
2. Zadpoor, A.A. Meta-biomaterials. *Biomater. Sci.* **2020**, *8*, 18–38. [CrossRef] [PubMed]
3. Granz, C.L.; Gorji, A. Dental stem cells: The role of biomaterials and scaffolds in developing novel therapeutic strategies. *World J. Stem Cells* **2020**, *12*, 897. [CrossRef] [PubMed]
4. Zakrzewski, W.; Dobrzyński, M.; Szymonowicz, M.; Rybak, Z. Stem cells: Past, present, and future. *Stem Cell Res. Ther.* **2019**, *10*, 68. [CrossRef] [PubMed]
5. Worku, M.G. Pluripotent and multipotent stem cells and current therapeutic applications. *Stem Cells Cloning Adv. Appl.* **2021**, *14*, 3. [CrossRef]
6. Sharpe, P.T. Dental mesenchymal stem cells. *Development* **2016**, *143*, 2273–2280. [CrossRef]
7. Hussein, A.M.; Darwish, Z.E.; Raslan, H.S.; Attia, M.A.; Abdel-Hamid, H.M. Dental stem cells (concepts and applications). *Alex. Dent. J.* **2021**, *46*, 66–71. [CrossRef]
8. Rodríguez-Lozano, F.J.; Bueno, C.; Insausti, C.L.; Meseguer, L.; Ramirez, M.C.; Blanquer, M.; Marin, N.; Martínez, S.; Moraleda, J.M. Mesenchymal stem cells derived from dental tissues. *Int. Endod. J.* **2011**, *44*, 800–806. [CrossRef]
9. Lan, X.; Sun, Z.; Chu, C.; Boltze, J.; Li, S. Dental pulp stem cells: An attractive alternative for cell therapy in ischemic stroke. *Front. Neurol.* **2019**, *10*, 824. [CrossRef]
10. Egusa, H.; Sonoyama, W.; Nishimura, M.; Atsuta, I.; Akiyama, K. Stem cells in dentistry–part I: Stem cell sources. *J. Prosthodont. Res.* **2012**, *56*, 151–165. [CrossRef]
11. Mercado-Rubio, M.D.; Pérez-Argueta, E.; Zepeda-Pedreguera, A.; Aguilar-Ayala, F.J.; Peñaloza-Cuevas, R.; Kú-González, A.; Rojas-Herrera, R.A.; Rodas-Junco, B.A.; Nic-Can, G.I. Similar Features, Different Behaviors: A Comparative In Vitro Study of the Adipogenic Potential of Stem Cells from Human Follicle, Dental Pulp, and Periodontal Ligament. *J. Pers. Med.* **2021**, *11*, 738. [CrossRef] [PubMed]
12. Chan, B.P.; Leong, K.W. Scaffolding in tissue engineering: General approaches and tissue-specific considerations. *Eur. Spine J.* **2008**, *17*, 467–479. [CrossRef] [PubMed]
13. Xu, Y.; Chen, C.; Hellwarth, P.B.; Bao, X. Biomaterials for stem cell engineering and biomanufacturing. *Bioact. Mater.* **2019**, *4*, 366–379. [CrossRef] [PubMed]
14. Baranwal, A.; Kumar, A.; Priyadharshini, A.; Oggu, G.S.; Bhatnagar, I.; Srivastava, A.; Chandra, P. Chitosan: An undisputed bio-fabrication material for tissue engineering and bio-sensing applications. *Int. J. Biol. Macromol.* **2018**, *110*, 110–123. [CrossRef] [PubMed]
15. Vinatier, C.; Guicheux, J. Cartilage tissue engineering: From biomaterials and stem cells to osteoarthritis treatments. *Ann. Phys. Rehabil. Med.* **2016**, *59*, 139–144. [CrossRef]
16. Anitua, E.; Troya, M.; Zalduendo, M. Progress in the use of dental pulp stem cells in regenerative medicine. *Cytotherapy* **2018**, *20*, 479–498. [CrossRef]
17. Martino, S.; D'Angelo, F.; Armentano, I.; Kenny, J.M.; Orlacchio, A. Stem cell-biomaterial interactions for regenerative medicine. *Biotechnol. Adv.* **2012**, *30*, 338–351. [CrossRef]
18. Galler, K.M.; Cavender, A.C.; Koeklue, U.; Suggs, L.J.; Schmalz, G.; D'Souza, R.N. Bioengineering of dental stem cells in a PEGylated fibrin gel. *Regen. Med.* **2011**, *6*, 191–200. [CrossRef]
19. Lambrichts, I.; Driesen, R.B.; Dillen, Y.; Gervois, P.; Ratajczak, J.; Vangansewinkel, T.; Wolfs, E.; Bronckaers, A.; Hilkens, P. Dental Pulp Stem Cells: Their Potential in Reinnervation and Angiogenesis by Using Scaffolds. *J. Endod.* **2017**, *43*, S12–S16. [CrossRef]
20. Asghari Sana, F.; Çapkın Yurtsever, M.; Kaynak Bayrak, G.; Tunçay, E.Ö.; Kiremitçi, A.S.; Gümüşderelioğlu, M. Spreading, proliferation and differentiation of human dental pulp stem cells on chitosan scaffolds immobilized with RGD or fibronectin. *Cytotechnology* **2017**, *69*, 617–630. [CrossRef]
21. Pecci-Lloret, M.P.; Vera-Sánchez, M.; Aznar-Cervantes, S.; García-Bernal, D.; Sánchez, R.O.; Pecci-Lloret, M.R.; Moraleda, J.M.; Cenis, J.L.; Rodríguez-Lozano, F.J. Analysis of the Adherence of Dental Pulp Stem Cells on Two-Dimensional and Three-Dimensional Silk Fibroin-Based Biomaterials. *J. Craniofac. Surg.* **2017**, *28*, 939–943. [CrossRef] [PubMed]
22. Núñez-Toldrà, R.; Martínez-Sarrà, E.; Gil-Recio, C.; Carrasco, M.Á.; Al Madhoun, A.; Montori, S.; Atari, M. Dental pulp pluripotent-like stem cells (DPPSC), a new stem cell population with chromosomal stability and osteogenic capacity for biomaterials evaluation. *BMC Cell Biol.* **2017**, *18*, 21. [CrossRef] [PubMed]
23. Yao, L.; Flynn, N. Dental pulp stem cell-derived chondrogenic cells demonstrate differential cell motility in type I and type II collagen hydrogels. *Spine J.* **2018**, *18*, 1070–1080. [CrossRef] [PubMed]

24. Louvrier, A.; Euvrard, E.; Nicod, L.; Rolin, G.; Gindraux, F.; Pazart, L.; Houdayer, C.; Risold, P.Y.; Meyer, F.; Meyer, C. Odontoblastic differentiation of dental pulp stem cells from healthy and carious teeth on an original PCL-based 3D scaffold. *Int. Endod. J.* **2018**, *51* (Suppl. S4), e252–e263. [CrossRef]
25. Soancă, A.; Lupse, M.; Moldovan, M.; Pall, E.; Cenariu, M.; Roman, A.; Tudoran, O.; Surlin, P.; Șorițău, O. Applications of inflammation-derived gingival stem cells for testing the biocompatibility of dental restorative biomaterials. *Ann. Anat. Anat. Anz. Off. Organ Anat. Ges.* **2018**, *218*, 28–39. [CrossRef]
26. Saberi, E.; Farhad-Mollashahi, N.; Sargolzaei Aval, F.; Saberi, M. Proliferation, odontogenic/osteogenic differentiation, and cytokine production by human stem cells of the apical papilla induced by biomaterials: A comparative study. *Clin. Cosmet. Investig. Dent.* **2019**, *11*, 181–193. [CrossRef]
27. Parthiban, S.P.; He, W.; Monteiro, N.; Athirasala, A.; França, C.M.; Bertassoni, L.E. Engineering pericyte-supported microvascular capillaries in cell-laden hydrogels using stem cells from the bone marrow, dental pulp and dental apical papilla. *Sci. Rep.* **2020**, *10*, 21579. [CrossRef]
28. Mansouri, N.; Al-Sarawi, S.; Losic, D.; Mazumdar, J.; Clark, J.; Gronthos, S.; O'Hare Doig, R. Biodegradable and biocompatible graphene-based scaffolds for functional neural tissue engineering: A strategy approach using dental pulp stem cells and biomaterials. *Biotechnol. Bioeng.* **2021**, *118*, 4217–4230. [CrossRef]
29. Birant, S.; Gokalp, M.; Duran, Y.; Koruyucu, M.; Akkoc, T.; Seymen, F. Cytotoxicity of NeoMTA Plus, ProRoot MTA and Biodentine on human dental pulp stem cells. *J. Dent. Sci.* **2021**, *16*, 971–979. [CrossRef]
30. Gu, Y.; Xie, X.; Zhuang, R.; Weir, M.D.; Oates, T.W.; Bai, Y.; Zhao, L.; Xu, H.H.K. A Biphasic Calcium Phosphate Cement Enhances Dentin Regeneration by Dental Pulp Stem Cells and Promotes Macrophages M2 Phenotype In Vitro. *Tissue Eng. Part A* **2021**, *27*, 1113–1127. [CrossRef]
31. Vagropoulou, G.; Trentsiou, M.; Georgopoulou, A.; Papachristou, E.; Prymak, O.; Kritis, A.; Epple, M.; Chatzinikolaidou, M.; Bakopoulou, A.; Koidis, P. Hybrid chitosan/gelatin/nanohydroxyapatite scaffolds promote odontogenic differentiation of dental pulp stem cells and in vitro biomineralization. *Dent. Mater.* **2021**, *37*, e23–e36. [CrossRef] [PubMed]
32. Hagar, M.N.; Yazid, F.; Luchman, N.A.; Ariffin, S.H.Z.; Wahab, R.M.A. Comparative evaluation of osteogenic differentiation potential of stem cells derived from dental pulp and exfoliated deciduous teeth cultured over granular hydroxyapatite based scaffold. *BMC Oral Health* **2021**, *21*, 263. [CrossRef] [PubMed]
33. Gendviliene, I.; Simoliunas, E.; Alksne, M.; Dibart, S.; Jasiuniene, E.; Cicenas, V.; Jacobs, R.; Bukelskiene, V.; Rutkunas, V. Effect of extracellular matrix and dental pulp stem cells on bone regeneration with 3D printed PLA/HA composite scaffolds. *Eur. Cell. Mater.* **2021**, *41*, 204–215. [CrossRef] [PubMed]
34. Zhang, R.; Li, C.-J.; Zhang, S.; Ma, X.-C.; Xiao, R.; Liu, H.-C. Effects of rhBMP-2 on Bone Formation Capacity of Rat Dental Stem/Progenitor Cells from Dental Follicle and Alveolar Bone Marrow. *Stem Cells Dev.* **2021**, *30*, 441–457. [CrossRef]
35. Atila, D.; Hasirci, V.; Tezcaner, A. Coaxial electrospinning of composite mats comprised of core/shell poly(methyl methacrylate)/silk fibroin fibers for tissue engineering applications. *J. Mech. Behav. Biomed. Mater.* **2022**, *128*, 105105. [CrossRef]
36. Zhang, Y.; Dou, X.; Zhang, L.; Wang, H.; Zhang, T.; Bai, R.; Sun, Q.; Wang, X.; Yu, T.; Wu, D.; et al. Facile fabrication of a biocompatible composite gel with sustained release of aspirin for bone regeneration. *Bioact. Mater.* **2022**, *11*, 130–139. [CrossRef]
37. Matichescu, A.; Ardelean, L.C.; Rusu, L.-C.; Craciun, D.; Bratu, E.A.; Babucea, M.; Leretter, M. Advanced biomaterials and techniques for oral tissue engineering and regeneration—A review. *Materials* **2020**, *13*, 5303. [CrossRef]
38. Tahmasebi, E.; Alam, M.; Yazdanian, M.; Tebyanian, H.; Yazdanian, A.; Seifalian, A.; Mosaddad, S.A. Current biocompatible materials in oral regeneration: A comprehensive overview of composite materials. *J. Mater. Res. Technol.* **2020**, *9*, 11731–11755. [CrossRef]
39. Zhang, S.; Yang, X.; Fan, M. BioAggregate and iR oot BP Plus optimize the proliferation and mineralization ability of human dental pulp cells. *Int. Endod. J.* **2013**, *46*, 923–929. [CrossRef]
40. Khan, R.; Khan, M.H. Use of collagen as a biomaterial: An update. *J. Indian Soc. Periodontol.* **2013**, *17*, 539–542. [CrossRef]
41. Lin, K.; Zhang, D.; Macedo, M.H.; Cui, W.; Sarmento, B.; Shen, G. Advanced collagen-based biomaterials for regenerative biomedicine. *Adv. Funct. Mater.* **2019**, *29*, 1804943. [CrossRef]
42. Prescott, R.S.; Alsanea, R.; Fayad, M.I.; Johnson, B.R.; Wenckus, C.S.; Hao, J.; John, A.S.; George, A. In vivo generation of dental pulp-like tissue by using dental pulp stem cells, a collagen scaffold, and dentin matrix protein 1 after subcutaneous transplantation in mice. *J. Endod.* **2008**, *34*, 421–426. [CrossRef] [PubMed]
43. Almushayt, A.; Narayanan, K.; Zaki, A.E.; George, A. Dentin matrix protein 1 induces cytodifferentiation of dental pulp stem cells into odontoblasts. *Gene Ther.* **2006**, *13*, 611–620. [CrossRef] [PubMed]
44. Rico-Llanos, G.A.; Borrego-González, S.; Moncayo-Donoso, M.; Becerra, J.; Visser, R. Collagen type I biomaterials as scaffolds for bone tissue engineering. *Polymers* **2021**, *13*, 599. [CrossRef] [PubMed]
45. Younes, I.; Rinaudo, M. Chitin and chitosan preparation from marine sources. Structure, properties and applications. *Mar. Drugs* **2015**, *13*, 1133–1174. [CrossRef] [PubMed]
46. Zhang, D.; Chen, Q.; Shi, C.; Chen, M.; Ma, K.; Wan, J.; Liu, R. Dealing with the Foreign-Body Response to Implanted Biomaterials: Strategies and Applications of New Materials. *Adv. Funct. Mater.* **2021**, *31*, 2007226. [CrossRef]
47. Husain, S.; Al-Samadani, K.H.; Najeeb, S.; Zafar, M.S.; Khurshid, Z.; Zohaib, S.; Qasim, S.B. Chitosan biomaterials for current and potential dental applications. *Materials* **2017**, *10*, 602. [CrossRef]

48. Kamal, A.; Khalil, E. Assessment of Human Dental Pulp Stem Cells with Chitosan Scaffold Versus Xenografts in Implant Osseointegration. An Experimental Study in a Rabbit Model. *Egypt. Dent. J.* **2018**, *64*, 3499–3509. [CrossRef]
49. Park, C.H.; Woo, K.M. Fibrin-Based Biomaterial Applications in Tissue Engineering and Regenerative Medicine. In *Biomimetic Medical Materials: From Nanotechnology to 3D Bioprinting*; Noh, I., Ed.; Springer: Singapore, 2018; Volume 1064, pp. 253–261. ISBN 978-981-13-0445-3.
50. Ducret, M.; Costantini, A.; Gobert, S.; Farges, J.C.; Bekhouche, M. Fibrin-based scaffolds for dental pulp regeneration: From biology to nanotherapeutics. *Eur. Cells Mater.* **2021**, *41*, 1–14. [CrossRef]
51. Bujoli, B.; Scimeca, J.C.; Verron, E. Fibrin as a multipurpose physiological platform for bone tissue engineering and targeted delivery of bioactive compounds. *Pharmaceutics* **2019**, *11*, 556. [CrossRef]
52. Noori, A.; Ashrafi, S.J.; Vaez-Ghaemi, R.; Hatamian-Zaremi, A.; Webster, T.J. A review of fibrin and fibrin composites for bone tissue engineering. *Int. J. Nanomed.* **2017**, *12*, 4937–4961. [CrossRef] [PubMed]
53. Bolhari, B.; Meraji, N.; Ghorbanzadeh, A.; Sarraf, P.; Moayeri, R. Applications of fibrin-based products in endodontics: A literature review. *Dent. Hypotheses* **2019**, *10*, 85.
54. Ahmed, T.A.E.; Dare, E.V.; Hincke, M. Fibrin: A versatile scaffold for tissue engineering applications. *Tissue Eng. Part B Rev.* **2008**, *14*, 199–215. [CrossRef] [PubMed]
55. Abbass, M.M.S.; El-Rashidy, A.A.; Sadek, K.M.; El Moshy, S.; Radwan, I.A.; Rady, D.; Dörfer, C.E.; Fawzy El-Sayed, K.M. Hydrogels and dentin–pulp complex regeneration: From the benchtop to clinical translation. *Polymers* **2020**, *12*, 2935. [CrossRef] [PubMed]
56. Moore, C.A.; Shah, N.N.; Smith, C.P.; Rameshwar, P. 3D bioprinting and stem cells. In *Somatic Stem Cells*; Springer: Berlin/Heidelberg, Germany, 2018; pp. 93–103.
57. Skeldon, G.; Lucendo-Villarin, B.; Shu, W. Three-dimensional bioprinting of stem-cell derived tissues for human regenerative medicine. *Philos. Trans. R. Soc. B Biol. Sci.* **2018**, *373*, 20170224. [CrossRef]
58. Han, J.; Kim, D.S.; Jang, H.; Kim, H.R.; Kang, H.W. Bioprinting of three-dimensional dentin–pulp complex with local differentiation of human dental pulp stem cells. *J. Tissue Eng.* **2019**, *10*, 2041731419845849. [CrossRef]
59. Enukashvily, N.I.; Dombrovskaya, J.A.; Kotova, A.V.; Semenova, N.; Karabak, I.; Banashkov, R.E.; Baram, D.; Paderina, T.; Bilyk, S.S.; Grimm, W.-D. Fibrin Glue Implants Seeded with Dental Pulp and Periodontal Ligament Stem Cells for the Repair of Periodontal Bone Defects: A Preclinical Study. *Bioengineering* **2021**, *8*, 75. [CrossRef]
60. Singh, A.; Elisseeff, J. Biomaterials for stem cell differentiation. *J. Mater. Chem.* **2010**, *20*, 8832–8847. [CrossRef]
61. Samavedi, S.; Poindexter, L.K.; Van Dyke, M.; Goldstein, A.S. *Synthetic Biomaterials for Regenerative Medicine Applications*; Elsevier Inc.: Amsterdam, The Netherlands, 2014; ISBN 9780123985231.
62. Kim, J.K.; Kim, H.J.; Chung, J.Y.; Lee, J.H.; Young, S.B.; Kim, Y.H. Natural and synthetic biomaterials for controlled drug delivery. *Arch. Pharm. Res.* **2014**, *37*, 60–68. [CrossRef]
63. Gaharwar, A.K.; Singh, I.; Khademhosseini, A. Engineered biomaterials for in situ tissue regeneration. *Nat. Rev. Mater.* **2020**, *5*, 686–705. [CrossRef]
64. Aguilar-Pérez, F.J.; Vargas-Coronado, R.F.; Cervantes-Uc, J.M.; Cauich-Rodríguez, J.V.; Rosales-Ibañez, R.; Rodríguez-Ortiz, J.A.; Torres-Hernández, Y. Titanium—Castor oil based polyurethane composite foams for bone tissue engineering. *J. Biomater. Sci. Polym. Ed.* **2019**, *30*, 1415–1432. [CrossRef] [PubMed]
65. Hanafy, A.K.; Shinaishin, S.F.; Eldeen, G.N.; Aly, R.M. Nano hydroxyapatite & mineral trioxide aggregate efficiently promote odontogenic differentiation of dental pulp stem cells. *Open Access Maced. J. Med. Sci.* **2018**, *6*, 1727–1731. [CrossRef] [PubMed]
66. Ahn, J.H.; Kim, I.R.; Kim, Y.; Kim, D.H.; Park, S.B.; Park, B.S.; Bae, M.K.; Kim, Y. Il The effect of mesoporous bioactive glass nanoparticles/graphene oxide composites on the differentiation and mineralization of human dental pulp stem cells. *Nanomaterials* **2020**, *10*, 620. [CrossRef]
67. Corral Nunez, C.; Altamirano Gaete, D.; Maureira, M.; Martin, J.; Covarrubias, C. Nanoparticles of bioactive glass enhance biodentine bioactivity on dental pulp stem cells. *Materials* **2021**, *14*, 2684. [CrossRef] [PubMed]
68. Wang, W.; Dang, M.; Zhang, Z.; Hu, J.; Eyster, T.W.; Ni, L.; Ma, P.X. Dentin regeneration by stem cells of apical papilla on injectable nanofibrous microspheres and stimulated by controlled BMP-2 release. *Acta Biomater.* **2016**, *36*, 63–72. [CrossRef]
69. Jamal, M.; Greish, Y.; Chogle, S.; Goodis, H.; Karam, S.M. Growth and Differentiation of Dental Stem Cells of Apical Papilla on Polycaprolactone Scaffolds. *Adv. Exp. Med. Biol.* **2018**, *1077*, 31–40. [CrossRef] [PubMed]
70. Alipour, M.; Aghazadeh, M.; Akbarzadeh, A.; Vafajoo, Z.; Aghazadeh, Z.; Raeisdasteh Hokmabad, V. Towards osteogenic differentiation of human dental pulp stem cells on PCL-PEG-PCL/zeolite nanofibrous scaffolds. *Artif. Cells Nanomed. Biotechnol.* **2019**, *47*, 3431–3437. [CrossRef]
71. Luo, L.; He, Y.; Jin, L.; Zhang, Y.; Guastaldi, F.P.; Albashari, A.A.; Hu, F.; Wang, X.; Wang, L.; Xiao, J.; et al. Application of bioactive hydrogels combined with dental pulp stem cells for the repair of large gap peripheral nerve injuries. *Bioact. Mater.* **2021**, *6*, 638–654. [CrossRef]
72. Jang, J.Y.; Park, S.H.; Park, J.H.; Lee, B.K.; Yun, J.H.; Lee, B.; Kim, J.H.; Min, B.H.; Kim, M.S. In Vivo Osteogenic Differentiation of Human Dental Pulp Stem Cells Embedded in an Injectable In Vivo-Forming Hydrogel. *Macromol. Biosci.* **2016**, *16*, 1158–1169. [CrossRef]
73. McMurray, R.J.; Dalby, M.J.; Tsimbouri, P.M. Using biomaterials to study stem cell mechanotransduction, growth and differentiation. *J. Tissue Eng. Regen. Med.* **2015**, *9*, 528–539. [CrossRef]

74. Ceccarelli, G.; Presta, R.; Benedetti, L.; Cusella De Angelis, M.G.; Lupi, S.M.; Rodriguez, Y.; Baena, R. Emerging Perspectives in Scaffold for Tissue Engineering in Oral Surgery. *Stem Cells Int.* **2017**, *2017*, 4585401. [CrossRef] [PubMed]
75. Naqvi, S.M.; McNamara, L.M. Stem cell mechanobiology and the role of biomaterials in governing mechanotransduction and matrix production for tissue regeneration. *Front. Bioeng. Biotechnol.* **2020**, *8*, 597661. [CrossRef] [PubMed]
76. Argentati, C.; Morena, F.; Tortorella, I.; Bazzucchi, M.; Porcellati, S.; Emiliani, C.; Martino, S. Insight into mechanobiology: How stem cells feel mechanical forces and orchestrate biological functions. *Int. J. Mol. Sci.* **2019**, *20*, 5337. [CrossRef] [PubMed]
77. D'Angelo, F.; Tiribuzi, R.; Armentano, I.; Kenny, J.M.; Martino, S.; Orlacchio, A. Mechanotransduction: Tuning Stem Cells Fate. *J. Funct. Biomater.* **2011**, *2*, 67–87. [CrossRef]
78. Xiao, E.; Chen, C.; Zhang, Y. The mechanosensor of mesenchymal stem cells: Mechanosensitive channel or cytoskeleton? *Stem Cell Res. Ther.* **2016**, *7*, 7–10. [CrossRef]
79. Wang, Y.; Xiao, B. The mechanosensitive Piezo1 channel: Structural features and molecular bases underlying its ion permeation and mechanotransduction. *J. Physiol.* **2018**, *596*, 969–978. [CrossRef]
80. Coste, B.; Mathur, J.; Schmidt, M.; Earley, T.J.; Ranade, S.; Petrus, M.J.; Dubin, A.E.; Patapoutian, A. Piezo1 and Piezo2 are essential components of distinct mechanically activated cation channels. *Science* **2010**, *330*, 55–60. [CrossRef]
81. He, L.; Ahmad, M.; Perrimon, N. Mechanosensitive channels and their functions in stem cell differentiation. *Exp. Cell Res.* **2019**, *374*, 259–265. [CrossRef]
82. Marrelli, M.; Codispoti, B.; Shelton, R.M.; Scheven, B.A.; Cooper, P.R.; Tatullo, M.; Paduano, F. Dental pulp stem cell mechanoresponsiveness: Effects of mechanical stimuli on dental pulp stem cell behavior. *Front. Physiol.* **2018**, *9*, 1685. [CrossRef]
83. Jin, Y.; Li, J.; Wang, Y.; Ye, R.; Feng, X.; Jing, Z.; Zhao, Z. Functional role of mechanosensitive ion channel Piezo1 in human periodontal ligament cells. *Angle Orthod.* **2015**, *85*, 87–94. [CrossRef]
84. Mousawi, F.; Peng, H.; Li, J.; Ponnambalam, S.; Roger, S.; Zhao, H.; Yang, X.; Jiang, L.H. Chemical activation of the Piezo1 channel drives mesenchymal stem cell migration via inducing ATP release and activation of P2 receptor purinergic signaling. *Stem Cells* **2020**, *38*, 410–421. [CrossRef] [PubMed]
85. Fels, B.; Bulk, E.; Pethő, Z.; Schwab, A. The role of TRP channels in the metastatic cascade. *Pharmaceuticals* **2018**, *11*, 48. [CrossRef] [PubMed]
86. Nelson, P.; Tran, T.D.N.; Zhang, H.; Zolochevska, O.; Figueiredo, M.; Feng, J.M.; Gutierrez, D.L.; Xiao, R.; Yao, S.; Penn, A.; et al. Transient receptor potential melastatin 4 channel controls calcium signals and dental follicle stem cell differentiation. *Stem Cells* **2013**, *31*, 167–177. [CrossRef] [PubMed]
87. Cui, L.; Xu, S.M.; Ma, D.D.; Wu, B.L. The effect of TRPM7 suppression on the proliferation, migration and osteogenic differentiation of human dental pulp stem cells. *Int. Endod. J.* **2014**, *47*, 583–593. [CrossRef] [PubMed]
88. Xiao, E.; Yang, H.Q.; Gan, Y.-H.H.; Duan, D.-H.H.; He, L.-H.H.; Guo, Y.; Wang, S.Q.; Zhang, Y. TRPM7 senses mechanical stimulation inducing osteogenesis in human bone marrow mesenchymal stem cells. *Stem Cells* **2015**, *33*, 615–621. [CrossRef]
89. Liu, Y.-S.; Liu, Y.-A.; Huang, C.-J.; Yen, M.-H.; Tseng, C.-T.; Chien, S.; Lee, O.K. Mechanosensitive TRPM7 mediates shear stress and modulates osteogenic differentiation of mesenchymal stromal cells through Osterix pathway. *Sci. Rep.* **2015**, *5*, 1–13. [CrossRef]
90. Kim, G.Y.; Lee, C.H. Antimicrobial susceptibility and pathogenic genes of Staphylococcus aureus isolated from the oral cavity of patients with periodontitis. *J. Periodontal Implant. Sci.* **2015**, *45*, 223–228. [CrossRef]
91. Yourek, G.; Hussain, M.A.; Mao, J.J. Cytoskeletal changes of mesenchymal stem cells during differentiation. *ASAIO J.* **2007**, *53*, 219–228. [CrossRef]
92. Du, Y.; Montoya, C.; Orrego, S.; Wei, X.; Ling, J.; Lelkes, P.I.; Yang, M. Topographic cues of a novel bilayered scaffold modulate dental pulp stem cells differentiation by regulating YAP signalling through cytoskeleton adjustments. *Cell Prolif.* **2019**, *52*, e12676. [CrossRef]
93. Collart-Dutilleul, P.Y.; Panayotov, I.; Secret, E.; Cunin, F.; Gergely, C.; Cuisinier, F.; Martin, M. Initial stem cell adhesion on porous silicon surface: Molecular architecture of actin cytoskeleton and filopodial growth. *Nanoscale Res. Lett.* **2014**, *9*, 1–10. [CrossRef]
94. Conserva, E.; Consolo, U.; Bellini, P. Adhesion and proliferation of human dental pulp stem cells on a laser microtextured implant surface: An in vitro study. *Oral Health Care* **2018**, *3*, 1–6. [CrossRef]
95. Bachhuka, A.; Delalat, B.; Ghaemi, S.R.; Gronthos, S.; Voelcker, N.H.; Vasilev, K. Nanotopography mediated osteogenic differentiation of human dental pulp derived stem cells. *Nanoscale* **2017**, *9*, 14248–14258. [CrossRef] [PubMed]
96. Marconi, G.D.; Fonticoli, L.; Della Rocca, Y.; Rajan, T.S.; Piattelli, A.; Trubiani, O.; Pizzicannella, J.; Diomede, F. Human periodontal ligament stem cells response to titanium implant surface: Extracellular matrix deposition. *Biology* **2021**, *10*, 931. [CrossRef] [PubMed]
97. Hasturk, O.; Ermis, M.; Demirci, U.; Hasirci, N.; Hasirci, V. Square prism micropillars on poly (methyl methacrylate) surfaces modulate the morphology and differentiation of human dental pulp mesenchymal stem cells. *Colloids Surf. B Biointerfaces* **2019**, *178*, 44–55. [CrossRef]
98. Ravindran, S.; Huang, C.C.; George, A. Extracellular matrix of dental pulp stem cells: Applications in pulp tissue engineering using somatic MSCs. *Front. Physiol.* **2014**, *4*, 395. [CrossRef]
99. Paduano, F.; Marrelli, M.; Alom, N.; Amer, M.; White, L.J.; Shakesheff, K.M.; Tatullo, M. Decellularized bone extracellular matrix and human dental pulp stem cells as a construct for bone regeneration. *J. Biomater. Sci. Polym. Ed.* **2017**, *28*, 730–748. [CrossRef]

100. Heng, B.C.; Zhu, S.; Xu, J.; Yuan, C.; Gong, T.; Zhang, C. Effects of decellularized matrices derived from periodontal ligament stem cells and SHED on the adhesion, proliferation and osteogenic differentiation of human dental pulp stem cells in vitro. *Tissue Cell* **2016**, *48*, 133–143. [CrossRef]
101. Bačáková, L.; Filová, E.; Rypáček, F.; Švorčík, V.; Starý, V. Cell Adhesion on Artificial Materials for Tissue Engineering. *Physiol. Res.* **2004**, *53*, S35–S45.
102. Lee, J.S.; Yi, J.K.; An, S.Y.; Heo, J.S. Increased osteogenic differentiation of periodontal ligament stem cells on polydopamine film occurs via activation of integrin and PI3K signaling pathways. *Cell. Physiol. Biochem.* **2014**, *34*, 1824–1834. [CrossRef]
103. Hung, C.J.; Hsu, H.I.; Lin, C.C.; Huang, T.H.; Wu, B.C.; Kao, C.T.; Shie, M.Y. The role of integrin αv in proliferation and differentiation of human dental pulp cell response to calcium silicate cement. *J. Endod.* **2014**, *40*, 1802–1809. [CrossRef]
104. Liu, J.; Jin, T.C.; Chang, S.; Czajka-Jakubowska, A.; Clarkson, B.H. Adhesion and growth of dental pulp stem cells (DPSCs) on enamel-like fluorapatite (FA) surfaces. *J. Biomed. Mater. Res. A* **2011**, *96*, 528–534. [CrossRef] [PubMed]
105. Yun, H.M.; Lee, E.S.; Kim, M.J.; Kim, J.J.; Lee, J.H.; Lee, H.H.; Park, K.R.; Yi, J.K.; Kim, H.W.; Kim, E.C. Magnetic nanocomposite scaffold-induced stimulation of migration and odontogenesis of human dental pulp cells through integrin signaling pathways. *PLoS ONE* **2015**, *10*, e0138614. [CrossRef] [PubMed]
106. Zhang, H.; Liu, S.; Zhou, Y.; Tan, J.; Che, H.; Ning, F.; Zhang, X.; Xun, W.; Huo, N.; Tang, L.; et al. Natural mineralized scaffolds promote the dentinogenic potential of dental pulp stem cells via the mitogen-activated protein kinase signaling pathway. *Tissue Eng.—Part A* **2012**, *18*, 677–691. [CrossRef] [PubMed]
107. Guo, T.; Cao, G.; Li, Y.; Zhang, Z.; Nör, J.E.; Clarkson, B.H.; Liu, J. Signals in Stem Cell Differentiation on Fluorapatite-Modified Scaffolds. *J. Dent. Res.* **2018**, *97*, 1331–1338. [CrossRef]
108. Lim, H.C.; Nam, O.H.; Kim, M.j.; El-Fiqi, A.; Yun, H.M.; Lee, Y.M.; Jin, G.Z.; Lee, H.H.; Kim, H.W.; Kim, E.C. Delivery of dexamethasone from bioactive nanofiber matrices stimulates odontogenesis of human dental pulp cells through integrin/BMP/mTOR signaling pathways. *Int. J. Nanomed.* **2016**, *11*, 2557–2567. [CrossRef]
109. Zhou, M.; Liu, N.X.; Shi, S.R.; Li, Y.; Zhang, Q.; Ma, Q.Q.; Tian, T.R.; Ma, W.J.; Cai, X.; Lin, Y.F. Effect of tetrahedral DNA nanostructures on proliferation and osteo/odontogenic differentiation of dental pulp stem cells via activation of the notch signaling pathway. *Nanomed. Nanotechnol. Biol. Med.* **2018**, *14*, 1227–1236. [CrossRef]
110. Crowder, S.W.; Leonardo, V.; Whittaker, T.; Papathanasiou, P.; Stevens, M.M. Material cues as potent regulators of epigenetics and stem cell function. *Cell Stem Cell* **2016**, *18*, 39–52. [CrossRef]
111. Long Wei, L.V.; Yun Song, L.I.U.; Ping Zhang, M.G.U.; Xiang Song, B.A.I.; Xiong, C.Y.; Zhou, Y.S. Transcriptomics and functional analysis of graphene-guided osteogenic differentiation of mesenchymal stem cells. *Chin. J. Dent. Res.* **2018**, *21*, 101–111.

*applied sciences*

MDPI

*Article*

# Digital Occlusion Analysis after Orthodontic Treatment: Capabilities of the Intraoral Scanner and T-Scan Novus System

**Dobromira Shopova [1,*], Desislava Bakova [2], Svetlana Yordanova [3], Miroslava Yordanova [3] and Todor Uzunov [4]**

1 Department of Prosthetic Dentistry, Faculty of Dental Medicine, Medical University of Plovdiv, 4000 Plovdiv, Bulgaria
2 Department of Healthcare Management, Faculty of Public Health, Medical University of Plovdiv, 4000 Plovdiv, Bulgaria
3 Department of Orthodontics, Faculty of Dental Medicine, Medical University of Plovdiv, 4000 Plovdiv, Bulgaria
4 Department of Prosthetic Dentistry, Faculty of Dental Medicine, Medical University of Sofia, 1431 Sofia, Bulgaria
* Correspondence: dent.shopova@gmail.com; Tel.: +359-887417078

**Abstract:** Digital technology is becoming increasingly popular in dentistry. The aim of this article is to demonstrate and compare the capabilities of two different digital approaches, namely, intraoral scanning and digital examination of occlusion, in the final analysis of occlusion after orthodontic treatment. The capabilities and limitations of both systems are emphasized to help clinicians determine which system to use in specific cases. Materials and methods: The study included 32 patients (15 males and 17 females) in the retention phase after orthodontic treatment. Patients were aged 15 to 28 years with a mean age of 18.62 years (±4.17), and 62.2% were aged under 18 years. At the beginning of the orthodontic treatment, 18 patients had Angle Class I and 14 had Angle Class II. Overall, 18 patients were treated without extractions and 14 with extractions, while 12 had impacted teeth. All patients wore an Essix retainer in the upper jaw and a fixed canine-to-canine retainer in the lower jaw. Intraoral scanning was performed using Trios color (3Shape, Copenhagen, Denmark, 2014), and digital occlusion imaging was performed using T-Scan Novus (Tekscan, Norwood, MA, USA, 2018). SPSS 23.0 was used to perform descriptive statistical analysis. Result and Conclusion: With the 3Shape system, the contacts are marked based on the proximity between dentitions. The T-Scan system measures the strength of the contacts, regardless of their area. Despite its many advantages, intraoral scanning is not a reliable method for recording occlusions. The results obtained are not incorrect, but they include limited parameters for analysis. The T-Scan system provides comprehensive results and allows analysis and treatment of occlusal dysfunctions. The T-Scan system can provide information on the first contact, strength of the contacts, contact distribution on each tooth, sequence of contacts, maximum bite force and maximum intercuspation, path of the lower jaw movement, and occlusion and disocclusion times as well as record videos with active sequences and distributions of the contacts. There is a good collaboration between intraoral scanning and digital occlusion determination.

**Keywords:** dentistry; digital impression; digital occlusion; intraoral scanning; 3Shape; T-Scan Novus; orthodontics

**Citation:** Shopova, D.; Bakova, D.; Yordanova, S.; Yordanova, M.; Uzunov, T. Digital Occlusion Analysis after Orthodontic Treatment: Capabilities of the Intraoral Scanner and T-Scan Novus System. *Appl. Sci.* **2023**, *13*, 4335. https://doi.org/10.3390/app13074335

Academic Editors: Vittorio Checchi and Andrea Scribante

Received: 18 February 2023
Revised: 20 March 2023
Accepted: 27 March 2023
Published: 29 March 2023



## 1. Introduction

Digital technology in dentistry is undergoing rapid development. Digital dental impressions made by intraoral scanners have many different applications and advantages over classic impressions, especially during the pandemic. These advantages include a lack of contact with the mucosa, comfort due to the lack of impression material, immediate visualization on the screen with the possibility of inspection and correction, real-time visualization, less time consumption, and easy and selective repeatability [1]. In contrast, conventional impressions require dentists to make a tray selection, perform an impression using different materials and methods depending on the specific case, disinfect the impression, ship it to the laboratory, pour the impression, and ultimately create a master model. The digital impression procedure has fewer steps, which includes software setup, scanning, digital shipping to the laboratory, and creating a digital master model [2]. Accuracy can be affected by various factors, such as operational and clinical differences (e.g., need for coating, larger scanner head, and specific distance from the target; absence of in-office milling units; difficulty in detecting deep margin lines in prepared teeth and/or in case of bleeding; and need for a learning curve) and cost (e.g., purchase and management costs) [3,4]. Accuracy is the consolidation of two elements, both essential and complementary: "trueness" and "precision." The term "trueness" refers to the ability of a measurement to match the actual value of the quantity being measured. Precision is defined as the ability of a measurement to be consistently repeated or, simply put, the ability of the scanner to produce repeatable results when applied in varied measurements of the same object [5].

Intraoral digital impression techniques can be discussed in terms of different dimensions, including the categories and principles of currently available intraoral digital impression apparatus; their operating characteristics; and a comparison of the operation, accuracy, and repeatability of intraoral digital impressions and conventional impressions [6]. Dental arches typically have different widths depending on personality traits (e.g., small, elongated, square, or narrow face; large, medium, or small head size, etc.) or age (child or adult), which can affect the precision of some intraoral scanners during the scanning of the whole jaws [7]. The scanning area and scanning accuracy are influenced by the type of intraoral scanner, scanning distance, and scanning angle selected to acquire the digital scans [8]. A new option is optical jaw-tracking systems, which can record mandibular motion during various treatment phases. The process allows occlusal adjustments using the patient's mandibular motion and facilitates the prosthetic design process, thus minimizing chair time at delivery [9]. This technique of optical jaw tracking for digital recording of the maxillomandibular relationship can visualize the maximum intercuspation and centric occlusion [10]. In a comparative research, Revilla-León et al. measured the accuracy (trueness and precision) of the maxillomandibular relationship at the centric relation position recorded using three different intraoral scanners with or without an optical jaw tracking system. Except for one intraoral scanner system, the optical jaw tracking system improved the trueness value [11]. An additional new software application can directly combine and merge three-dimensional cone beam computed tomography (CBCT) and electronic jaw motion tracking (JMT) information. This examination can improve the treatment of bruxism and temporomandibular disorders (TMD) [12].

Orthodontic treatment is aimed at improving not only the aesthetics but also the function. Achieving a balanced occlusion with uniform contacts without blockages is necessary to attain normal masticatory function and muscle balance [13,14]. Andrew's six keys to occlusion, which include molar relationship, crown angulation, crown inclination, no rotation, no spaces, and flat occlusal planes, are utilized in orthodontics [15]. A retention phase is usually necessary after active orthodontic tooth movement to maintain teeth in a new ideal esthetic and functional relationship and prevent their inherent tendency to return to their previous position [16]. Bonded or removable retainer can be used in the retention phase [17]. Fixed and removable retainers show similar effectiveness in maintaining stability outcomes [18]. The number of follow-up visits during the retention phase is affected by the practitioner's experience, whether vacuum-formed retainers were used, whether the orthodontist considered the presence of third molars or special-need patients when choosing the type of retainer, and to whom the orthodontist attributed responsibility during the retention phase [19].

Several occlusal analyzers are available for registering the occlusal relationships between dental arches. These indicators can be categorized into qualitative and quantitative indicators, with quantitative indicators being capable of measuring tooth contact events. Qualitative indicators include articulating paper, film and silk, occlusal spray, metallic shim stock film, and high spot indicator. In contrast, quantitative indicators include the T-Scan occlusal analysis system and virtual dental patient [20,21]. Articulation paper is the most accessible means of inspecting and visualizing occlusal contacts. However, it carries a risk of error as extensive plane contact is not always strong, with single-point contacts being more powerful [22]. T-Scan Novus is an objective analysis tool that can determine both the force and timing, making it superior to articulating paper, which can only determine the location [23]. The T-Scan occlusal analysis system records and analyzes bite force distribution, indicating its relative intensity and occlusal timing. The balance plot, time display, and comparison screen are the three ways in which occlusal contacts can be recorded and analyzed [24,25].

T-Scan 10 (2018), the newest version of the T-Scan system, has improved software details that benefit implant treatment. The previous version had artifacts in the frontal area, but T-Scan 10 can remove sensor artifacts due to overlapping front teeth. The software features of T-Scan 10 include analyzing occlusal function and an implant warning tool. Digital models can easily be uploaded, and T-Scan data can be overlayed onto an STL digital arch scan [26].

In one comparative study, three different techniques (intraoral and laboratory scanners, T-Scan III system, and the conventional classical method with articulating paper) were compared, and intraoral scanners showed reliability in occlusion registration when compared to the current gold standard [27]. In clinical demonstrations, intraoral scanning ends with an occlusion scan (bite registration). The accuracy of scanners differs depending on the correct scanning technique (every brand has a scheme and consequence of scanning steps) and the number of images (a large number of images can make the file heavy). Digital T-Scan analysis provides details of occlusion evolution, such as a digital timeline, contact sequence, intensity, and type of contacts between the left and right sides at every moment as a video recording as well as parameters such as occlusion and disocclusion times, which are very important in bruxism treatment [28,29]. In a comparative survey, the highest occlusal contact area values were detected using the T-Scan and the lowest using the 3D surface scan [30].

Digital technologies play a part in teledentistry. A digital impression is an initial unit of the whole process [31]. It allows minimal patient contact with the treating dentist. Dental technicians do not have any contact with saliva or blood from the patient, which can be potentially dangerous [32]. Telemedicine clinics and health phone applications were very popular during the COVID-19 pandemic and continue to develop. In awake bruxism, it is possible to identify 70% of symptoms through the different frequencies of behavior provided by the app [33,34]. T-Scan computerized occlusal analysis technology eliminates the process of subjective interpretation of occlusal contacts obtained using articulating paper marks, precisely pinpoints the excessively forceful contact locations, and displays them for analysis of the occlusal force distribution [35]. Among the dynamic occlusal parameters (occlusion and disocclusion times) evaluated, centric slide and balancing side interferences have been found to be highly influential in the etiology of temporomandibular disorders (TMD) [36]. Some general diseases, such as multiple sclerosis and osteoarthritis, can affect the evolution of TMDs [37,38].

This article aims to demonstrate the capabilities of two different digital approaches, namely, intraoral scanning and digital examination of occlusion with T-Scan Novus system, in the final analysis of occlusion after orthodontic treatment. The capabilities and limitations of both systems are emphasized so that clinicians can easily be guided on which system to use in different cases.

## 2. Materials and Methods

A total of 32 subjects (15 men and 17 women) who were in the retention phase after completing orthodontic treatment were included in the study. Patients were aged 15 to 28 years with a mean age of 18.62 ($\pm$4.17), and 62.2% were aged under 18 years. At the beginning of their orthodontic treatment, 18 patients had an intermaxillary relation in the canine's zone Angle Class I, while 14 had Angle Class II. A total of 18 patients underwent treatment without extractions and 14 underwent treatment with extractions, while 12 had impacted teeth, as shown in Table 1. The average age was 17.34 (±3.71) for men and 19.12 (±6.02) for women. The average duration of treatment was 27.68 months (±6.46) for men and 29.12 (±2.98) for women. All patients wore an Essix retainer on the upper dental arch and a fixed canine-to-canine retainer on the lower dental arch.

**Table 1.** Distribution of patients according to Angle class, extractions, and impacted teeth.

| | | Extractions | | Impacted Teeth | |
|---|---|---|---|---|---|
| | | No | Yes | No | Yes |
| Angel_class | Angle Class I | 12 | 6 | 12 | 6 |
| | Angle Class II | 6 | 8 | 8 | 6 |
| Total | | 18 | 14 | 20 | 12 |

The norm for completion of orthodontic treatment, regardless of whether it involves extraction or not, is the achievement of an orthognathic bite, coincidence of the midlines of the upper and lower jaw, multiple contacts, and Angle Class I. This was also the reason for conducting the study on orthodontically treated patients with balanced occlusion. The presented methodology can be used in many cases, such as to detect traumatic areas after prosthetic treatment, implant placement, bruxism patients with the help of occlusion and disocclusion time values, temporomandibular joint (TMJ) disorders, asymmetrical lower jaw movement due to blockage, etc. [20,24,30].

Intraoral scanning was performed using Trios Standard Pod (3Shape, Copenhagen, Denmark, 2014). The workflow included scanning the upper and lower dental arches and the right and left bites. The information was formatted and saved as an STL file using the specialized 3Shape Unite (2021) software. The same clinician performed the scans with the two devices.

For more precise analysis, digital imaging of the occlusion relationship was performed using T-Scan Novus (Tekscan, Norwood, United States, 2018). The system comprises of a sensor, sensor frame, handle, cable, and system unit. The pressure-sensitive sensor is placed in a holder (frame) towards the device and is positioned between the dental arches. The patient is in an upright position with the back of the dental chair at the maximum straight position, and the head is straight without touching the headrest. The proper technique requires the position of the holder being parallel to the floor. The pin of the sensor frame is situated between the upper central incisors. The patient closes their mouth to ensure complete contact (Figure 1). For better visualization, intraoral scans were preimported. Without intraoral scans, the first step before digital measurement of the occlusion is to measure and fill the frontal teeth's mesiodistal size and add information about the dental status (especially missing teeth). The clinician needs articulation paper to find the corresponding contact of the digital image. Preimportation of the intraoral scans shortens the clinical time. Here, contact points are positioned on the tooth surfaces of the screen image and can easily be found in the patient's mouth. Licensed software version 10.0.40 (T-Scan 10, Tekscan, 2022) was used.

Before starting the examination, both digital systems require the entry of dental status, which minimizes contact misplacement. Importing a scan from one system to the other also reduces the potential for error.

The statistical package SPSS version 23.0 was used to perform statistical computations. The patients' demographic characteristics were analyzed using descriptive statistics. Counts and percentages were used for categorical variables. The mean and standard deviation were used for the occlusal force percentage of the four zones of first contact. Microsoft Office 2016 was used for tables and figures.

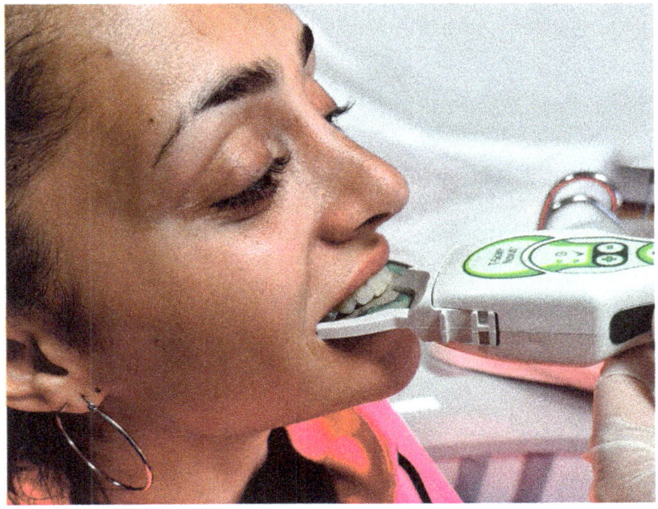

**Figure 1.** Positioning the T-Scan device in the patient's mouth.

## 3. Results

Based on intraoral imaging and occlusion scans (right and left), the 3Shape software generates a color map of the occlusal contacts. Therefore, it is necessary to ensure that the patient does not relax their lower jaw during the occlusion scan. The areas marked in red on the map are the densest, followed by yellow areas 1 mm apart and green areas 2 mm apart. The symmetrical distribution of the contacts can be used as an indication of proper scanning of the dental arches without any deviations or unilaterally stronger contacts (Figure 2A).

The T-Scan system also produces a color map, but it is based on the pressure on the sensor and only real contacts are counted. The color marks correspond to the strength of the contacts, with strong contacts in red, followed by yellow, green, and weak contacts in blue. Pressure information on each tooth is automatically outputted by the quadrants (frontal right and left, distal right and left). Preliminary importing of the digital impressions allows the software to place the contacts in their exact places on the tooth surfaces. Without them, it is necessary to use articulation paper to transfer information to the patient's mouth (Figure 2B).

Both digital systems can determine the occlusal contacts. This study used the same digital impressions but interpreted them with different systems. The 3Shape system marks only the densest contacts, which does not necessarily mean they are the strongest. This system visualizes based on proximity. On the other hand, the T-Scan system measures the strength of the contacts, which is easily demonstrated by bar charts of different colors. Figures 3A,B and 4A,B show the dense contacts according to 3Shape, the first contact according to T-Scan, and the strength of the contacts according to T-Scan. The following results can be seen (the pictures are examples; the patient was randomly selected, and the pictures are intended to show the differences between the two systems, not to draw conclusions):

- The tight contact of tooth 13 according to the 3Shape system is the first contact according to the T-Scan system;
- The tight contact of tooth 14 according to the 3Shape system is moderately strong (light blue marking) according to the T-Scan system;
- The tight contact of tooth 15 according to the 3Shape system is the strongest (yellow marking) according to the T-Scan system;

- The tight contacts of teeth 26 and 27 according to the 3Shape system are moderately strong (green marking) according to the T-Scan system;
- All contacts in the 3Shape system have the same markings, but the difference between them can be analyzed only by the T-Scan system;
- The percentage distribution of the strength of the contacts in the dental arch on the single teeth or on the quadrants can be visualized only by the T-Scan system;
- The T-Scan system generates a video and shows the sequence and strength of the contacts in great detail, combined with the movement of the lower jaw;
- The T-Scan system notes occlusion and disocclusion times, which are important parameters in the examination and treatment of patients with parafunction;
- The movement of the lower jaw and its direction and shape can also be documented only through the T-Scan system.

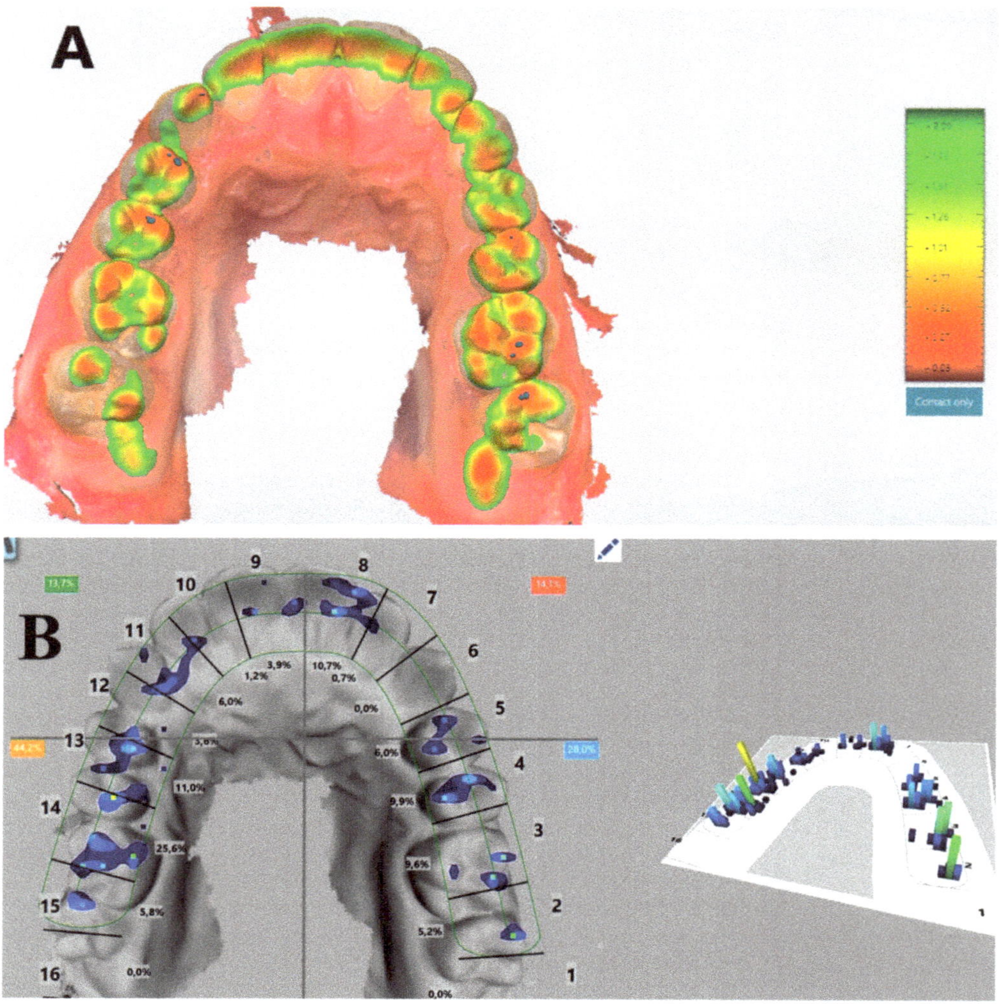


**Figure 2.** (**A**) Occlusion map from intraoral scanner Trios (3Shape, 2014); (**B**) occlusion map from T-Scan Novus (Tekscan, 2018).

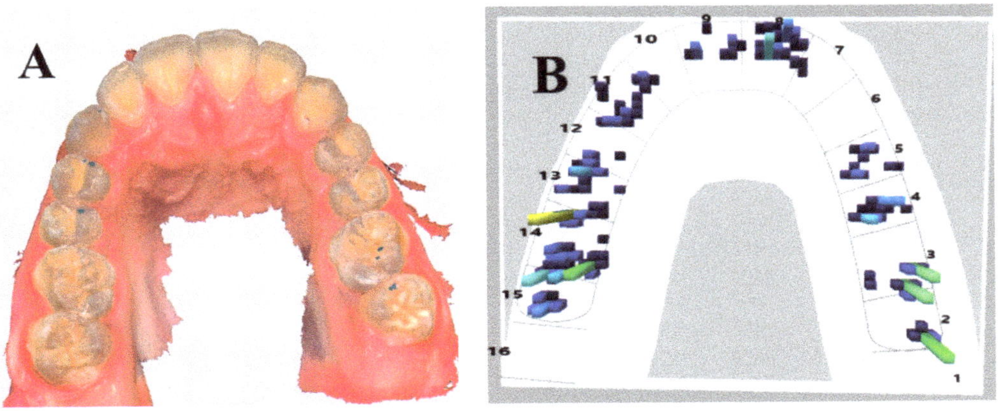


**Figure 3.** (**A**) Complete contacts according to the Trios system. The system detects contacts in only four points: the mesial surface of the first upper right premolar, the mesial surface of the second upper right premolar, the central area of the first upper left molar, and the mesial surface of the second upper left molar. (**B**) Occlusal diagram according to the T-Scan system. Almost symmetrical contacts exist except for the upper left lateral incisor and canine area.

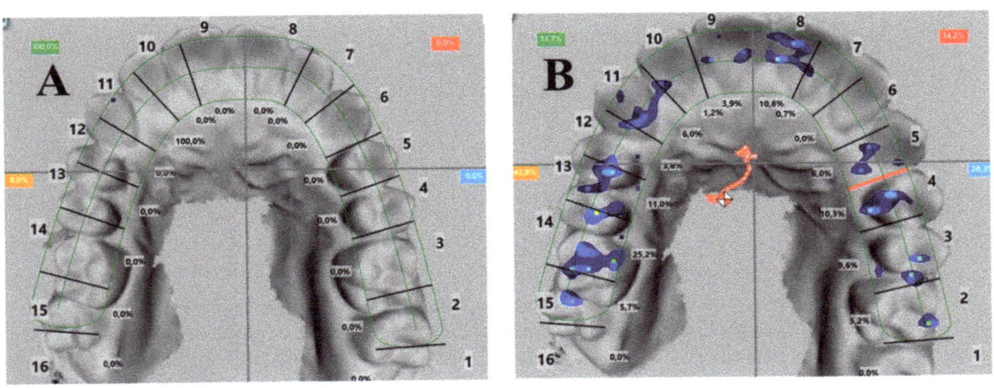


**Figure 4.** (**A**) First contact (T-Scan system) on the upper right canine. (**B**) Quadrant distribution and lower jaw movement (T-Scan system). The system divides the dentition into four quadrants: left and right frontal and left and right distal. The force distribution is shown on each tooth. The path of the lower jaw movement is also presented.

To better visualize the differences, the particular indicators are shown in Table 2. The purpose of the table is not to reject intraoral scanning; on the contrary, it is a necessity in modern dentistry to indicate its possibilities. For standard treatment, these possibilities are absolutely sufficient. For more specific treatment (such as bruxism and occlusion trauma), the help of the T-Scan system is needed.

The T-Scan system can only determine the first contact in central occlusion. The results are presented in Table 3. In rare cases, there may not be only one first contact. In two of our measurements, we observed a double first contact but with different pressures:

- Male, 17 years old, right frontal zone 32.6%, left distal zone 67.4%;
- Female, 26 years old, left frontal zone 41.2%, left distal zone 58.8%.

**Table 2.** Comparison between intraoral scanning and digital occlusion determination with the T-Scan system.

| Type of System<br>Comparative Indicator | Trios Intraoral Scan<br>(3Shape System) | T-Scan Novus<br>(Tekscan) |
|---|---|---|
| Occlusal map | Yes | Yes |
| Distance between the upper and lower jaws | Yes | No |
| Strength of the contacts | No | Yes |
| Contact distribution on each tooth (in%) | No | Yes |
| Sequence of the contacts | No | Yes |
| First contact | No | Yes |
| Maximum bite force | No | Yes |
| Maximum intercuspation | No | Yes |
| Occlusion | Virtual articulator with possible and probable movements | Video of real movements, dynamic occlusion |
| Scheme of lower jaw movement | No | Yes |
| Occlusion and disocclusion times | No | Yes |

**Table 3.** Comparison of zones of the first contact between males and females as determined by the T-Scan system.

| Zone | Male (N = 15) | | Female (N = 17) | |
|---|---|---|---|---|
| | Mean ± SD | Number of Cases | Mean ± SD | Number of Cases |
| Right distal zone | 46.67 ± 1.65 | 7 | 47.06 ± 1.78 | 8 |
| Right frontal zone | 6.67 ± 0.23 | 1 | 5.88 ± 0.34 | 1 |
| Left frontal zone | 6.67 ± 0.23 | 1 | 0 ± 0.12 | 0 |
| Left distal zone | 40.00 ± 1.52 | 6 | 47.06 ± 1.78 | 8 |

## 4. Discussion

The purpose of orthodontic treatment is threefold: morphological norm, optimal aesthetics, and functional balance. The study was performed on an orthodontically treated patient who achieved a balanced occlusion, meeting the orthodontic criteria for successful treatment, including overjet and overbite in norm, Angle Class I, with multiple contacts, without blockages, sprouted tubercles, and Godon's phenomenon [15]. After orthodontic treatment, the teeth in the dental arches were arranged and leveled according to rules similar to the arrangement of artificial teeth in full dentures. The strongest contacts were 2.03 ± 1.57 per denture, and in the most distal zone, the total strength in the maximum intercuspation averaged 99.39 ± 0.66% [39]. Cases of partial or complete edentulism in children are rare and are most often genetically determined. In these cases, orthodontic and prosthetic treatment is combined. The clinical protocol includes orthodontic treatment of the existing teeth, placement of fixed or removable structures, and implants after the completion of body growth (18 years of age) [40,41].

According to Trpevska et al., evidence supports the T-Scan system as a quick and precise method for identifying the distribution of tooth contacts. It can be a promising clinical diagnostic screening device for determining and improving occlusion after diverse dental treatments [42]. The different Angle classes show many nonideal occlusal function characteristics, including Class I. The apparent "ideal occlusion" does not always form an ideal occlusal function. Digital occlusal analysis using the T-Scan system helps diagnose the different variations of malocclusion [43].

Qadeer's study explored measured excursive movement occlusal contact parameters and their association with temporomandibular disorder symptoms between non- and post-orthodontic subjects. Statistically significant differences were observed, with 72.7% working and 27.3% nonworking side contacts seen in the group without orthodontic treatment. In contrast, in the group after orthodontic treatment, near-equal 54.7% working and 45.3% nonworking side contacts were seen. Canine guidance was observed in 60% of the nontreated group and 24% in the post-treated group. TMD symptoms were most commonly presented (72%) among patients after orthodontics. The digital occlusal analysis is a neutral diagnostic method that identifies the location and balance of lower jaw movements after orthodontic treatment [44]. According to Thumati, the T-Scan system can be used in a treatment protocol [45].

Some anatomical features can influence precision. The different widths of dental arches can affect the accuracy of scans. In a clinical trial with Trios scanners (3Shape), no significant differences were found between width and accuracy. The scanning technique is more important than the shape and length [7]. According to a literature review by Morsy et al., virtual interocclusal records with intraoral scanners presented acceptable results for diagnostic precision, with sensitivity of 0.76, specificity of 0.80, diagnostic odds ratios of 14.77, area under the summary receiver operator characteristic of 0.87, cut-off point of 80, positive likelihood ratio of 3.66, and negative likelihood ratio of 0.31. The pooled data for trueness and precision were within acceptable limits. The studies included in the review reported accurate occlusion for fixed restorations fabricated using virtual interocclusal records with intraoral scanners. Furthermore, most of the research on trueness based on virtual occlusal contact zone reported acceptable accuracy [46]. Together with other technologies and computerized devices, intraoral scanning represents one of the most important instruments introduced in dental clinical practice, and future studies are needed in order to understand the possibilities and limitations of these new technologies [47,48].

An alternative to intraoral is extraoral scanning. They are usually applied in cases where the clinician does not have an intraoral scanner available or prefers to work with conventional impression methods. An extraoral scan is a laboratory scan of an impression or plaster cast. Precision of extraoral scanning is acceptable in scanning any scope of arch region [49]. In a comparative study, the extraoral scanners showed substantially higher precision measurements for cross-arch measurement. Surface topography did not correlate to precision; rather, precision correlated with the scanning mechanism. For quadrant scanning, both intraoral and extraoral scanners are recommended, but extraoral scanners are recommended for full-arch scanning [50].

The accuracy and reproducibility of occlusal marking through the T-Scan system are still uncertain. A preliminary study was conducted on four specific points loaded on a sensor by applying weights from 0.1 to 10 kg. The results showed that certain insensitive zones were caused by anatomical features, the most sensitive area was measured from 0.1 to 2.1 kg, and the device was more suitable for recording within lower loads. Although the system has certain shortcomings in terms of reproducibility, it contributes to achieving diagnosis and treatment of occlusal contacts for quantitative estimation [25]. T-Scan can be used in the case completion process. After the orthodontic appliance is removed, changes in occlusion result from "settling" because teeth can move freely in the periodontium. Despite subsequent treatment, a visually "perfect" Angle Class I relationship and ideal occlusal contacts are often not the result of tooth movement alone. Creating simultaneous and uniform contacts after the removal of a fixed appliance can be achieved using T-Scan data to optimize the final occlusal contact pattern. The software's force distribution and timing indicators (the two- and three-dimensional force views, percentage of force per tooth, per quadrant, per half-arch, the center of force, and the occlusion and disocclusion time) help obtain an ideal occlusal force distribution during the completion of the case [51,52].

Through a virtual procedure, the T-Scan system detects occlusal contacts and intraoral scanners obtain the occlusal surfaces. After aligning the three-dimensional occlusal surface and the T-Scan registration, the resulting contacts are projected onto the patient's occlusal surfaces, producing occlusal forces over time. The results received with this procedure demonstrate the relevance of integrating different tools and software and the complete integration of this procedure into a dental digital workflow [25].

Classical occlusal analysis using articulation paper only provides some necessary information to achieve balanced occlusal contacts. Intraoral scanners, on the other hand, can provide similar information for clinical examinations. Due to the possibility of multiple magnifications and views from different angles (including from inside the mouth and the throat), the analysis is much more accurate and thorough. Digital T-Scan analysis can also provide additional valuable information, including force intensity, the moment of first contact, and localization of severe traumatic contact, which can be used for analysis and treatment [28,29]. According to Fraile et al., intraoral scanners appear reliable in intermaxillary occlusal contact registration compared to intra- and extraoral digital scanners and T-Scan III system [27].

Other studies comparing intraoral scanning and T-Scan in natural dentition confirm our results. Their conclusion is that T-Scan is a reliable method for measuring occlusal contact area but 3D surface scans are not. Occlusal registration shows high validity [29].

Intraoral scanning can be a great method of checking occlusion in general. The T-Scan methodology is only aimed at determining occlusion. In addition to diagnostics, it can also be used for treatment by establishing preliminary contacts and overloading certain areas, which is especially important in the integration of implants, treatment of bruxism, and TMJ diseases [53–55].

*Research Limitation*

The limitations of the present study included the sample size of 32 patients, all of whom were treated with the straight wire technique (MBT system). The patients wore an upper Essix retainer and a fixed lower canine-to-canine retainer.

Operator experience appears to be an important factor in the overall evaluation of intraoral scanners [56]. One possible limitation for intraoral scans can be the size of the scanner head. Due to the conical shape of the head, it may be difficult to reach the posterior molar areas in adolescents with a small oral cavity [57]. Most of the existing limitations can be overcome with experience and good clinical skills. However, higher-quality studies are essential for orthodontists to properly interpret data, evaluate new findings, compare the results to existing evidence, and form an up-to-date and objective opinion [58].

Another limitation is the technical characteristics of the T-Scan device. It has been shown that thinner occlusal registration materials provide more consistent records of contact points. T-Scan sensors are made as thin as possible (0.1 mm) to meet technological demands, but they are still relatively thicker than occlusal indicators such as articulating silk. The sensors can be damaged when forces are concentrated over a small area, such as a sharp tooth cusp. The T-Scan system can reproduce occlusal interferences only exceeding 0.6 mm in dimension [59].

## 5. Conclusions

The 3Shape system marks contacts based on proximity between dentitions, while the T-Scan system measures the strength of contacts regardless of their area. Despite its many advantages, intraoral scanning is unreliable for recording occlusion. Although the results obtained are correct, they include limited parameters for analysis. In contrast, the T-Scan system provides comprehensive results and allows the analysis and treatment of occlusal dysfunctions. The T-Scan system can provide information about the first contact, strength of contacts, contact distribution on each tooth, sequence of contacts, maximum bite force and maximum intercuspation, scheme of the lower jaw movement, and occlusion and disocclusion times. There is a good collaboration between intraoral scanning and digital occlusion determination.

The research team's future plans include deepening and covering other perspectives in the study of the two digital systems.

**Author Contributions:** Conceptualization, D.B. and S.Y.; methodology, D.S. and T.U.; software, M.Y.; validation, D.B. and S.Y.; formal analysis, D.B.; investigation, D.S. and M.Y.; resources, D.B.; data curation, S.Y.; writing—original draft preparation, D.S. and M.Y.; writing—review and editing, D.S. and D.B.; visualization, T.U.; supervision, T.U.; project administration, D.S.; funding acquisition, D.S. All authors have read and agreed to the published version of the manuscript.

**Funding:** This study was funded by Grant No 13/2020, Medical University of Plovdiv, Bulgaria.

**Institutional Review Board Statement:** The study was conducted according to the guidelines of the Declaration of Helsinki and was approved by the Ethics Committee of the Medical University of Plovdiv, Bulgaria, protocol №3/20.05.2021.

**Informed Consent Statement:** Informed consent was obtained from all patients involved in the study. Written informed consent was obtained from the patients to publish this paper.

**Data Availability Statement:** Intraoral scanning were conducted at the CAD/CAM Center Dental Medicine at the Research Institute, Medical University of Plovdiv, Bulgaria.

**Conflicts of Interest:** The authors declare no conflict of interest.

## Abbreviations

| | |
|---|---|
| TMJ | temporomandibular joint |
| TMD | temporomandibular disorders |
| MBT system | McLaughlin, Bennett, Trevisi (by the names of the creators) |
| CBCT | cone beam computed tomography |
| JMT | jaw motion tracking |

## References


1. Zimmermann, M.; Mehl, A.; Mörmann, W.H.; Reich, S. Intraoral scanning systems—A current overview. *Int. J. Comput. Dent.* **2015**, *18*, 101–129.
2. Patzelt, S.B.; Lamprinos, C.; Stampf, S.; Att, W. The time efficiency of intraoral scanners: An in vitro comparative study. *J. Am. Dent. Assoc.* **2014**, *145*, 542–551. [CrossRef]
3. Aswani, K.; Wankhade, S.; Khalikar, A.; Deogade, S. Accuracy of an intraoral digital impression: A review. *J. Indian Prosthodont. Soc.* **2020**, *20*, 27. [CrossRef]
4. Mangano, F.; Gandolfi, A.; Luongo, G.; Logozzo, S. Intraoral scanners in dentistry: A review of the current literature. *BMC Oral Health* **2017**, *17*, 1–11. [CrossRef] [PubMed]
5. Imburgia, M.; Logozzo, S.; Hauschild, U.; Veronesi, G.; Mangano, C.; Mangano, F.G. Accuracy of four intraoral scanners in oral implantology: A comparative in vitro study. *BMC Oral Health* **2017**, *17*, 92. [CrossRef] [PubMed]
6. Ting-Shu, S.; Jian, S. Intraoral digital impression technique: A review. *J. Prosthodont.* **2015**, *24*, 313–321. [CrossRef] [PubMed]
7. Kaewbuasa, N.; Ongthiemsak, C. Effect of different arch widths on the accuracy of three intraoral scanners. *J. Adv. Prosthodont.* **2021**, *13*, 205. [CrossRef] [PubMed]
8. Button, H.; Kois, J.C.; Barmak, A.B.; Zeitler, J.M.; Rutkunas, V.; Revilla-León, M. Scanning accuracy and scanning area discrepancies of intraoral digital scans acquired at varying scanning distances and angulations among 4 different intraoral scanners. *J. Prosthet. Dent.* **2023**, in press. [CrossRef] [PubMed]
9. Bedrossian, E.A.; Bedrossian, E.; Kois, J.C.; Revilla-León, M. Use of an optical jaw-tracking system to record mandibular motion for treatment planning and designing interim and definitive prostheses: A dental technique. *J. Prosthet. Dent.* **2022**, *in press*. [CrossRef]
10. Revilla-León, M.; Zeitler, J.M.; Kois, J.C. Digital maxillomandibular relationship and mandibular motion recording by using an optical jaw tracking system to acquire a dynamic virtual patient. *J. Prosthet. Dent.* **2022**, in press. [CrossRef]
11. Revilla-León, M.; Fernández-Estevan, L.; Barmak, A.B.; Kois, J.C.; Pérez-Barquero, J.A. Accuracy of the maxillomandibular relationship at centric relation position recorded by using 3 different intraoral scanners with or without an optical jaw tracking system: An in vivo pilot study. *J. Dent.* **2023**, *132*, 104478. [CrossRef] [PubMed]
12. He, S.; Kau, C.H.; Liao, L.; Kinderknecht, K.; Ow, A.; Abou Saleh, T. The use of a dynamic real-time jaw tracking device and cone beam computed tomography simulation. *Ann. Maxillofac. Surg.* **2016**, *6*, 113. [PubMed]
13. Mahony, D. Refining occlusion with muscle balance to enhance long-term orthodontic stability. *J. Clin. Pediatr. Dent.* **2005**, *29*, 93–98. [CrossRef] [PubMed]
14. Davies, S.J.; Gray RM, J.; Sandler, P.J.; O'Brien, K.D. Orthodontics and occlusion. *Br. Dent. J.* **2001**, *191*, 539–549. [CrossRef]
15. McLaughlin, R.P.; Bennett, J.C. Evolution of treatment mechanics and contemporary appliance design in orthodontics: A 40-year perspective. *Am. J. Orthod. Dentofac. Orthop.* **2015**, *147*, 654–662. [CrossRef] [PubMed]
16. Littlewood, S.J.; Kandasamy, S.; Huang, G. Retention and relapse in clinical practice. *Aust. Dent. J.* **2017**, *62*, 51–57. [CrossRef]

17. Heymann, G.C.; Grauer DA, N.; Swift, E.J., Jr. Contemporary approaches to orthodontic retention. *J. Esthet. Restor. Dent.* **2012**, *24*, 83–87. [CrossRef]
18. Al-Moghrabi, D.; Littlewood, S.J.; Fleming, P.S. Orthodontic retention protocols: An evidence-based overview. *Br. Dent. J.* **2021**, *230*, 770–776. [CrossRef]
19. Bibona, K.; Shroff, B.; Best, A.M.; Lindauer, S.J. Factors affecting orthodontists' management of the retention phase. *Angle Orthod.* **2014**, *84*, 225–230. [CrossRef]
20. Devi, S.; Nallaswamy, D.; Venugopalan, S. Prosthetic Occlusal Analyzers—A Comprehensive Review. *Int. J. Dent. Oral Sci.* **2021**, *8*, 3550–3554.
21. Babu, R.R.; Nayar, S.V. Occlusion indicators: A review. *J. Indian Prosthodont. Soc.* **2007**, *7*, 170.
22. Carey, J.; Craig, M.; Kerstein, R.B.; Radke, J. Determining a relationship between applied occlusal load and articulation paper mark area. *Open Dent. J.* **2007**, *1*, 1–7. [CrossRef]
23. Available online: https://www.tekscan.com/products-solutions/systems/t-scan-novus (accessed on 9 February 2023).
24. Cerna, M.; Ferreira, R.; Zaror, C.; Navarro, P.; Sandoval, P. Validity and reliability of the T-Scan® III for measuring force under laboratory conditions. *J. Oral Rehabil.* **2015**, *42*, 544–551. [CrossRef] [PubMed]
25. Solaberrieta, E.; Etxaniz, O.; Otegi, J.R.; Brizuela, A.; Pradies, G. Customized procedure to display T-Scan occlusal contacts. *J. Prosthet. Dent.* **2017**, *117*, 18–21. [CrossRef]
26. Kerstein, R.B. Current applications of computerized occlusal analysis in dental medicine. *Gen. Dent.* **2001**, *49*, 521–530. [PubMed]
27. Fraile, C.; Ferreiroa, A.; Romeo, M.; Alonso, R.; Pradíes, G. Clinical study comparing the accuracy of interocclusal records, digitally obtained by three different devices. *Clin. Oral Investig.* **2021**, *26*, 4663–4668. [CrossRef]
28. Buduru, S.; Mesaros, A.; Talmaceanu, D.; Baru, O.; Ghiurca, R.; Cosgarea, R. Occlusion in the digital era: A report on 3 cases. *Med. Pharm. Rep.* **2019**, *92* (Suppl. S3), S78. [CrossRef]
29. Kerstein, R.B. The Evolution of the T-Scan I System From 1984 to the Present Day T-Scan 10 System. In *Handbook of Research on Clinical Applications of Computerized Occlusal Analysis in Dental Medicine*; IGI Global: Hershey, PA, USA, 2020; pp. 1–54.
30. Ayuso-Montero, R.; Mariano-Hernandez, Y.; Khoury-Ribas, L.; Rovira-Lastra, B.; Willaert, E.; Martinez-Gomis, J. Reliability and validity of T-scan and 3d intraoral scanning for measuring the occlusal contact area. *J. Prosthodont.* **2020**, *29*, 19–25. [CrossRef]
31. Shopova, D.; Yordanova, M.; Yordanova, S. The Digital Impression As An Initial Unit Of Modern Dental Medicine-Literature Review. *Knowl.-Int. J.* **2020**, *38*, 797–801.
32. Shopova, D.; Bakova, D.; Yordanova, M.; Yordanova, S. Teledentistry Methods In Orthodontics And Prosthetic Dentistry During COVID-19 Pandemic. *Knowl.-Int. J.* **2021**, *49*, 667–672.
33. Reddy, L.K.V.; Madithati, P.; Narapureddy, B.R.; Ravula, S.R.; Vaddamanu, S.K.; Alhamoudi, F.H.; Minervini, G.; Chaturvedi, S. Perception about Health Applications (Apps) in Smartphones towards Telemedicine during COVID-19: A Cross-Sectional Study. *J. Pers. Med.* **2022**, *12*, 1920. [CrossRef]
34. Ron, B.V.; Cisneros, V.M.; Troncoso, P.P.; Tates, M.R.; Lalvay, E.A.; Bajaña, L.C.; Balladares, A.O. Monitoring of awake bruxism by intelligent app. *F1000Research* **2022**, *11*, 479.
35. Komali, G.; Ignatius, A.V.; Srivani, G.S.; Anuja, K. T-scan system in the management of temporomandibular joint disorders–A review. *J. Indian Acad. Oral Med. Radiol.* **2019**, *31*, 252–256.
36. Haralur, S.B. Digital Evaluation of Functional Occlusion Parameters and their Association with Temporomandibular Disorders. *J. Clin. Diagn. Res.* **2013**, *7*, 1772–1775. [CrossRef]
37. Minervini, G.; Mariani, P.; Fiorillo, L.; Cervino, G.; Cicciù, M.; Laino, L. Prevalence of temporomandibular disorders in people with multiple sclerosis: A systematic review and meta-analysis. *CRANIO®* **2022**, 1–9. [CrossRef] [PubMed]
38. Minervini, G.; Del Mondo, D.; Russo, D.; Cervino, G.; D'Amico, C.; Fiorillo, L. Stem cells in temporomandibular joint engineering: State of art and future persectives. *J. Craniofacial Surg.* **2022**, *33*, 2181–2187. [CrossRef]
39. Dimova-Gabrovska, M.I. Protocol for clinical articulation of complete dentures in maximum intercuspation. *Stomatologiia* **2019**, *98*, 45–49. [CrossRef]
40. Dimitrova, D.; Andreeva, R.; Dimova-Gabrovska, M. Application of aesthetic crowns in children patients. *Varna Med. Forum* **2018**, *7*, 141–145. [CrossRef]
41. Dimova-Gabrovska, M.; Dimitrova, D.; Mitronin, V.A. Removable prosthetic treatment in children-literature review. *J. IMAB–Annu. Proceeding Sci. Pap.* **2018**, *24*, 2172–2176. [CrossRef]
42. Trpevska, V.; Kovacevska, G.; Benedeti, A.; Jordanov, B. T-Scan III system diagnostic tool for digital occlusal analysis in orthodontics–a modern approach. *Prilozi* **2014**, *35*, 155–160. [CrossRef]
43. Koval, S.; Kerstein, R.; Radke, J. Characteristics of static and excursive occlusal parameters in subjects seeking orthodontic treatment using t-scan 9 digital occlusal analysis. *Adv. Dent. Technol. Tech.* **2021**, *3*, 87–99.
44. Doh, R.M.; Kim, J.E.; Nam, N.E.; Shin, S.H.; Lim, J.H.; Shim, J.S. Evaluation of Dimensional Changes during Postcuring of a Three-Dimensionally Printed Denture Base According to the Curing Time and the Time of Removal of the Support Structure: An In Vitro Study. *Appl. Sci.* **2021**, *11*, 10000. [CrossRef]
45. Vitale, M.C.; Gallo, S.; Pascadopoli, M.; Alcozer, R.; Ciuffreda, C.; Scribante, A. Local anesthesia with SleeperOne S4 computerized device vs traditional syringe and perceived pain in pediatric patients: A randomized clinical trial. *J. Clin. Pediatr. Dent.* **2023**, *47*, 82–90.

46. Su, T.S.; Sun, J. Comparison of repeatability between intraoral digital scanner and extraoral digital scanner: An in-vitro study. *J. Prosthodont. Res.* **2015**, *59*, 236–242. [CrossRef]
47. Lee, S.J.; Kim, S.W.; Lee, J.J.; Cheong, C.W. Comparison of intraoral and extraoral digital scanners: Evaluation of surface topography and precision. *Dent. J.* **2020**, *8*, 52. [CrossRef]
48. Qadeer, S.; Yang, L.; Sarinnaphakorn, L.; Kerstein, R.B. Comparison of closure occlusal force parameters in post-orthodontic and non-orthodontic subjects using T-Scan®III DMD occlusal analysis. *CRANIO®* **2016**, *34*, 395–401. [CrossRef]
49. Thumati, P. Digital analysis of occlusion using T-Scan III in orthodontics. *J. Indian Orthod. Soc.* **2016**, *50*, 196–201. [CrossRef]
50. Morsy, N.; El Kateb, M. Accuracy of intraoral scanners for static virtual articulation: A systematic review and meta-analysis of multiple outcomes. *J. Prosthet. Dent.* **2022**, in press. [CrossRef]
51. Cohen-Levy, J. Orthodontic T-Scan Applications. *Handb. Res. Comput. Occlusal Anal. Technol. Appl. Dent. Med.* **2015**, 523–561. [CrossRef]
52. Cohen-Levy, J. Orthodontic Monitoring and Case Finishing With the T-Scan System. *Handb. Res. Clin. Appl. Comput. Occlusal Anal. Dent. Med.* **2020**, 1057–1124. [CrossRef]
53. Shopova, D.; Mladenov, K. Case Report: A digital workflow in the treatment of bruxism in a young patient. *F1000Research* **2022**, *10*, 894. [CrossRef]
54. Shopova, D.; Bozhkova, T.; Yordanova, S.; Yordanova, M. Case Report: Digital analysis of occlusion with T-Scan Novus in occlusal splint treatment for a patient with bruxism. *F1000Research* **2021**, *10*, 915. [CrossRef]
55. Dimova-Gabrovska, M. Algorithm for computerized analysis of static, dynamic and functional occlusion in patients with bruxism and bruxomania. *Comptes Rendus De L'Académie Bulg. Des Sci.* **2019**, *72*, 259–266.
56. Park, H.R.; Park, J.M.; Chun, Y.S.; Lee, K.N.; Kim, M. Changes in views on digital intraoral scanners among dental hygienists after training in digital impression taking. *BMC Oral. Health* **2015**, *15*, 151. [CrossRef] [PubMed]
57. Liczmanski, K.; Stamm, T.; Sauerland, C.; Blanck-Lubarsch, M. Accuracy of intraoral scans in the mixed dentition: A prospective non-randomized comparative clinical trial. *Head Face Med.* **2020**, *16*, 1–7. [CrossRef]
58. Christopoulou, I.; Kaklamanos, E.G.; Makrygiannakis, M.A.; Bitsanis, I.; Perlea, P.; Tsolakis, A.I. Intraoral scanners in Orthodontics: A critical review. *Int. J. Environ. Res. Public Health* **2022**, *19*, 1407. [CrossRef] [PubMed]
59. Jain, R.; Jabbal, R.; Bindra, S.; Aggarwal, S.; Jain, R. T-Scan a digital pathway to occlusal perfection: A review. *Ann. Prosthodon. Restor. Dent.* **2015**, *1*, 32–35.

*applied sciences*

MDPI

*Article*

# Pain Perception during Orthodontic Treatment with Fixed Appliances

**Cristian Doru Olteanu [1], Sorana-Maria Bucur [2,*], Manuela Chibelean [3], Eugen Silviu Bud [3,*], Mariana Păcurar [3,*] and Dana Gabriela Feștilă [1]**

[1] Orthodontic Department, Faculty of Dental Medicine, Iuliu Hațieganu University of Medicine and Pharmacy, 8 Babeș Str., 400012 Cluj-Napoca, Romania; cristidolteanu@yahoo.com (C.D.O.); dana.festila@umfcluj.ro (D.G.F.)

[2] Faculty of Medicine, Dimitrie Cantemir University of Târgu Mureș, 3-5 Bodoni Sandor Str., 540545 Târgu Mureș, Romania

[3] Orthodontic Department, Faculty of Dentistry, George Emil Palade University of Medicine, Pharmacy, Science and Technology, 540142 Târgu Mureș, Romania; manuela.chibelean@umfst.ro

* Correspondence: bucursoranamaria@gmail.com (S.-M.B.); eugen.bud@umfst.ro (E.S.B.); mariana.pacurar@umfst.ro (M.P.)

**Abstract:** The present study aimed to determine the intensity of pain perception in patients undergoing fixed orthodontic treatment. We analyzed the severity of pain concerning four routine procedures: the placement of separating elastics, ring cementations, arch activations, and elastic tractions. Our study consisted of a sample of 100 patients between 12 and 35 years old during the initial months of orthodontic treatment with fixed appliances. The patients completed a questionnaire meant to assess their pain sensation perception. The study sample was divided according to age and sex. By determining the intensity of pain felt during the four orthodontic procedures, we found that the most painful one was the ring cementation in all four age groups. The therapeutic-arch-activation procedure ranked second, with a higher mean value (2.66) in the 18–24 age group; the least painful was considered the elastic traction procedure, with a higher value (1.33) in the group over 30 years old. The most painful period was during the first 3–4 days after procedures. Most patients showed moderate pain after following the studied orthodontic interventions and required analgesic medication, the most frequently used being Nurofen, ketonal or paracetamol. The level of pain felt was significantly higher in men than in women. Patients suffer differently from the intensity of perceived pain as they grow older.

**Keywords:** pain perception; fixed appliances; orthodontic treatment

**Citation:** Olteanu, C.D.; Bucur, S.-M.; Chibelean, M.; Bud, E.S.; Păcurar, M.; Feștilă, D.G. Pain Perception during Orthodontic Treatment with Fixed Appliances. *Appl. Sci.* **2022**, *12*, 6389. https://doi.org/10.3390/app12136389

Academic Editors: Mary Anne Melo and George Eliades

Received: 21 May 2022
Accepted: 20 June 2022
Published: 23 June 2022



## 1. Introduction

The high incidence of dento-maxillary anomalies and patients' desire to improve facial appearance and esthetics have increased the number of patients seeking orthodontic treatment, especially with fixed appliances. Recent studies have shown that people, especially adolescents and adults, prefer to undergo a treatment with clear aligners to safeguard esthetics. Unfortunately, only a small number of them can afford the costs of this more comfortable and esthetic treatment type [1,2].

Pain sensation and masticatory discomfort are the most common side effects of orthodontic treatment. For efficient patient compliance and favorable outcomes, the orthodontist should inform patients about these aspects before starting treatment and should evaluate their motivation and potential risks. Moreover, it is ethically important to inform the patient about potential side effects of treatment, and it should be part of the patient's informed consent [3]. Orthodontic tooth displacement induces specific inflammatory reactions of the periodontium and the dental pulp that stimulate the release of various biochemical mediators, thus causing the sensation of pain [4,5]. Generally, the action of orthodontic appliances consists of a change in the balance of the preexisting dentofacial forces, by triggering new ones or by favoring and selectively directing the action of natural forces.

Orthodontic forces depend on the properties of the appliances' materials (elasticity of wires/rubber rings, etc.), the construction particularities, and its interrelation with the dento-maxillary system [6–8]. The essential coordinates in orthodontic biomechanics are the orthodontic force, the weight-bearing area, and the application area, forming De *Nèvrezé*'s triad [9]. Force applied to the tooth crown is transmitted through the root to the periodontal ligament and the alveolar bone. For tooth displacement, alveolar bone resorption should occur in response to this stress; for the tooth to remain firmly attached, bone deposits should also develop to maintain the integrity of the attachment mechanism [10–13].

The International Association for the Study of Pain (IASP) defines pain as an unpleasant sensory and emotional experience associated with actual or potential tissue damage [14]. On the other hand, psychogenic pain is the pain generated by pure concurrent psychological factors strictly related to the person concerned or the environment in which that person lives. Psychogenic pain determined by the patient's psycho-emotional condition does not have a somatic origin [15]. Since pain is a subjective experience, we cannot evaluate it by indirect methods. In the case of children who cannot provide conclusive answers, the following parameters might be assessed:

- Physiological parameters: pulse, blood pressure, and sweating;
- Behavioral parameters: facial expressions (closed eyes, open mouth, dilated nostrils, hollow tongue), high-pitched crying, and body movements (kicking, closed fists) [16]. Still, there are some scales to determine pain intensity.
    1. Verbal scales—used at the time of presentation or during treatment, which classifies pain in 3, 5 or 7 grades: absent/weak/mild/moderate/intense/severe/extreme pain [15].
    2. Visual analog scales—these consist of a line with a length of 10 cm, oriented vertically/horizontally, whose extremes are two terms: "no pain" and "the greatest possible pain" [17].
    3. Numerical scales—in these cases, the patient is asked to quantify pain using numerical values between 0 and 10 or 0 and 100 (0 representing no pain and 10/100 extreme pain). These scales are easier to understand, providing at the same time a better description of pain intensity, and frequently replace verbal/visual scales [17].
    4. Behaviorally anchored scales—these quantify the intensity of pain based on its effect on behavior and describe the impact of pain on daily activities [17].

The study aimed to evaluate the intensity of pain perception in patients undergoing fixed orthodontic treatment. We analyzed the severity of pain concerning four routine procedures: the placement of separating elastics, ring cementation, arch ligation, and elastic traction. We wanted to determine which of these fixed orthodontic procedures causes pain to the patient, what is the pain intensity, and how long after performing the procedure does the intensity of the pain reach a maximum in order to be able to prepare them mentally for the appearance of pain and to indicate the appropriate medication. Determining which was the most used medication in fighting pain was also an objective of the study.

## 2. Materials and Methods

The current study was conducted at "Algocalm" Clinic of Târgu Mureș, Romania. A sample of 100 patients, children and adults aged 12–35 years with a good health status, were evaluated during the initial months of orthodontic treatment with fixed appliances. They were asked to complete a questionnaire to assess pain sensation perception. Thus, the patients answered what best fitted their perception of pain; using the numerical evaluation scale of our multiple-choice questionnaire (Appendix A), they could accurately assess the intensity level of pain [18]. Other pain implications, such as which was the most painful period after the procedure, when was the pain more intense, which medication was more effective in fighting pain, and which was the most painful orthodontic procedure, were studied.

Informed consent was obtained from all the adult subjects involved in the study. For minor patients, informed consent was obtained from one of the parents. All the tested parameters were applied to both children and adults.

For the statistical analysis and the interpretation of the results, Microsoft Excel 2010 and GNU PSPP (Program for Statistical Analysis of Sampled Data) software programs version 1.5.3 (https://www.gnu.org/software/pspp/) were used, and the statistical $p$-value (representing the probability of a statistical test, being the lowest value of the significance level $\alpha$ for which the information extracted from the sample was significant) was determined using the Student $t$-test as well as the ANOVA results.

## 3. Results

Our sample included 100 patients divided into four age groups: 12–18 years (22%), 18–24 years (29%), 24–30 years (32%), and over 30 years (17%).

Distribution of pain intensity depending on the number of patients: the Numerical Pain Rating Scale ranged from 0 to 10 (0 being no pain, and 10 being extreme pain). Figure 1 shows the distribution of patients according to the age limits we have chosen. Figure 2 shows that of all 100 subjects included in the study, only 1 patient chose 2 as the lowest value, most of the patients chose the values 5 and 6 for pain intensity, and only 4 patients chose the highest value, 10. Following the calculations performed, the total mean of pain for the entire sample was 5.76.

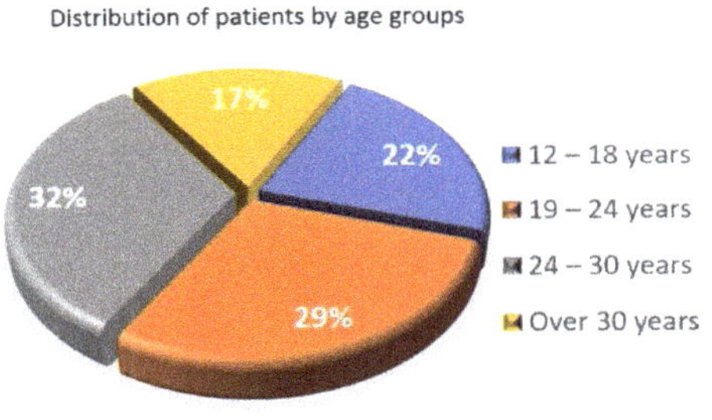


**Figure 1.** Distribution of patients by age groups.

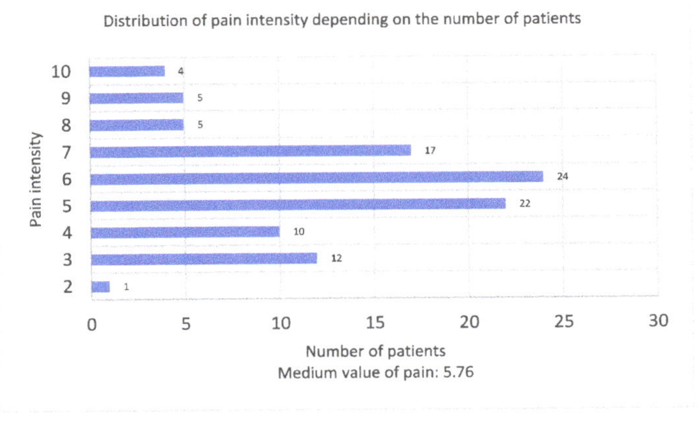


**Figure 2.** Distribution of pain intensity depending on the number of patients.

Distribution of patients depending on the period perceived as most painful: in the following diagram (Figure 3), the most painful period perceived by the subjects included in the study is analyzed. A significant number of them (29) chose the first 24 h as the most painful period, while the majority (40) selected the first 3–4 days as the most painful ones.

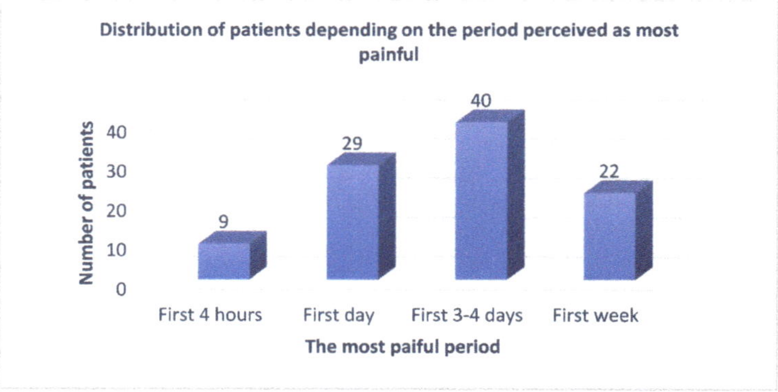


**Figure 3.** Distribution of patients depending on the period perceived as most painful.

Figure 4 shows that the perceived pain was significantly higher for the patients who needed pre-medication before interventions than for those who took no medication. At the same time, we may see that the mean pain value in men was higher than in women in both situations (with or without pre-medication).

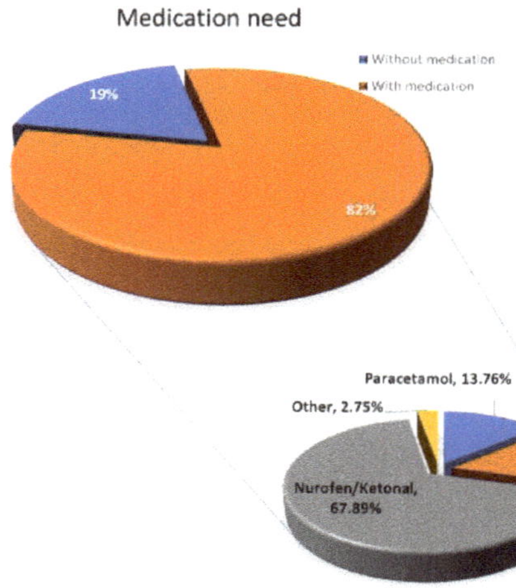


**Figure 4.** Distribution of patients depending on the type and the need for medication.

The perception of pain is different in our group depending on age, as is indicated by the Student *t*-test value obtained: $t = 1.94$, $p < 0.01$. We admit that people suffer the intensity of perceived pain differently as they grow older.

Concerning the need for medication after placement of orthodontic appliances, we can see that only 19% of the entire studied sample did not consider self-medication as necessary, whilst the vast majority, of 81%, chose to take medication to relieve the sensation of pain. Among those who used self-medication, almost 68% selected Ibuprofen, 15.6% chose Metamizole, 13.7% Paracetamol (Acetaminophen), and about 3% chose other drugs such as Codeine.

Figure 5 shows that for the females in the studied sample, the mean pain value was significantly lower than the mean value for the males.

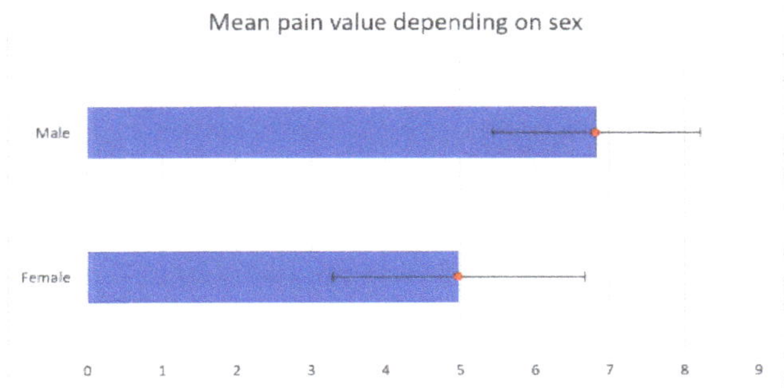


**Figure 5.** Graphical representation of pain value depending on sex.

There are differences in pain perception depending on gender, as indicated by the ANOVA results: F = 33.6, $p < 0.01$. Males suffered more than women from orthodontic procedures (interventions).

The diagram below (Figure 6) shows that the mean pain value varied during both daytime and night-time throughout the first 24 h.

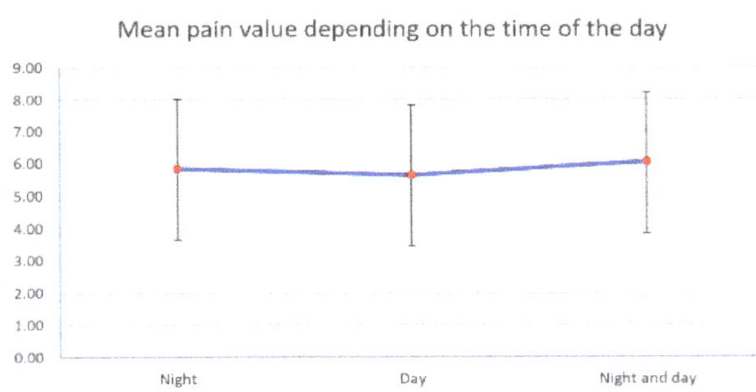


**Figure 6.** Graphical representation of pain value depending on the time of the day.

By analyzing the intensity of pain during the four most frequent orthodontic procedures, we may see that the most painful one was ring cementation in all four age groups, with a higher value for the group aged 18–24 years old (m = 2.83). The therapeutic-arch-activation procedure ranked second, with a higher mean value of 2.66 in the 18–24 age group, and the least painful was considered the elastic traction procedure, with a higher value of 1.33 in the group over 30 years old (Table 1, Figure 7).

**Table 1.** Pain intensity during the orthodontic procedures depending on age.

| Procedure | Age Group | Mean | *p* Value |
|---|---|---|---|
| Elastic separation | 12–18 | 2.09 | 0.04 |
| Ring cementation | 18–24 | 2.21 | 0.00 |
| Arch activation | 24–30 | 2.14 | 0.00 |
| Elastic traction | >30 | 1.07 | 0.04 |

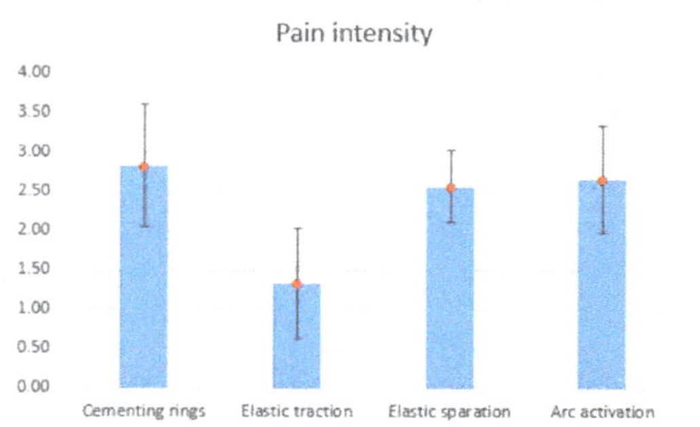


**Figure 7.** Graphical representation of pain intensity/procedure.

## 4. Discussion

The evaluation of pain is relevant for orthodontic treatments. Pain management supposes using specific verbal and non-verbal techniques to calm the patient and help them cope better with the pain [19]. Remarkable progress in pain study and mechanisms has been made over the past years. The visual analog scale, VAS, assesses the intensity of sensory pain and demonstrates that a non-invasive evaluation method is easy to use. Its disadvantage is the one-dimensional analysis of pain that is very complex and has many more particularities, even in usual social activities such as playing sports or meeting friends, attending school, etc. Interpersonal relations represent one of the most studied psychology issues. Social psychology concerns the relations between an individual and others [11].

Orthodontic forces should be applied 24 h/day to produce the most effective tooth displacement rate [20]. Evidence-based findings suggest that an orthodontic force action of at least 6 h/day is required to achieve minimal displacement. An optimal tooth displacement coefficient is considered to be of 1 mm/month. This movement may depend on the following factors:

- The force applied—both small and large forces cause tooth displacement, but in the case of smaller intensity forces that reduce and avoid periodontal ligament hyalinization, the displacement coefficient is bigger;
- The patient's age can influence the displacement coefficient; thus, in the case of adults, the tooth displacement rate is lower than in children due to the increased alveolar bone density and the diminution of cell response effectiveness [12].

We chose the age limit of 12, when permanent teeth are present in the oral cavity, and the correction of spacing/crowding is much easier. After 12 years, tooth displacement is assisted by facial development, and complete orthodontic treatment can be performed within a reasonable period of 18–24 months if the patient is compliant [21].

It is the age when behavioral disorders start to develop through self-neglect or, on the contrary, through a significant increase in interest in physical appearance, thus requiring a correction of dento-maxillary anomalies by orthodontic treatments, mainly for aesthetic considerations [22,23]. Following the calculations performed, the total mean pain value for the entire sample was 5.76. Specialized studies have reported that 8% of the studied samples, or about every 10th patient, discontinue orthodontic treatment because of the pain felt during the initial stages [24,25].

Regarding the period perceived as most painful, scientific studies mention that, generally, pain intensity increases over time from 4 h to 24 h after orthodontic procedures but decreases to normal after the first week [25–27]. Other studies report that pain perception starts several hours after putting on the orthodontic forces (with arch ligation to the brackets) and lasts about five days [28,29].

Most of the patients experienced moderate pain, with a pain level ranging between 5 and 7, and a mean value of 5.76.

After the placement of orthodontic appliances, if the patients considered medication as necessary, they were informed to select their own ones, excluding aspirin and Algocalmin, which have been shown to inhibit tooth movement, as proven in other studies [30]. The patients selected their medication based on previous experiences regarding pain release. According to other researchers, on the first days after each orthodontic appointment, patients take analgesics for pain caused by the dental appliances used for tooth displacement [21,31].

Regarding the mean pain value depending on age groups, the Student test performed showed that the $p$-value = 0.02642366, which is lower than the threshold $\alpha = 0.05$; hence, $p$ is statistically significant, and we may say that the pain perception depends on age.

Our results demonstrated that the mean pain value was different between the two sexes, regardless of age groups.

Studies show that the effect of age on the perception of the sensation of pain during orthodontic treatment is difficult to compare. Most authors suggest that adult subjects perceive a higher pain level than young subjects [26,27]. The 18–24 age group is usually associated with a higher degree of emotional disorders, which might explain the higher level of pain perception in this age group [9].

Some studies indicate that the male sex tolerates pain easily, considering the female sex more fragile and sensitive to the perception of the pain sensation caused by fixed orthodontic appliances [29,31]; other studies show no statistically significant difference between the two sexes [21].

Other authors such as Nandi et al. [32] showed that women more frequently present postoperative pain. Different explanations have been proposed for this: one of them [26] is based on the biological differences between the sexes. These refer to differences in the reproductive organs, which involve hormonal fluctuations associated with changes in serotonin and noradrenaline and an increase in the prevalence of pain during the menstrual cycle [21]. Ethical approaches interfere with pain perception in some cases [3]. On the other hand, one study [26] shows that the mean pain values were generally higher during the day than during the night, and reached a peak only during the first night, causing insomnia in the case of some patients (18%).

## 5. Conclusions

Most patients showed moderate pain following the studied orthodontic procedures.

1. The period perceived as most painful by patients treated with fixed orthodontic appliances was during the first 3–4 days after placement.
2. Most patients required analgesic medication during the fixed orthodontic treatment, the most frequent being Nurofen, ketonal, and paracetamol.
3. The mean value of the pain sensation felt was significantly higher in the case of the male sex compared to the female sex in all four age groups. Patients suffer the intensity of perceived pain differently as they grow older.
4. The most painful procedure was represented by ring cementation in all age groups, with the highest pain intensity in the 18–24 age group.
5. In cases where the clinical situation and the treatment plan allow, the cemented rings should be replaced with orthodontic tubes. If not, we will have to recommend an analgesic medication, especially 3 to 4 days after putting in the fixed orthodontic appliance.

**Author Contributions:** Conceptualization, C.D.O. and S.-M.B.; methodology, S.-M.B.; software, E.S.B.; validation, M.P., S.-M.B. and D.G.F.; formal analysis, M.C.; investigation, C.D.O., E.S.B. and D.G.F.; resources, M.P.; data curation, M.C. and E.S.B.; writing—original draft preparation, S.-M.B.; writing—review & editing, S.-M.B.; visualization, M.C.; supervision, D.G.F. All authors have read and agreed to the published version of the manuscript.

**Funding:** This research received no external funding.

**Institutional Review Board Statement:** The study was conducted according to the guidelines of the Declaration of Helsinki, and approved by the Ethics Committee of SC Algocalm SRL, Targu-Mures, Romania, 917/06.05.2021.

**Informed Consent Statement:** Informed consent was obtained from all subjects involved in the study. For minor patients, informed consent was obtained from one of the parents.

**Data Availability Statement:** Data supporting reported results can be found by contacting Cristian Doru Olteanu, cristidolteanu@yahoo.com.

**Conflicts of Interest:** The authors declare no conflict of interest.

## Appendix A

*Questionnaire*

Evaluation of the perception of the pain sensation during the initial stages of orthodontic treatment with fixed appliances. Personal data will be used strictly for academic purposes, while respecting confidentiality!

1. Name:
2. Age:
   (a) 12 to 18 years
   (b) 18 to 24 years
   (c) 24 to 30 years
   (d) over 30 years
3. Sex:
   (a) male
   (b) female
   (c) other
4. General health status:
   (a) Good

Affected (mention the disease, e.g., allergies, heart diseases, diabetes, bleeding disorders, leukemia, juvenile rheumatoid arthritis, renal failure, endocarditis, cystic fibrosis).

5. The most painful period was:
   (a) the first 4 h
   (b) the first day
   (c) the first 3–4 days
   (d) the first week
6. Pain was more intense:
   (a) during the day
   (b) at night
   (c) during the day and the night
7. Mention the level of the perceived pain on a numerical scale from 0 to 10 (0 being no pain and 10 being extreme pain):

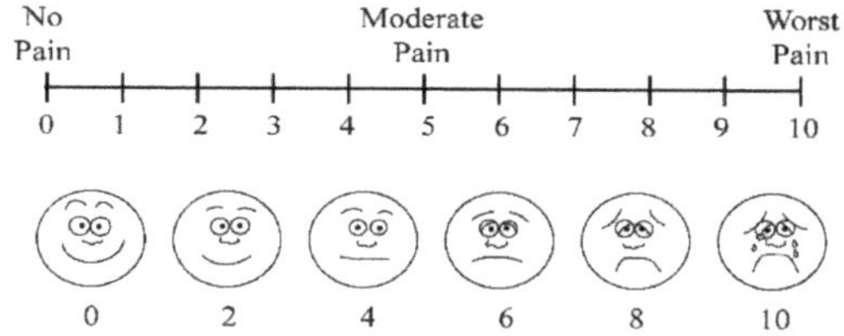


**Figure A1.** Visual representation of pain perception.

8. The drugs administered for pain relief were: Which was the most effective in fighting pain
    (a) Ketonal/Ibuprofen/Nurofen
    (b) Metamizole
    (c) Paracetamol
    (d) Other (mention them)
9. Mention the most painful procedure:
    (a) ring cementation
    (b) use of separating elastics
    (c) arch activation
    (d) elastic traction

    Date, Signature

## References


1. Alansari, R.A. Youth Perception of Different Orthodontic Appliances. *Patient Prefer. Adher.* **2020**, *14*, 1011–1019. [CrossRef] [PubMed]
2. Fujiyama, K.; Honjo, T.; Suzuki, M.; Matsuoka, S.; Deguchi, T. Analysis of pain level in cases treated with Invisalign aligner: Comparison with fixed edgewise appliance therapy. *Prog. Orthod.* **2014**, *15*, 64. [CrossRef] [PubMed]
3. Bucur, S.M.; Chibelean, M.; Pacurar, M.; Sita, D.D.; Zetu, I.N. Ethical considerations in Orthodontics and Dentofacial Orthopaedics. *Rev. Rom. Bioet.* **2014**, *12*, 80–84.
4. Yamaguchi, M.; Fukasawa, S. Is Inflammation a Friend or Foe for Orthodontic Treatment?: Inflammation in Orthodontically Induced Inflammatory Root Resorption and Accelerating Tooth Movement. *Int. J. Mol. Sci.* **2021**, *22*, 2388. [CrossRef]
5. D'Apuzzo, F.; Nucci, L.; Delfino, I.; Portaccio, M.; Minervini, G.; Isola, G.; Serino, I.; Camerlingo, C.; Lepore, M. Application of Vibrational Spectroscopies in the Qualitative Analysis of Gingival Crevicular Fluid and Periodontal Ligament during Orthodontic Tooth Movement. *J. Clin. Med.* **2021**, *10*, 1405. [CrossRef]
6. Mansour, A.Y. A comparison of orthodontic elastic forces: Focus on reduced inventory. *J. Orthod. Sci.* **2017**, *6*, 136–140. [CrossRef]
7. Nucera, R.; Gatto, E.; Borsellino, C.; Aceto, P.; Fabiano, F.; Matarese, G.; Perillo, L.; Cordasco, G. Influence of bracket-slot design on the forces released by superelastic nickel-titanium alignment wires in different deflection configurations. *Angle Orthod.* **2014**, *84*, 541–547. [CrossRef]
8. McNamara, C.; Drage, K.J.; Sandy, J.R.; Ireland, A.J. An evaluation of clinicians' choices when selecting archwires. *Eur. J. Orthod.* **2010**, *32*, 54–59. [CrossRef]
9. Foster, T.D. *A Textbook of Orthodontics*, 3rd ed.; Blackwell Scientific Publications: Boston, MA, USA, 1990; pp. 123–129.
10. Proffit, W.R.; Fields, H.W., Jr. *1992 Contemporary Orthodontics*, 2nd ed.; Mosby Year Book: Mount Joy, PA, USA, 1992; pp. 12–18.
11. D'Apuzzo, F.; Cappabianca, S.; Ciavarella, D.; Monsurrò, A.; Silvestrini-Biavati, A.; Perillo, L. Biomarkers of Periodontal Tissue Remodeling during Orthodontic Tooth Movement in Mice and Men: Overview and Clinical Relevance. *Sci. World J.* **2013**, *2013*, 105873. [CrossRef]
12. Miles, T.S.; Nauntofte, B.; Svensson, P. *Clinical Oral Physiology*; Quintessence Publishing Co., Ltd.: New Malden, UK, 2004; pp. 45–61.
13. Jeon, H.H.; Teixeira, H.; Tsai, A. Mechanistic Insight into Orthodontic Tooth Movement Based on Animal Studies: A Critical Review. *J. Clin. Med.* **2021**, *10*, 1733. [CrossRef]
14. Raja, S.N.; Carr, D.B.; Cohen, M.; Finnerup, N.B.; Flor, H.; Gibson, S.; Keefe, F.J.; Mogil, J.S.; Ringkamp, M.; Sluka, K.A.; et al. The revised International Association for the Study of Pain definition of pain: Concepts, challenges, and compromises. *Pain* **2020**, *161*, 1976–1982. [CrossRef] [PubMed]
15. Grassia, V.; Rotolo, R.P.; Nucci, L.; D'Apuzzo, F.; Perillo, L. Bullying and malocclusion in adolescence: A case report. *South Eur. J. Orthod. Dentofac. Res.* **2020**, *7*, 17–20. [CrossRef]
16. Patel, V. Non-completion of Active Orthodontic Treatment. *Br. J. Orthod.* **1992**, *19*, 47–54. [CrossRef] [PubMed]
17. Bergius, M.; Berggren, U.; Kiliaridis, S. Experience of pain during an orthodontic procedure. *Eur. J. Oral Sci.* **2002**, *110*, 92–98. [CrossRef]
18. Available online: https://assessment-module.yale.edu/im-palliative/visual-analogue-scale (accessed on 3 April 2021).
19. Asiry, M.A. Biological aspects of orthodontic tooth movement: A review of literature. *Saudi J. Biol. Sci.* **2018**, *25*, 1027–1032. [CrossRef] [PubMed]
20. Anthonappa, R.P.; Ashley, P.; Bonetti, D.L.; Lombardo, G.; Riley, P. Non-pharmacological interventions for managing dental anxiety in children. *Cochrane Database Syst. Rev.* **2017**, *2017*, CD012676. [CrossRef]
21. Scheurer, P.A.; Firestone, A.R.; Burgin, W.B. Perception of pain as a result of orthodontic treatment with fixed appliances. *Eur. J. Orthod.* **1996**, *18*, 349–357. [CrossRef]
22. Fernandes, L.M.; Skoglund, L. Pain and discomfort experienced after placement of a conventional or a superelastic NiTi aligning archwire. A randomized clinical trial. *J. Orofac. Orthop.* **1998**, *59*, 331–339. [CrossRef]
23. Aslihan, M.E.; Dincer, B. Perception of pain during orthodontic treatment with fixed appliances. *Eur. J. Orthod.* **2004**, *26*, 79–85.
24. Rakhshan, H.; Rakhshan, V. Pain and discomfort perceived during the initial stage of active fixed orthodontic treatment. *Saudi Dent. J.* **2015**, *27*, 81–87. [CrossRef]

25. White, L.W. Pain and cooperation in orthodontic treatment. *J. Clin. Orthod.* **1984**, *18*, 572–575. [PubMed]
26. Krishnan, V. Orthodontic pain: From causes to management—A review. *Eur. J. Orthod.* **2007**, *29*, 170–179. [CrossRef] [PubMed]
27. Bergius, M.; Kiliardis, S.; Berggren, U. Pain in orthodontics: A review and discussion of the literature. *J. Orofac. Orthop.* **2000**, *61*, 125–137. [CrossRef] [PubMed]
28. Bud, E.; Vlasa, A.; Chibelean, M.; Martha, K.; Păcurar, M.; Bud, A.; Esian, D. Factors Associated with Pain Intensity in Patients Undergoing Orthodontic Treatment Based on Mini-Implants. *J. Interdiscip. Med.* **2021**, *6*, 74–81. [CrossRef]
29. Ingersoll, D.B. *Behavioral Aspects in Dentistry*; Appleton Century Crofts: Norwalk, CT, USA, 1982; pp. 14–32.
30. Olteanu, C.D.; Şerbănescu, A.; Boşca, A.B.; Mihu, C.M. Orthodontic tooth movement following analgesic treatment with Aspirin and Algocalmin. An experimental study. *Rom. J. Morphol. Embryol.* **2015**, *56*, 1339–1344.
31. Arias, O.R.; Marquez-Orozco, M.C. Aspirin, acetaminophen, and ibuprofen: Their effects on orthodontic tooth movement. *Am. J. Orthod. Dentofac. Orthop.* **2006**, *130*, 364–370. [CrossRef]
32. Nandi, M.; Schreiber, K.L.; Martel, M.O.; Cornelius, M.; Campbell, C.M.; Haythornthwaite, J.A.; Smith, M.T.; Wright, J.; Aglio, L.S.; Strichartz, G.; et al. Sex differences in negative affect and postoperative pain in patients undergoing total knee arthroplasty. *Biol. Sex Differ.* **2019**, *10*, 23. [CrossRef]

applied sciences

MDPI

Article

# The Fourth Cervical Vertebra Anterior and Posterior Body Height Projections (*Vba*) for the Assessment of Pubertal Growth Spurt

**Roberto Cameriere [1], Luz Andrea Velandia Palacio [2], Enita Nakaš [3], Ivan Galić [4,*], Hrvoje Brkić [5,6,*], Danijela Kalibović Govorko [7], Daniel Jerković [4], Liliana Jara [2] and Luigi Ferrante [8]**

1 AgEstimation Project, Department of Medicine and Health Sciences "Vincezo Tiberio", University of Molise, 86100 Campobasso, Italy
2 Research Center Dental Department, Institución Universitaria Colegios de Colombia (UNICOC), Bogota 250001, Colombia
3 Department of Orthodontics, School of Dental Medicine, University of Sarajevo, 71000 Sarajevo, Bosnia and Herzegovina
4 Departments of Oral Surgery, School of Medicine, University Hospital of Split, University of Split, 21000 Split, Croatia
5 Department of Dental Anthropology and Chair of Forensic Dentistry, School of Dental Medicine, University of Zagreb, 10000 Zagreb, Croatia
6 Faculty of Dental Medicine, University of Lisbon, 1649-004 Lisbon, Portugal
7 Department of Orthodontics, School of Medicine, University Hospital of Split, University of Split, 21000 Split, Croatia
8 Center of Epidemiology, Biostatistics, and Medical Information Technology, Department of Biomedical Sciences and Public Health, Polytechnic University of Marche, Via Conca 71, 60020 Torrette di Ancona, Italy
* Correspondence: igalic@mefst.hr (I.G.); brkic@sfzg.hr (H.B.); Tel.: +385-2155-7700 (I.G.); +385-1480-2166 (H.B.)

**Featured Application: Roberto Cameriere and Ivan Galić equally contributed to this paper.**

**Abstract:** This paper aims to propose a statistical model to assess pubertal growth spurt using the ratio of the anterior height projection to the posterior (*Vba*) of the fourth cervical vertebra body (C4) on cephalograms and to calculate the residual proportion of skeletal maturation and the time for the pubertal growth spurt to end for a given *Vba*. A sample of 538 cephalograms from healthy-living children aged between 5 and 15 years was analyzed. A segmented regression model was used to explain the different *Vba* stages relative to the pubertal growth spurt. In addition, the time to achieve skeletal maturation was evaluated for a given *Vba* between the beginning ($Vba_1$) and the end ($Vba_2$) of the pubertal growth spurt. A longitudinal sample of 25 males and 25 females was analyzed to validate the proposed method. The values of *Vba* corresponding to higher pubertal development rate ranged from $Vba_1$ = 0.677 (95%CI, 0.644–0.711) to $Vba_2$ = 0.966 (95%CI, 0.905–1.028) and from $Vba_1$ = 0.669 (95%CI, 0.645–0.693) to $Vba_2$ = 1.073 (95%CI, 1.044–1.101) in males and females, respectively. The validation process results showed that our model did not produce any incorrect forecasts. The proposed method estimates the beginning and the end of the pubertal growth spurt together with the residual proportion of skeletal maturation for a given *Vba*.

**Keywords:** dental age; skeletal age; cervical vertebrae; pubertal growth spurt; segmented regression; dental growth; AgEstimation

**Citation:** Cameriere, R.; Velandia Palacio, L.A.; Nakaš, E.; Galić, I.; Brkić, H.; Kalibović Govorko, D.; Jerković, D.; Jara, L.; Ferrante, L. The Fourth Cervical Vertebra Anterior and Posterior Body Height Projections (*Vba*) for the Assessment of Pubertal Growth Spurt. *Appl. Sci.* **2023**, *13*, 1819. https://doi.org/10.3390/app13031819

Academic Editor: Vittorio Checchi

Received: 10 January 2023
Revised: 28 January 2023
Accepted: 29 January 2023
Published: 31 January 2023



## 1. Introduction

Dynamics and timing of dental and skeletal maturation in growing children are fundamental in orthodontic treatment planning; they provide clinical information on how and when a patient should start using maxillary orthopedic appliances or indicate the necessity for orthognathic surgery [1–3]. Growth and development assessments use individual indicators or developmental stages to describe the changes that occur during life.

Indicators can vary from height and weight gain, development of sexual characteristics, menarche in women, and assessment of mental maturity [4]. Since chronological age is an unreliable way to estimate pubertal growth spurt because of the high variability among individuals in its timing of initiation, duration, and amount during children's growth, several other approaches have been used [5–10].

X-ray of the hand and wrist to assess skeletal maturity has been a standard procedure in clinical orthodontics to assess whether a person is skeletally mature or determine the possibilities of planned therapy [11]. The most straightforward approach to assessing the development of the hand and wrist is to compare the X-ray image with the available Atlas of the development of the hand and wrist [12]. According to Greulich and Pyle, the Atlas of skeletal development of the hand and wrist contains images of the hand and wrist of normal healthy children from birth to adulthood with an age interval of 3 years [13]. Hagg and Taranger [12] studied the skeletal stages of the hand and wrist to indicate a pubertal growth spurt. They concluded that specific skeletal indicators, the ulnar sesamoid of the metacarpophalangeal joint of the first finger, the epiphyses of the middle and distal phalanges of the third finger, and the distal epiphysis of the radius might indicate the onset, peak, and end of the pubertal growth spurt [12]. Bjork et al. [4], in their method for epidemiological registration of malocclusion, defined two stages of the eruption of deciduous teeth, five stages of the eruption of permanent anterior teeth, and four stages of the eruption of permanent molars. Björk and Helm [14] showed that dental stages from Bjork et al. [4], close to the timing of maximum pubertal growth in height, DS4, all canines, and premolars fully erupted, and DS $M_2$, all second molars fully erupted, were of little value as criteria of pubertal peak comparing to ossification of the ulnar sesamoid at the metacarpophalangeal joint of the thumb or menarche. The timing of the eruption of permanent teeth is more dependent on local factors such as loss of deciduous teeth or crowding [15].

Historically, the most common method for assessment of skeletal maturation was an analysis of hand–wrist radiograph, used later by Fishman [16], who related specific skeletal maturity indicator stages to pubertal growth spurt. Furthermore, Lamparski [17] claimed that the use of the cervical vertebrae was as valid as the hand–wrist bones to assess skeletal maturation and described a new approach based on the changes in the shape of five cervical vertebrae. His study designed a series of standards of cervical vertebral maturation (CVM), separating male and female participants concerning chronological age and skeletal maturation [17]. Hassel and Farman [18] modified Lamparski's method and proved that CVM was acceptably accurate and helpful in estimating an individual's skeletal maturity and residual growth potential, as well as the hand–wrist method. Studies from Baccetti [1] and Franchi [19] further demonstrated that CVM method is useful as a biological indicator for both mandibular and somatic maturation.

Hassel and Farman [18] modified Lamparski's method and demonstrated the changes in the shape of cervical vertebrae in each stage of skeletal growth, proving to be acceptably accurate and valuable for estimating skeletal maturity and residual growth potential of an individual as the hand–wrist method. Finally, Baccetti et al. [1] and Franchi et al. [19] showed that the cervical vertebral maturation method is useful as a biological indicator for both mandibular and somatic maturation. Their study was critical due to the use of longitudinal data from radiographs and because their method was based on changes in the annual increase in total mandibular length instead of comparison with hand–wrist skeletal age [1,19].

Dental age estimation methods in children can help assess the development of the dentition, whether it is accelerated or delayed, and the effect of specific therapeutic procedures in oncology patients. In addition, they can be used in research on the growth and development of twins, the effect of hormone replacement therapy, or in estimating age in persons without the possibility of identification [20–25]. In the development of permanent teeth, their exchange with milk teeth is essential, as the lower and upper molars and front incisors sprout first, and tooth sprouting takes place until 21–23 years of age [26]. In addition to age assessment based on the number of permanent teeth in the mouth, more reliable methods of dental age assessment are based on the analysis of radiographic images, and so far, several methods have been presented that mainly assess tooth development in stages. The most commonly used methods that use developed stages are Demirjian, Willems, Haavikko, and Chaillet [27–30]. If a strong association of dental development with skeletal development were to be proven, some of the values used to assess tooth development could be taken as a reference or even the first choice in diagnosing the pubertal growth spurt. Dental scans are a mandatory part of the protocol when planning orthodontic therapy so that they can assess the expected or completed pubertal growth spurt [31].

The atlas or staging systems generally used in estimating the development regularly contain a set of longitudinal figures of different ossification stages, which typically do not stand on accurate measurements with definite orientation points [32]. Cameriere et al. introduced another approach for studying dental and skeletal development for age estimation by specific lengths or area measurements of the apposition of secondary dentine in dental radiographs and the ossification of the carpal skeleton in hand and wrist radiographs [33–49].

Cameriere et al. [40] and Gulsahi et al. [50] published articles where the heights of the anterior and posterior sides of the C4 vertebral body from lateral cephalograms in individuals aged 5–15 years were used to estimate the chronological age with forensic purposes. The ratio of heights or *Vba* has shown a correlation to chronological age and was recognized as a potential indicator for age estimation in this age range [40]. After Bayes calibration, the mean absolute errors (MAEs) were 1.34 years with standard deviation (SD) of 0.95 years and 1.01 years (SD 0.71 years), and the mean inter-quartile ranges (MIQRs) of the calibrating distribution were 2.32 years (SD, 0.25 years) and 1.72 years (SD, 0.39 years) in males and females, respectively [40]. Gulsahi et al. [50] also investigated the correlation of age and *Vba* on the Turkish sample, and after Bayes calibration, MAEs were 0.879 years and 0.906 years (mean interquartile ranges (MIQR.s) 1.290 and 1.435 years) in males and females, respectively.

According to published results of the usefulness of *Vba* in the specific age span of development when adolescent growth spurt occurs, we decided to study the values of *Vba*, particularly the distributions of its minimum and maximum, during adolescence.

The aims of this study were, therefore, to evaluate the ratio of the anterior height projection to the posterior (*Vba*) of the fourth cervical vertebra body (C4) on cephalograms and its relationship with a pubertal growth spurt and to propose a statistical model based on segmented regression to calculate the residual proportion of the skeletal maturation for a given *Vba* and the time for the pubertal growth spurt to end for a given *Vba*.

The proposed model will be validated using longitudinal data from the Michigan Growth Center supported by the American Association of Orthodontists Foundation (AAOF).

## 2. Materials and Methods

This cross-sectional observational study evaluated 527 lateral cephalograms previously taken for dental diagnoses and pretreatment planning. All participants were healthy individuals aged between 5 and 15 years who lived in Croatia and without a recorded history of genetic or developmental anomalies of the skeleton. The study was conducted by the ethical standards laid down by the Declaration of Helsinki [51].

The age and sex distribution for each age category of the sample are presented in Figure 1.

In addition, the following data were recorded for each subject: dates of birth and of the radiograph, sex, as reported on the radiograph, and ancestry as reported by either self or family. The observers were blinded to information on the subject's sex and age.

The radiographs were processed according to the method of Cameriere et al. [40]. The ratio of the anterior height projection to the posterior (A/B = *Vba*), Figure 2, was used first to correlate with the different moments of the pubertal growth spurt and second, to propose a method that can quantitatively determine the beginning and the end of the pubertal growth spurt in an individual.

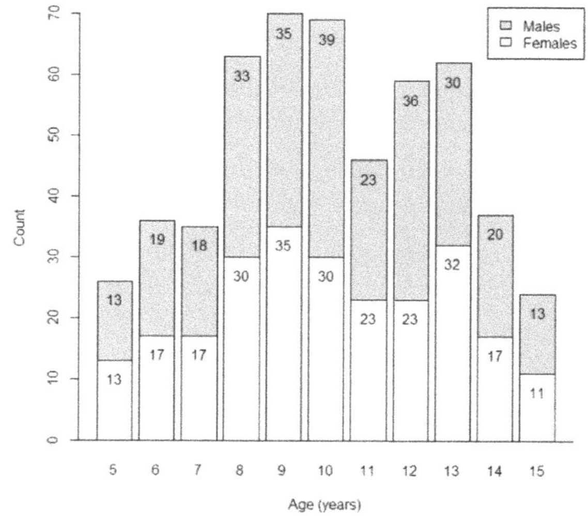


**Figure 1.** Frequency distribution of the sample by sex and age cohort.

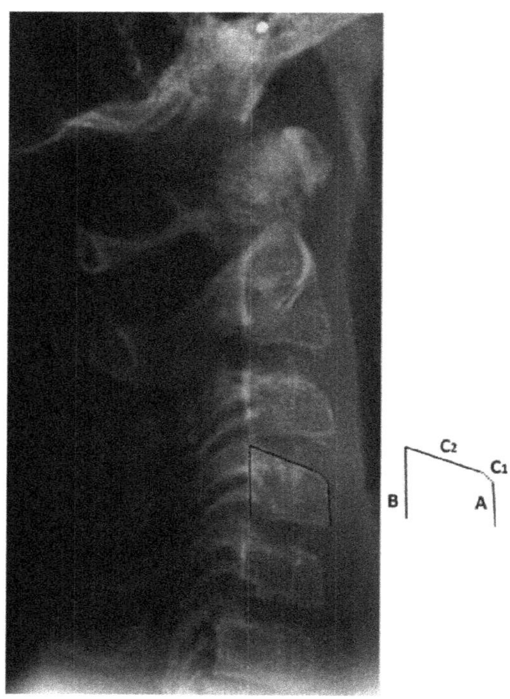


**Figure 2.** An example of the anterior (A) and the posterior (B) sides of the fourth cervical vertebral body. The anterior side of the body is measured up to the point where the anterior side (A) curves (C1) towards the superior side (C2) of the vertebral body.

We evaluated lateral cephalograms from 50 subjects (25 males and 25 females) to validate the proposed model. The lateral cephalograms of the subjects belong to the Michigan Growth Center and include the subset of subjects with at least four radiographs. For each subject, the number of observations ranged from 4 to 6, totaling 227 radiographs.

*Statistical Analysis*

Thirty randomly selected lateral cephalograms were reanalyzed after two weeks to assess the intra-observer repeatability and inter-observer reliability of *Vba* by the same observer and a second one, respectively. The intra-class correlation coefficient (ICC) was used to evaluate intra- and inter-observer agreement [52].

According to the results in this study and reported by Cameriere et al. [40], we considered that C4 development presented as *Vba* increment is not constant concerning age, but it seems to follow three distinct phases with increment in the intermediate phase.

The nonlinear relationship between *Vba* and actual age suggests fitting data using a segmented regression model, which allows us to estimate two breakpoints, $\tau_1$ and $\tau_2$ and both regression coefficients characterize the interval of ages with higher pubertal development rate [53]. The proposed segmented regression model to fit the data is:

$$Vba = \beta_0 + \beta_1 \cdot age + \beta_2 \cdot (age - \tau_1)_+ + \beta_3 \cdot (age - \tau_2)_+ \quad (1)$$

where $\beta_i$, $i = 0, \ldots 3$, are the regression coefficients, and $(x)_+$ is equal to $x$ if $x$ is positive and 0 otherwise. The meanings of the regression coefficients are: $\beta_0$ is the intercept of the piecewise linear curve with the vertical axis (see Figure 3), i.e., it is the mean *Vba* value at age = 0; $\beta_1$ is the "left" slope, i.e., the growth rate when age < $\tau_1$; the sum $\beta_1 + \beta_2$ is the "central" slope, i.e., the growth rate of *Vba* when the individual age belongs to the interval $(\tau_1, \tau_2)$; finally, the sum $\beta_1 + \beta_2 + \beta_3$ is the "right" slope, namely the slope when age > $\tau_2$) and it is the growth rate of *Vba* when individual's age is greater than $\tau_2$.

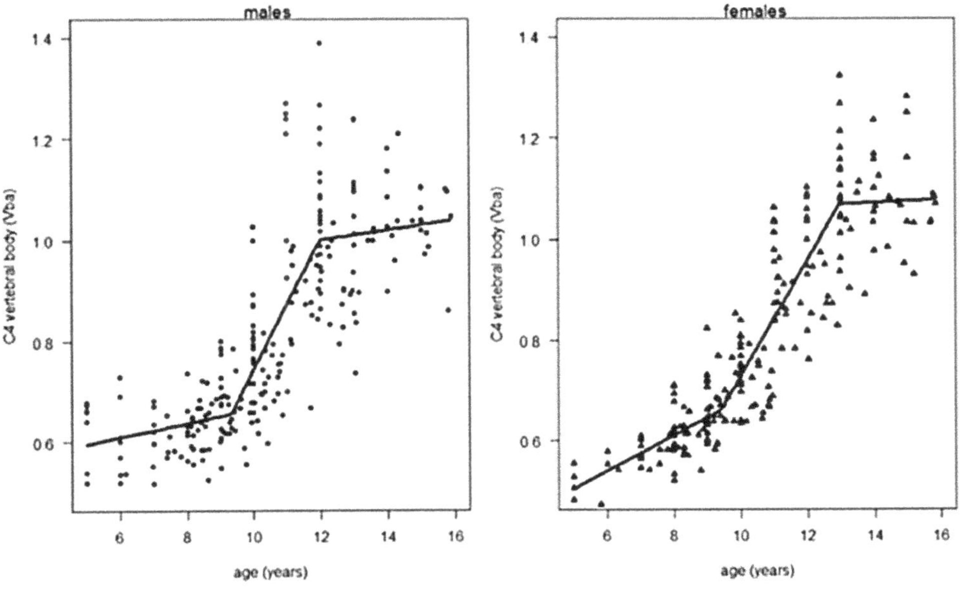


**Figure 3.** The distribution of the proportions of the anterior and posterior sides of the C4 vertebral body (*Vba*) as the function of age for males (**left**) and females (**right**) subjects with segmented regression plots.

Fitting the model to the data, we estimated the regression coefficients and two breakpoints. Furthermore, we estimated the values of *Vba* corresponding to the two breakpoints, $Vba_1$ and $Vba_2$ (spurts), and, for a given value of *Vba*, the residual proportion of maturation of the C4 vertebral body, $\theta$. Considering that $Vba_1$ and $Vba_2$ are the random variables normally distributed, the residual proportion of maturation, $\theta$, is also a random variable, but it is not normally distributed. Consequently, for each value of *Vba*, we reported the median, the first, and the third quartile of $\theta$.

Concerning the validation process, for the *k*-th subject ($k$ = 1, ... N), the gathered information can be summarized considering the set $\mathcal{I}_k = \{(a_i, Vba_i), i = 1, \ldots n_k\}$, where $a_i$ is the age of the subject at the *i*-th radiograph, $Vba_i$ is the corresponding *Vba* value, and $n_k$ is the number of radiographs of the *k*-th subject.

Since our model allowed us to estimate the beginning of the pubertal spurt, $\tau_1$, and the corresponding *Vba* value, $Vba_1$, we can consider $\eta_1 = \min\{Vba_i\colon Vba_i \geq v\}$, i.e., the first radiograph of the subject with *Vba* value greater than $Vba_1$, and $t_1$, the corresponding age of the subject. Subsequently, we evaluated the residual proportion of maturation of the C4 vertebral body $\theta_k = Vba_2 - \eta_1$, and $\Delta\tau$, the time elapsed from $\eta_1$ to $Vba_2$.

Finally, we estimated the expected age for the end of the spurt, $t_2 = t_1 + \Delta\tau$, for the *k*-th subject, the value $\alpha = \min\{a_i\colon a_i \geq t_2, i = 1, \ldots n_k\}$ and $\eta_2$, the corresponding *Vba* value obtained using equation (1): $\eta_2 = Vba(\alpha)$.

If $\eta_2$ belonged to the 95% CI for $Vba_2$, the forecast of the expected end of the pubertal spurt for the *k*-th subject was considered correct (C). If $\eta_2$ resulted in less than the lower limit of the 95% CI for $Vba_2$, but the next observed *Vba* value of the subject, say $\eta_3$, belonged to the 95% CI for $Vba_2$, the forecast was considered slightly underestimated (U). If none of the above conditions was verified, the estimate was considered an incorrect forecast (I). Statistical analyses were performed with the R statistical program [54].

## 3. Results

There were no statistically significant intra-observer differences between paired sets of measurements on re-examined lateral cephalograms, ICC = 0.97 (95%CI, 0.95–0.98). A similar result was obtained considering the agreement between the two observers, ICC = 0.93 (95%CI, 0.89–0.96).

The parameter estimates of the segmented model used to fit the data for both males and females are listed in Table 1, with their standard errors.

**Table 1.** Parameter estimates of the segmented regression model (1) were used to fit the data separately for males and females.

| Coefficients | Males | | Females | |
|---|---|---|---|---|
| | Estimate | Se | Estimate | Se |
| $\beta_0$ | 0.441 | 0.056 | 0.394 | 0.048 |
| $\beta_1$ | 0.024 | 0.007 | 0.028 | 0.006 |
| $\beta_2$ | 0.145 | 0.030 | 0.086 | 0.009 |
| $\beta_3$ | −0.154 | 0.030 | −0.112 | 0.017 |
| cut-offs | | | | |
| $\tau_1$ | 9.679 | 0.213 | 9.384 | 0.241 |
| $\tau_2$ | 11.391 | 0.235 | 13.02 | 0.247 |

The segmented regression equations explained 73% and 86% of the total variance of *Vba* for males and females, respectively.

For males, the two breakpoints, characterizing the higher pubertal development rate, lasted for 1.71 years with a *Vba* increasing rate (slope of the curve) of 0.169 years$^{-1}$ (se = 0.029 years$^{-1}$), Figure 3. The values of *Vba* corresponding to the beginning and the end of the growth spurt were $Vba_1$ = 0.676 (95%CI, 0.642–0.711) and $Vba_2$ = 0.966 (95%CI, 0.905–1.028).

For females, the two breakpoints, characterizing the higher pubertal development rate, lasted for 3.76 years with a *Vba* increasing rate (slope of the curve) of 0.114 years$^{-1}$ (se = 0.007 years). The values of *Vba*, corresponding to the beginning and end of the higher pubertal development rate, were $Vba_1$ = 0.658 (95%CI, 0.634–0.682) and $Vba_2$ = 1.073 (95%CI, 1.044–1.101) respectively. Table 2 reported, for some different values of *Vba*, the corresponding median values of $\theta$ (%) and the median of the time elapsed to the end of the pubertal spurt $\Delta\tau$ (years) with the first and third quartile of its distribution.

**Table 2.** Median, first, and third quartile of the distribution of the residual proportion of the maturation, $\theta$ (%), and the time elapsed to the end of the pubertal spurt, $\Delta\tau$ (years), for the given ratio of projections of the anterior and posterior heights of the C4 vertebral body (*Vba*) in males and females.

| *Vba* | $\theta$ (%) | | | $\Delta\tau$ (Years) | | | *Vba* | $\theta$ (%) | | | $\Delta\tau$ (Years) | | |
|---|---|---|---|---|---|---|---|---|---|---|---|---|---|
| | Q1 | Median | Q3 | Q1 | Median | Q3 | | Q1 | Median | Q3 | Q1 | Median | Q3 |
| **Males** | | | | | | | **Females** | | | | | | |
| 0.67 | 0.95 | 0.99 | 1.00 | 1.57 | 1.81 | 2.10 | 0.65 | 0.99 | 1.00 | 1.03 | 3.55 | 3.73 | 3.92 |
| 0.69 | 0.88 | 0.93 | 0.97 | 1.47 | 1.69 | 1.97 | 0.67 | 0.94 | 0.96 | 0.98 | 3.38 | 3.55 | 3.73 |
| 0.71 | 0.81 | 0.86 | 0.91 | 1.36 | 1.57 | 1.84 | 0.69 | 0.90 | 0.92 | 0.93 | 3.21 | 3.37 | 3.55 |
| 0.73 | 0.75 | 0.80 | 0.85 | 1.25 | 1.46 | 1.71 | 0.71 | 0.85 | 0.87 | 0.88 | 3.04 | 3.19 | 3.36 |
| 0.75 | 0.68 | 0.73 | 0.78 | 1.14 | 1.34 | 1.57 | 0.73 | 0.80 | 0.82 | 0.84 | 2.86 | 3.02 | 3.18 |
| 0.77 | 0.61 | 0.67 | 0.72 | 1.03 | 1.22 | 1.44 | 0.75 | 0.75 | 0.77 | 0.79 | 2.69 | 2.84 | 2.99 |
| 0.79 | 0.55 | 0.60 | 0.66 | 0.92 | 1.10 | 1.31 | 0.77 | 0.70 | 0.72 | 0.74 | 2.52 | 2.66 | 2.81 |
| 0.81 | 0.48 | 0.54 | 0.60 | 0.81 | 0.98 | 1.18 | 0.79 | 0.66 | 0.67 | 0.69 | 2.35 | 2.48 | 2.63 |
| 0.83 | 0.41 | 0.47 | 0.53 | 0.70 | 0.87 | 1.05 | 0.81 | 0.61 | 0.63 | 0.64 | 2.18 | 2.31 | 2.44 |
| 0.85 | 0.35 | 0.41 | 0.47 | 0.59 | 0.75 | 0.93 | 0.83 | 0.56 | 0.58 | 0.60 | 2.00 | 2.13 | 2.26 |
| 0.87 | 0.28 | 0.35 | 0.41 | 0.48 | 0.63 | 0.80 | 0.85 | 0.51 | 0.53 | 0.55 | 1.83 | 1.95 | 2.08 |
| 0.89 | 0.21 | 0.28 | 0.34 | 0.37 | 0.51 | 0.67 | 0.87 | 0.46 | 0.48 | 0.50 | 1.66 | 1.77 | 1.89 |
| 0.91 | 0.15 | 0.22 | 0.28 | 0.25 | 0.39 | 0.55 | 0.89 | 0.41 | 0.43 | 0.45 | 1.49 | 1.60 | 1.71 |
| 0.93 | 0.08 | 0.15 | 0.22 | 0.14 | 0.28 | 0.42 | 0.91 | 0.37 | 0.38 | 0.40 | 1.31 | 1.42 | 1.53 |
| 0.95 | 0.01 | 0.09 | 0.16 | 0.02 | 0.16 | 0.30 | 0.93 | 0.32 | 0.34 | 0.36 | 1.14 | 1.24 | 1.35 |
| | | | | | | | 0.95 | 0.27 | 0.29 | 0.31 | 0.96 | 1.06 | 1.16 |
| | | | | | | | 0.97 | 0.22 | 0.24 | 0.26 | 0.79 | 0.88 | 0.98 |
| | | | | | | | 0.99 | 0.17 | 0.19 | 0.21 | 0.61 | 0.71 | 0.80 |

The results of the validation process are synthesized in Table 3. It shows that our model did not produce any incorrect forecast. Furthermore, although the difference between males and females is not statistically significant, the number of correct forecasts in sampled males is almost twice that of females.

**Table 3.** The frequency distribution of the forecasts of the expected end of the spurt periods using regression model (1) for the 50 subjects belongs to the Michigan Growth Center.

| Sex | Forecast | | |
|---|---|---|---|
| | C | U | I |
| Males | 17 | 8 | 0 |
| Females | 9 | 16 | 0 |

Abbreviation: C, correct forecast; U, slightly underestimated forecast; I, incorrect forecast.

## 4. Discussion

In our study, we analyzed the ratio of the anterior and posterior sides of C4 (*Vba*), and our findings showed the variability of time and the incremental span of *Vba* in the circumpubertal period of life. Therefore, we hypothesized that this incremental span of *Vba* was a potential indicator of the beginning and the end of the pubertal growth spurt and skeletal development.

Segmental regression analysis detected specific *Vba* values at the beginning and the end of the pubertal growth spurt in males and females, which also determined the specific age interval of the spurt in the tested population. The spurt began at nine years and three months old in females and was ahead of males for over four months. The mean ending of the spurt was at twelve years and nine months and was delayed in males for over fourteen months. Different regression models, Bayesian approach, and response surface methodology with statistical potentials in other topics may be a potential statistical tool for fitting an assumed experimental model to data obtained under the chosen design [7,55–59].

One of the limitations of qualitative vertebral cervical methods is identifying the different stages or shapes. Nestman et al. [60] studied CVM reproducibility and observed poor concordance and difficulties in classifying the shapes of C3 and C4 vertebral bodies as trapezoidal, rectangular horizontal, square, or rectangular vertical. Because of those difficulties, the method's reproducibility was tested for clinical use in determining the timing of orthodontic treatment. However, Perinetti et al. [61] reported that visual assessment of CVM appears accurate and repeatable, but stages 4 and 5 require a more careful evaluation. Furthermore, in a systematic review of the reliability of the CVM method to predict pubertal spurt, the authors concluded that although there was a good correlation between hand–wrist and CVM methods, there was a low level of evidence. Therefore, the reliability of the method remained uncertain [62].

The previous observations suggest the need for improvement of current methods by using a different approach that relies more on quantitative measurements rather than comparison based on stages. For example, when comparing *Vba* visually to the CVM stages, it is possible to observe that *Vba* values close to $Vba_1$ correspond to a trapezoidal shape or CVMS II, while *Vba* values of $Vba_2$ or close to 1.00 are more rectangular and, therefore, similar to CVM III. However, the CVM and Cervical Vertebral Maturation Stage (CVMS) methods can only show the stage of the evaluated patient.

The studies that have observed the morphological changes of the cervical vertebral bodies during growth from lateral cephalograms describe a consistent shift from a trapezoidal shape in the initial stages of maturation to a more rectangular shape related to the final stages of maturation [16,17]. Such variations in cervical vertebral body shapes suggest a relationship between the proportions of the posterior and anterior sides of the cervical bodies and the beginning and end of the pubertal growth spurt; the C4 vertebral body was chosen because it is usually clearly visible in the lateral cephalograms. Björk and Helm investigated the age at maximum height growth at puberty in Danish children to determine whether the maximal growth spurt had been reached or passed. They compared the maximum increase in height with age at ossification of the sesamoid of the thumb, and menarche, two specific stages of tooth development: all canines and premolars fully erupted, and all second molars fully erupted. They showed that the maximum growth in height was $18 \pm 3.0$ months and ossification of the ulnar sesamoid of the thumb $21 \pm 3.0$ months ahead in girls compared to boys. The gender difference in tooth development was significantly smaller, with the full eruption of the occlusal level of the canines and premolars being attained only $2 \pm 5.2$ months earlier in girls, while the full eruption of the second molars was earlier in girls by $6 \pm 4.7$ months. The ulnar sesamoid of the thumb was ossified by an average of 12 months before maximum pubertal growth in females and nine months before in males and preceded or coincided with maximum pubertal growth for both sexes.

From a clinical perspective, it would be helpful to obtain more precise information on the residual amount of growth just by calculating an easy-to-measure single variable such as *Vba* since this was not possible with current CVM or CVMS methods. Furthermore, our intra-observer and inter-observer reliability results show excellent concordance due to the ease of measuring precise and visible projections and calculating their proportion, making the method straightforward and practical.

The possible application of dental development analysis to assess pubertal growth spurt compared to skeletal development was compared by Bittencourt et al. [31] in a systematic review and meta-analysis. In the analyzed articles, the authors used skeletal methods according to Greulich-Pyle and Fishman and dental methods according to Nolla, Demirjian, and Moorrees [25]. Half of the research in the meta-analysis indicates a strong correlation between tooth development and skeletal development, identifying the lower canine as the tooth that correlates the most with skeletal development. However, they pragmatically concluded that it is not possible to assess pubertal growth spurt by tooth development [31].

For orthodontic clinicians, the measurements of the posterior and anterior projections of body heights from C4 vertebrae and their ratio *Vba* would allow them to estimate the amount of time remaining for the growth spurt to occur or to determine if it has already passed. However, similar to other growth indicators, it must be used considering the individual variations and using additional information since no method has complete diagnostic reliability in identifying the pubertal growth spurt [27,45,63].

The longitudinal sample of cephalograms taken from the Michigan Growth Center to test the method presented positive results showing no incorrect predictions. However, it suggests that future studies should verify them using a larger sample of longitudinal data with the *Vba* measurement and evaluate the method and its specific cut-offs of *Vba* with other skeletal methods on different samples to test its applicability in clinical practice.

## 5. Conclusions

This study analyzed the ratio of the anterior height projection to the posterior of the C4 vertebral body or *Vba* during childhood, where preadolescence and adolescence occurred, and proved the applicability of *Vba* for estimating the beginning and end of the pubertal growth spurt and in a specific population. Based on the observations, the proposed method estimated the starting cut-off value of *Vba*, $Vba_1$, and the ending cut-off value, $Vba_2$, of the higher pubertal development rate and the residual proportion of *Vba* of C4 maturation, $\theta$ (%), with their standard errors.

The specific results suggest that the cut-off value of *Vba* breakpoints and $\theta$ (%) need to be validated on other available C4 samples of different ethnic and geographical specificities.

**Author Contributions:** Conceptualization, R.C., I.G. and L.F.; methodology, L.F., E.N. and D.K.G.; statistics, L.F.; validation, L.A.V.P. and L.J.; writing—original draft preparation, E.N., I.G., D.J. and L.A.V.P.; writing—reviewing and editing, I.G., L.A.V.P. and H.B. All authors have read and agreed to the published version of the manuscript.

**Funding:** This research was funded by Croatian Science Foundation, grant number IP-2020-02-9423.

**Institutional Review Board Statement:** Not applicable.

**Informed Consent Statement:** Not applicable.

**Conflicts of Interest:** The authors declare no conflict of interest.

## References

1. Baccetti, T.; Franchi, L.; McNamara, J.A., Jr. An improved version of the cervical vertebral maturation (CVM) method for the assessment of mandibular growth. *Angle Orthod.* **2002**, *72*, 316–323. [CrossRef] [PubMed]
2. Baccetti, T.; Franchi, L.; McNamara, J.A., Jr. Treatment and posttreatment craniofacial changes after rapid maxillary expansion and facemask therapy. *Am. J. Orthod. Dentofac. Orthop.* **2000**, *118*, 404–413. [CrossRef] [PubMed]
3. Ball, G.; Woodside, D.; Tompson, B.; Hunter, W.S.; Posluns, J. Relationship between cervical vertebral maturation and mandibular growth. *Am. J. Orthod. Dentofac. Orthop.* **2011**, *139*, e455–e461. [CrossRef]
4. Björk, A.; Krebs, A.; Solow, B. A method for epidemiological registration of malocclusion. *Acta Odontol. Scand.* **1964**, *22*, 27–41. [CrossRef] [PubMed]
5. O'Reilly, M.T.; Yanniello, G.J. Mandibular growth changes and maturation of cervical vertebrae—A longitudinal cephalometric study. *Angle Orthod.* **1988**, *58*, 179–184. [CrossRef]
6. So, L.L. Skeletal maturation of the hand and wrist and its correlation with dental development. *Aust. Orthod. J.* **1997**, *15*, 1–9.
7. Yuan, J.T.; Furdock, R.J.; Benedick, A.; Liu, R.W. Estimating Skeletal Maturity by Segmented Linear Modeling of Key AP Knee Radiographic Parameters. *J. Pediatr. Orthop.* **2022**, *42*, 169–173. [CrossRef] [PubMed]
8. Sahin, R.; Kazadal, C. The Relationship Between Ossification in Metacarpophalangeal Sesamoids of the Thumb and the Period of Puberty: A Radiographic Study. *Medeni. Med. J.* **2022**, *37*, 300–305. [CrossRef]

9. Paschoini, V.L.; Nunes, D.C.; Matias, M.; Nahás-Scocate, A.C.R.; Feres, M.F.N. Accuracy of dental calcification stages for the identification of craniofacial pubertal growth spurt: Proposal of referral parameters. *Eur. Arch. Paediatr. Dent.* **2022**, 1–9. [CrossRef] [PubMed]
10. Szemraj-Folmer, A.; Wojtaszek-Słomińska, A.; Racka-Pilszak, B.; Kuc-Michalska, M. Assessment of the duration of the pubertal growth spurt in patients with skeletal open bite: A cross-sectional study. *J. Orofac. Orthop.* **2021**, *82*, 92–98. [CrossRef]
11. Al Khal, H.A.; Wong, R.W.; Rabie, A.B. Elimination of hand-wrist radiographs for maturity assessment in children needing orthodontic therapy. *Skelet. Radiol.* **2008**, *37*, 195–200. [CrossRef]
12. Hagg, U.; Taranger, J. Skeletal stages of the hand and wrist as indicators of the pubertal growth spurt. *Acta Odontol. Scand.* **1980**, *38*, 187–200. [CrossRef] [PubMed]
13. Dahlberg, P.S.; Mosdol, A.; Ding, Y.; Bleka, O.; Rolseth, V.; Straumann, G.H.; Skjerven-Martinsen, M.; Delaveris, G.J.M.; Vist, G.E. A systematic review of the agreement between chronological age and skeletal age based on the Greulich and Pyle atlas. *Eur. Radiol.* **2019**, *29*, 2936–2948. [CrossRef]
14. Bjork, A.; Helm, S. Prediction of the age of maximum puberal growth in body height. *Angle Orthod.* **1967**, *37*, 134–143. [CrossRef]
15. Fekonja, A. Evaluation of the eruption of permanent teeth and their association with malocclusion. *Clin. Exp. Dent. Res.* **2022**, *8*, 836–842. [CrossRef] [PubMed]
16. Fishman, L.S. Maturational patterns and prediction during adolescence. *Angle Orthod.* **1987**, *57*, 178–193. [CrossRef] [PubMed]
17. Lamparski, D.G. Skeletal age assessment utilizing cervical vertebrae. *Am. J. Orthod.* **1975**, *67*, 458–459. [CrossRef]
18. Hassel, B.; Farman, A.G. Skeletal maturation evaluation using cervical vertebrae. *Am. J. Orthod. Dentofac. Orthop.* **1995**, *107*, 58–66. [CrossRef]
19. Franchi, L.; Baccetti, T.; McNamara, J.A., Jr. Mandibular growth as related to cervical vertebral maturation and body height. *Am. J. Orthod. Dentofac. Orthop.* **2000**, *118*, 335–340. [CrossRef]
20. Thomas, L.A.; Thomas, L.R.; Balla, S.B.; Gopalaiah, H.; Kanaparthi, A.; Sai Sravanthi, G.; Palla, A.; Galic, I. Above or below 14 years? An orthopantomographic study based on chronological course of eruption of mandibular premolars and second molars in a sample of south Indian children. *Leg. Med.* **2021**, *48*, 101814. [CrossRef] [PubMed]
21. Kelmendi, J.; Cameriere, R.; Kocani, F.; Galic, I.; Mehmeti, B.; Vodanovic, M. The third molar maturity index in indicating the legal adult age in Kosovar population. *Int. J. Leg. Med.* **2018**, *132*, 1151–1159. [CrossRef]
22. Rozylo-Kalinowska, I.; Kalinowski, P.; Kozek, M.; Galic, I.; Cameriere, R. Validity of the third molar maturity index I(3M) for indicating the adult age in the Polish population. *Forensic Sci. Int.* **2018**, *290*, 352.e1–352.e6. [CrossRef] [PubMed]
23. Balla, S.B.; Banda, T.R.; Galic, I.; Naga, N.M.; Naishadham, P.P. Validation of Cameriere's third molar maturity index alone and in combination with apical maturity of permanent mandibular second molar for indicating legal age of 14 years in a sample of South Indian children. *Forensic Sci. Int.* **2019**, *297*, 243–248. [CrossRef] [PubMed]
24. Balla, S.B.; Chinni, S.S.; Galic, I.; Alwala, A.M.; Machani, P.; Cameriere, R. A cut-off value of third molar maturity index for indicating a minimum age of criminal responsibility: Older or younger than 16 years? *J. Forensic Leg. Med.* **2019**, *65*, 108–112. [CrossRef] [PubMed]
25. da Luz, L.C.P.; Anzulovic, D.; Benedicto, E.N.; Galic, I.; Brkic, H.; Biazevic, M.G.H. Accuracy of four dental age estimation methodologies in Brazilian and Croatian children. *Sci. Justice* **2019**, *59*, 442–447. [CrossRef] [PubMed]
26. Galic, I.; Pacifici, A.; Carbone, D.; Pacifici, L.; Jeroncic, A.; Cameriere, R. Age estimation by the Cameriere's normalized measurements (CNM) of the single permanent mandibular tooth on a panoramic radiograph. *Leg. Med.* **2017**, *26*, 65–72. [CrossRef]
27. Brkic, H.; Galic, I.; Vodanovic, M.; Dumancic, J.; Mehdi, F.; Anic Milosevic, S. The Cameriere, Haavikko, Demirjian, and Willems methods for the assessment of dental age in Croatian children. *Int. J. Leg. Med.* **2022**, *136*, 1685–1696. [CrossRef] [PubMed]
28. Galic, I.; Vodanovic, M.; Jankovic, S.; Mihanovic, F.; Nakas, E.; Prohic, S.; Galic, E.; Brkic, H. Dental age estimation on Bosnian-Herzegovinian children aged 6–14 years: Evaluation of Chaillet's international maturity standards. *J. Forensic Leg. Med.* **2013**, *20*, 40–45. [CrossRef] [PubMed]
29. Galic, I.; Vodanovic, M.; Cameriere, R.; Nakas, E.; Galic, E.; Selimovic, E.; Brkic, H. Accuracy of Cameriere, Haavikko, and Willems radiographic methods on age estimation on Bosnian-Herzegovian children age groups 6–13. *Int. J. Leg. Med.* **2011**, *125*, 315–321. [CrossRef] [PubMed]
30. Dadgar, S.; Hadian, H.; Ghobadi, M.; Sobouti, F.; Rakhshan, V. Correlations among chronological age, cervical vertebral maturation index, and Demirjian developmental stage of the maxillary and mandibular canines and second molars. *Surg. Radiol. Anat.* **2021**, *43*, 131–143. [CrossRef]
31. Bittencourt, M.V.; Cericato, G.; Franco, A.; Girão, R.; Lima, A.P.B.; Paranhos, L. Accuracy of dental development for estimating the pubertal growth spurt in comparison to skeletal development: A systematic review and meta-analysis. *Dentomaxillofac. Radiol.* **2018**, *47*, 20170362. [CrossRef] [PubMed]
32. Wittschieber, D.; Vieth, V.; Wierer, T.; Pfeiffer, H.; Schmeling, A. Cameriere's approach modified for pelvic radiographs: A novel method to assess apophyseal iliac crest ossification for the purpose of forensic age diagnostics. *Int. J. Leg. Med.* **2013**, *127*, 825–829. [CrossRef]
33. Cameriere, R.; Brogi, G.; Ferrante, L.; Mirtella, D.; Vultaggio, C.; Cingolani, M.; Fornaciari, G. Reliability in age determination by pulp/tooth ratio in upper canines in skeletal remains. *J. Forensic Sci.* **2006**, *51*, 861–864. [CrossRef]

34. Cameriere, R.; Cingolani, M.; Giuliodori, A.; De Luca, S.; Ferrante, L. Radiographic analysis of epiphyseal fusion at knee joint to assess likelihood of having attained 18 years of age. *Int. J. Leg. Med.* **2012**, *126*, 889–899. [CrossRef] [PubMed]
35. Cameriere, R.; Cunha, E.; Wasterlain, S.N.; De Luca, S.; Sassaroli, E.; Pagliara, F.; Nuzzolese, E.; Cingolani, M.; Ferrante, L. Age estimation by pulp/tooth ratio in lateral and central incisors by peri-apical X-ray. *J. Forensic Leg. Med.* **2013**, *20*, 530–536. [CrossRef] [PubMed]
36. Cameriere, R.; De Angelis, D.; Ferrante, L.; Scarpino, F.; Cingolani, M. Age estimation in children by measurement of open apices in teeth: A European formula. *Int. J. Leg. Med.* **2007**, *121*, 449–453. [CrossRef]
37. Cameriere, R.; Ferrante, L.; Cingolani, M. Age estimation in children by measurement of open apices in teeth. *Int. J. Leg. Med.* **2006**, *120*, 49–52. [CrossRef]
38. Cameriere, R.; Ferrante, L.; De Angelis, D.; Scarpino, F.; Galli, F. The comparison between measurement of open apices of third molars and Demirjian stages to test chronological age of over 18 year olds in living subjects. *Int. J. Leg. Med.* **2008**, *122*, 493–497. [CrossRef]
39. Cameriere, R.; Ferrante, L.; Mirtella, D.; Cingolani, M. Carpals and epiphyses of radius and ulna as age indicators. *Int. J. Leg. Med.* **2006**, *120*, 143–146. [CrossRef] [PubMed]
40. Cameriere, R.; Giuliodori, A.; Zampi, M.; Galic, I.; Cingolani, M.; Pagliara, F.; Ferrante, L. Age estimation in children and young adolescents for forensic purposes using fourth cervical vertebra (C4). *Int. J. Leg. Med.* **2015**, *129*, 347–355. [CrossRef]
41. Cameriere, R.; Scendoni, R.; Ferrante, L.; Mirtella, D.; Oncini, L.; Cingolani, M. An Effective Model for Estimating Age in Unaccompanied Minors under the Italian Legal System. *Healthcare* **2023**, *11*, 224. [CrossRef]
42. Zolotenkova, G.V.; Rogachev, A.I.; Pigolkin, Y.I.; Edelev, I.S.; Borshchevskaya, V.N.; Cameriere, R. Age Classification in Forensic Medicine Using Machine Learning Techniques. *Sovrem. Tekhnol. V Meditsine* **2022**, *14*, 15–22. [CrossRef]
43. Spinas, E.; Melis, G.; Zerman, N.; De Luca, S.; Cameriere, R. Age Assessment in Children and Adolescents by Measuring the Open Apices in Teeth: A New Sardinian Formula. *Dent. J.* **2022**, *10*, 50. [CrossRef]
44. Scendoni, R.; Ribeiro, I.L.A.; Cingolani, M.; Giovagnoni, A.; Curzi, M.; Fedeli, P.; Cameriere, R. A new analytical cut-off point for determining 18 years of age using MRI on medial clavicular epiphysis. *Leg. Med.* **2022**, *54*, 102010. [CrossRef]
45. Pereira, C.P.; Belo, C.; Sardinha, J.; Santos, R.; Salvado, F.; Cameriere, R. Quantitative and Qualitative Approaches for Dental Age Assessment in Sub Adult Portuguese Population: European Regression Formula and Demirjian Stages. *Acta Stomatol. Croat.* **2022**, *56*, 288–298. [CrossRef] [PubMed]
46. Kihara, E.; Galic, I.; Nyamunga, D.; Mehdi, F.; Velandia Palacio, L.A.; Cameriere, R. Validation of the Italian, European, North German, Malaysian, and South African black formulas on Cameriere method using panoramic radiographs in Kenyan children. *Int. J. Leg. Med.* **2022**, *136*, 1495–1506. [CrossRef]
47. Angelakopoulos, N.; De Luca, S.; Oliveira-Santos, I.; Ribeiro, I.L.A.; Bianchi, I.; Balla, S.B.; Kis, H.C.; Jimenez, L.G.; Zolotenkova, G.; Yusof, M.Y.P.; et al. Third molar maturity index (I(3M)) assessment according to different geographical zones: A large multi-ethnic study sample. *Int. J. Leg. Med.* **2022**. [CrossRef] [PubMed]
48. Palmela Pereira, C.; Rodrigues, A.; Santos, A.; Salvado, F.; Santos, R.; Cameriere, R. Cut-off for the legal ages in the Portuguese Population by Third Maturity Index: Measures of Accuracy. *Arch. Oral Biol.* **2021**, *125*, 105089. [CrossRef]
49. Angelakopoulos, N.; Galic, I.; Balla, S.B.; Kis, H.C.; Gomez Jimenez, L.; Zolotenkova, G.; Mohd Yusof, M.Y.P.; Hadzic Selmanagic, A.; Pandey, H.; Palmela Pereira, C.; et al. Comparison of the third molar maturity index (I(3M)) between left and right lower third molars to assess the age of majority: A multi-ethnic study sample. *Int. J. Leg. Med.* **2021**, *135*, 2423–2436. [CrossRef]
50. Gulsahi, A.; Cehreli, S.B.; Galic, I.; Ferrante, L.; Cameriere, R. Age estimation in Turkish children and young adolescents using fourth cervical vertebra. *Int. J. Leg. Med.* **2020**, *134*, 1823–1829. [CrossRef] [PubMed]
51. World Medical, A. World Medical Association Declaration of Helsinki: Ethical principles for medical research involving human subjects. *JAMA* **2013**, *310*, 2191–2194. [CrossRef]
52. Ferrante, L.; Cameriere, R. Statistical methods to assess the reliability of measurements in the procedures for forensic age estimation. *Int. J. Leg. Med.* **2009**, *123*, 277–283. [CrossRef]
53. Muggeo, V.M. Estimating regression models with unknown break-points. *Stat. Med.* **2003**, *22*, 3055–3071. [CrossRef]
54. R Core Team R. *R: A Language and Environment for Statistical Computing*; R Core Team R.: Vienna, Austria, 2020.
55. Sodeifian, G.; Ansari, K. Optimization of Ferulago Angulata oil extraction with supercritical carbon dioxide. *J. Supercrit. Fluids* **2011**, *57*, 38–43. [CrossRef]
56. Sodeifian, G.; Ardestani, N.S.; Sajadian, S.A.; Ghorbandoost, S. Application of supercritical carbon dioxide to extract essential oil from Cleome coluteoides Boiss: Experimental, response surface and grey wolf optimization methodology. *J. Supercrit. Fluids* **2016**, *114*, 55–63. [CrossRef]
57. Faragalli, A.; Skrami, E.; Bucci, A.; Gesuita, R.; Cameriere, R.; Carle, F.; Ferrante, L. Combining Bayesian Calibration and Copula Models for Age Estimation. *Int. J. Environ. Res. Public Health* **2023**, *20*, 1201. [CrossRef]
58. Cameriere, R.; De Luca, S.; Soriano Vazquez, I.; Kis, H.C.; Pigolkin, Y.; Kumagai, A.; Ferrante, L. A full Bayesian calibration model for assessing age in adults by means of pulp/tooth area ratio in periapical radiography. *Int. J. Leg. Med.* **2021**, *135*, 677–685. [CrossRef] [PubMed]
59. Ferrante, L.; Skrami, E.; Gesuita, R.; Cameriere, R. Bayesian calibration for forensic age estimation. *Stat. Med.* **2015**, *34*, 1779–1790. [CrossRef]

60. Nestman, T.S.; Marshall, S.D.; Qian, F.; Holton, N.; Franciscus, R.G.; Southard, T.E. Cervical vertebrae maturation method morphologic criteria: Poor reproducibility. *Am. J. Orthod. Dentofac. Orthop.* **2011**, *140*, 182–188. [CrossRef]
61. Perinetti, G.; Perillo, L.; Franchi, L.; Di Lenarda, R.; Contardo, L. Maturation of the middle phalanx of the third finger and cervical vertebrae: A comparative and diagnostic agreement study. *Orthod. Craniofac. Res.* **2014**, *17*, 270–279. [CrossRef]
62. Santiago, R.C.; de Miranda Costa, L.F.; Vitral, R.W.; Fraga, M.R.; Bolognese, A.M.; Maia, L.C. Cervical vertebral maturation as a biologic indicator of skeletal maturity. *Angle Orthod.* **2012**, *82*, 1123–1131. [CrossRef]
63. Perinetti, G.; Contardo, L. Reliability of Growth Indicators and Efficiency of Functional Treatment for Skeletal Class II Malocclusion: Current Evidence and Controversies. *BioMed Res. Int.* **2017**, *2017*, 1367691. [CrossRef]

applied sciences

MDPI

Article

# Multiscale Evaluation of Jaw Geometry Reproduction Obtained Via the Use of Selected Orthodontic Materials in Dental Implants and Orthodontics—In Vitro Case Study

**Michał Jakubowicz, Bartosz Gapiński *, Lidia Marciniak-Podsadna, Michał Mendak, Patryk Mietliński and Michał Wieczorowski**

Division of Metrology and Measurement Systems, Institute of Mechanical Technology, Faculty of Mechanical Engineering, Poznan University of Technology, 5 M. Skłodowska-Curie Square, 60-965 Poznan, Poland
* Correspondence: bartosz.gapinski@put.poznan.pl

**Abstract:** In this paper, the multiscale analysis of the reproduction accuracy of jaw geometry obtained via the use of selected orthodontic materials is discussed. Impressions were made from two types of impression material. An accuracy assessment of the model geometry mapping was performed using noncontact systems, including a fringe projection optical 3D scanner, computed tomography, and a focus variation microscope. Measurements were made in three modes for comparison, as were the silicone and polyether impression materials. These modes were a jaw model and impression, an impression and plaster model, and plaster and jaw models. The research results are presented as colorful maps of deviations. Data analysis showed that deviations were the smallest in the case of silicone and that the best fit occurred between the silicone impression and the plaster model. The conducted research confirmed the validity of the assumptions considering the use of multiscale analysis for geometric analysis. The use of modern multiscale measurement methods allows for shorter and more efficient prosthetic operations. At present, these devices are expensive and complicated to use, but developments in technology should simplify the process, and prosthetic professionals should be aware of the possibilities described in the paper.

**Keywords:** biomedical engineering; focus variation microscope; fringe projection optical 3D scanner; multiscale analysis; orthodontics material; X-ray computed tomography

**Citation:** Jakubowicz, M.; Gapiński, B.; Marciniak-Podsadna, L.; Mendak, M.; Mietliński, P.; Wieczorowski, M. Multiscale Evaluation of Jaw Geometry Reproduction Obtained Via the Use of Selected Orthodontic Materials in Dental Implants and Orthodontics—In Vitro Case Study. *Appl. Sci.* **2023**, *13*, 6932. https://doi.org/10.3390/app13126932

Academic Editor: Vittorio Checchi

Received: 25 February 2023
Revised: 2 June 2023
Accepted: 4 June 2023
Published: 8 June 2023



## 1. Introduction

Currently, implantoprosthetic orthodontics and other fields of dentistry are experiencing rapid progression [1–5]. These implants use dental models created based on a matrix of impressions [6] and are produced when it is necessary to use braces to correct malocclusion, insert implants, crowns, or bridges.

The main task of the impression is to accurately reproduce the shape, size, and position of the teeth in dental arches in order to produce the most accurate model on the corresponding matrix. Consequently, impression materials should fulfil a number of conditions. Requirements for such materials among doctors and dental technicians include environmental inertness, ease of preparation, adequate flow properties, appropriate and short setting time in the mouth, the possibility of adjusting the setting time, easy release of the impression, the accurate reproduction of details, resistance to the negative effects of body fluids, low cost of the materials and instrumentation used, ease of disinfection, compatibility with casting materials, and obtaining plaster models with a smooth surface [7–11]. For the patient, it is important that the impression material has a pleasant taste and is nontoxic, stays in the mouth for a short time, and is quickly and easily removed from the mouth [12].

In order to meet the requirements of patients and to enable the dentist and technician to reliably do their jobs, it is important to implement modern technologies that speed up and streamline prosthetic operations. This measure will allow the finished product to be made without the need for additional processing. Full standardization of operations, however, is hampered by the great diversity of clinical cases. This diversity often requires additional machining of pre-prepared prostheses. The use of modern technology through multiscale digitization will allow the design and manufacture of work in a way that reduces the need for the postprocessing and correction of finished dental prostheses. In this way, the patient's final visit to the dentist's office during the denture seating process will be significantly reduced.

A very important issue is the geometric accuracy of the mapped jaw [13,14]. The geometric accuracy of the impression is influenced by a great number of factors: the impression technique, the impression method, the type of impression tray, and the types and properties of the impression compounds [15,16]. Accurate reproduction of the jaw geometry, position, and shape of the teeth are very important to precisely match components produced by technicians who are not in direct contact with the patient or the teeth and other anatomical structures situated in the patient's mouth. Aesthetics and comfort are very important to the patient [17]. More than a dozen materials are available on the market with different properties, applications, and mapping accuracy.

The most commonly used impression materials are increasingly being replaced by other methods of mapping jaw geometry [18,19]. One of these methods is the use of an oral scanner [20–23], which allows precise digital models of the dentition to be made without the need to use impression materials [24]. Optical scanners with various digitization techniques included in CAD/CAM systems are also used in dentistry [21]. Most of these systems are used for scanning models in prosthetic laboratories. In recent years, digital imaging techniques have evolved greatly, enabling the development of new systems capable of capturing three-dimensional images of prepared teeth in the patient's mouth [25,26]. Nevertheless, the most popular and widely used methods in dental practice continue to employ classic impression materials.

The authors in [27] presented 3D scanning methods commonly used in dentistry. The authors also described the advantages of using these methods. The authors in [28] presented a literature review on the application of micro-CT in bioengineering applications. The use of micro-CT for bone analysis was presented in [29,30]. However, an analysis of recent literature did not find a comprehensive research approach for the multiscale evaluation of jaw geometry reproduction using a 3D scanner, micro-CT, or focus variation microscope. Such data fusion is a novel approach that could provide many benefits to dental science.

Accuracy analyses of materials used in dental implants and orthodontics have been performed. Studies on the accuracy of geometry mapping were presented, for example, by the authors in [31–35]. These studies, however, were primarily directed towards macroscale geometry analysis. Microscale measurements were directed at determining the surface roughness parameters of orthodontic arches made of different materials [9].

Length and angle metrology has also been undergoing intensive development for many years. This development is linked to the Industry 4.0 strategy in which angle metrology indirectly fits [36]. One of the key trends in 4.0 metrology is the use of multisensor and multiscale analysis [36–38]. The use of different sensors makes it possible to acquire data using different techniques. Each sensor provides a different set of information, and the combination of these data gives full multiscale information [39]. All this information is based on coordinate metrology, which is a technique that involves measuring geometric features. While this technique is commonly associated with largescale measurements considered to be macro, it also applies to smaller scales such as the nano- and microscale, where this method can measure surface irregularities, as well as the intermediate (meso-) scale, where it can measure the transition between irregularities and geometric features. As dimensions become smaller, the boundaries between scales become blurry, and it is important to analyze the object being measured across all scales to obtain a complete picture.

Therefore, metrological verification must include measuring geometric features and shapes, as well as surface roughness, to provide a holistic view of the object being measured.

The aim of the research presented in this article was to confirm the desirability of using state-of-the-art measuring CMs operating at different scales to comprehensively evaluate the representation of jaw geometry obtained using selected orthodontic materials. Such a comprehensive approach has not been presented before, which is the novelty of this article. The increasing demands of patients and the expectations of dentists and dental technicians mean that extensive multiscale examinations should become a common procedure in the near future. The use of a multiscale approach to measurement allows the fusion of data describing different areas of information. Macroscale measurements describe the jaw geometry, the shape and position of individual teeth, as well as the position of teeth relative to each other. The micro-CT examination also allows the impression to be measured together with the jaw model and evaluated without physical separation. Due to its resolution, this method also allows the evaluation of details "invisible" to a 3D scanner. On the other hand, the measurement of surface topography with a focus variation microscope allows a very precise evaluation of the surface for all types of elements measured. The complete data include a set of triangle meshes (STLs) that can be interconnected, enabling the microscale data to be position-defined (specific position) using the macroscale data. This approach also allows the impression material to be assessed in relation to "large flat" tooth surfaces and hard-to-reach areas.

## 2. Materials and Methods

The primary objective of the presented research task was to analyze the representation accuracy of the geometric features of the human jaw obtained with selected orthodontic materials using contactless measurement methods on a macro- and microscale. For this purpose, photogrammetric methods, computed tomography, and noncontact methods for measuring surface topography were used. Other goals were to apply reverse engineering and rapid prototyping technology to obtain a model of the jaws [40]. The final result is a multiscale analysis directly in line with the idea of Industry 4.0.

This type of research can significantly contribute to new advanced diagnostic methods and allow the construction of implants and prostheses of cartilage–skeletal elements to be accelerated and greatly simplified.

The scope of the present research was as follows:

- Measurements of the jaw model geometry (photogrammetric method, micro-CT);
- Preparation of impressions with selected types of orthodontic impression compounds;
- Measurements of the impression geometry obtained using the photogrammetric method;
- Application of reverse engineering to obtain digital models of the examined jaws;
- Application of rapid prototyping technology (3D printing) to obtain models;
- Casting of plaster models of the jaws using dental plaster;
- Measurements of impression geometry obtained using nonmedical computed tomography;
- Measurements of the obtained plaster models and models obtained via 3D printing;
- Surface structure measurements of selected dental impressions and gypsum models.

The dentition geometry obtained via orthodontic impression materials, photogrammetric measurement systems that allow imaging, and evaluation of the entire element surface on a macroscale are very effective at verifying reproduction accuracy [41–44]. Photogrammetric methods refer to the techniques used for obtaining measurements and information about objects and features from photographs or images. Such techniques are noncontact, nondestructive, and nonintrusive methods of data acquisition that have many applications in various fields. Length metrology involves measuring elements of the characteristic features of an object encoded in the form of markers and points, lines, or stripes projected onto the object. Photogrammetric measurement methods work on the principle of triangulation, so the geometric relationships present in a triangle are used to measure distance [45,46].

Photogrammetric methods make it possible to measure the geometric features of individual elements made of different materials such as the jaw model, the orthodontic impression, and the obtained plaster model of the dentition [47].

It should be emphasized that dental plaster, which reproduces the arrangement of the jaw based on the orthodontic impressions made, is subject to shrinkage and deformation during drying and may be damaged during the separation of the plaster model from the impression [48,49]. In this case, spatial analysis of plaster models of the jaws without separating them from the impression is possible through the use of a CT scanner [50,51]. Tomographic measurements are carried out using X-rays that are attenuated as they pass through the object under examination, creating an X-ray image. Computed tomography has been used in medicine since the 1970s. However, only micro-CT offers resolutions suitable for the analyses presented in this article [52]. It is possible to evaluate the components in an assembly and virtually detach them, which allows assessment of the actual adhesion of the impression materials to the tooth surface. Unfortunately, micro-CT is not adapted to the examination of a living person like a classic CT device, so studies conducted on applied models were necessary. During the examination, a series of images were taken at different angular positions to obtain a spatial image [53]. The study used a micro-CT device, which allows for data with better resolution than that under commonly used medical CT scanners [54]. Based on the volumetric image (after a thoroughly prepared calibration [55]), it becomes possible to analyze both the geometric deformation of surfaces under examination and the reproduction accuracy shape of the dentition by means of a plaster material. For some applications, optical scanners and computed tomographs give very similar results, as demonstrated by comparative analysis [56].

An important aspect of a jaw mapping evaluation with impression materials is measurements describing the surface structure on a microscale [9]. Such measurements provide evidence of mapped surface quality [57], which has a significant impact on the aesthetics of the fabrication of, for example, dental prostheses. Assessment of the surface structure linked to microscale shape analysis is made possible by focal differentiation microscopy. The principle of focus variation microscopy is based on using the sharpness of a surface image in an optical microscope to assess the change in surface roughness. The object to be measured is illuminated with a light with suitable modulation, transmitted through the optics and focused on the surface to be measured. The reflected light is returned through the optics and recorded by a digital detector searching for the focused beam. The image of the surface is shaped by the optical system allowing both photometric (brightness, color, etc.) and geometric (distance and shape) information to be obtained. An integral feature of this method is the existence of a focused image surface (FIS), defined as a surface formed by a cloud of points for which the camera lens allows a focused light beam to be obtained. According to the principles and theory of geometrical optics, there is a direct relationship between the shape of the real object and the shape of its image focus surface, making it possible to derive the shape of the object surface (or its irregularities) from the shape of the FIS [57].

Figure 1 shows a general block diagram of the measurement path incorporating the three noncontact measurement methods that form the basis of the multiscale analysis presented in this article. Based on measurements, the data obtained in the form of a point cloud were further processed and optimized. The point clouds corresponding to the measurement data were subjected to a polygonization process. This process involves building a model in the form of a triangle mesh with vertices located at each point in the set, thereby generating files in the STL format and creating 3D models of the measured objects. Digitalization of each object using an optical scanner produced multiple individual scans that had to be automatically combined using an intelligent algorithm based on surface matching and a combination of reference points to obtain the most complete model possible. For the measured impression data obtained to be compared with the jaw model and the plaster models, they had to undergo an inversion operation, i.e., a symmetrical outward extension along the vertical axis. This ensured that all measurements were for convex objects.

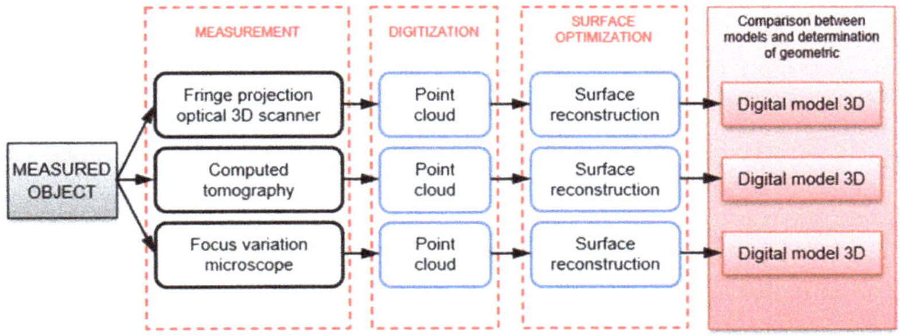


**Figure 1.** General block diagram of the measurement path including the three contactless measurement methods that form the basis of the multiscale analysis.

Two software programs were used to analyze the obtained measurement data. The macroscale analysis was carried out using the GOM Inspect Professional (GOM GmbH, Braunschweig, Germany) program, while the microscale analysis was carried out using the MountainsMap (Digital Surf® Headquarters, Besançon, France) software. The results of the comparisons are presented in the form of a color map, where deviations in inspection points are represented by a scale. A diagram of the measurements and analyses carried out is shown in Figure 2. As can be seen, the entire research task was divided into a series of analyses, from which four main stages of work were identified. The following paper presents a synthesis and selected examples of the completed research.

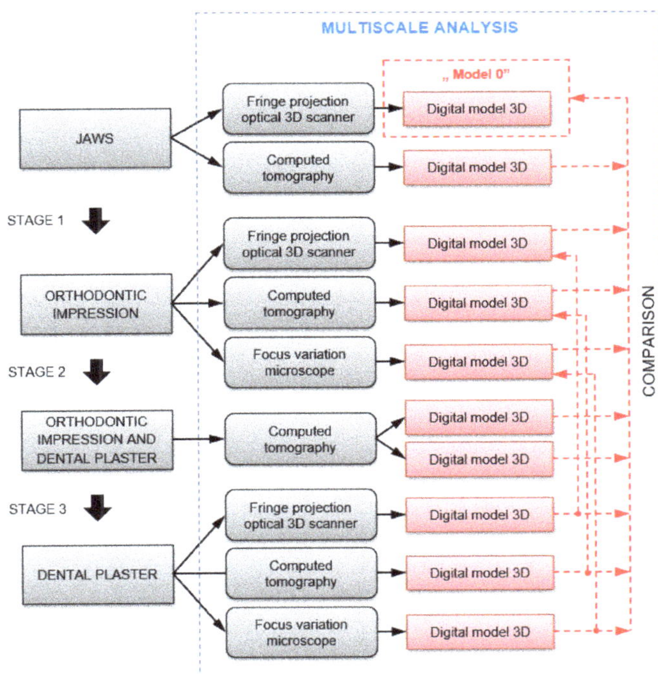


**Figure 2.** Flow chart of the measurements and analyses carried out.

## 3. Results and Discussion

The research presented in this paper was based on a dental model of the upper part of the human jaw (Figure 3). Prior to use, the model was measured using an GOM ATOS Core 185 (GOM GmbH, Braunschweig, Germany) photogrammetric measurement system, which was adopted as the base model in the further comparative analyses "Model 0". Additionally, the base model was digitized using a GE Phoenix v | tome | x s240 (Waygate Technologies, Wunstorf, German) micro-CT device to complete the measurement information with surfaces inaccessible to scanning with structured light.

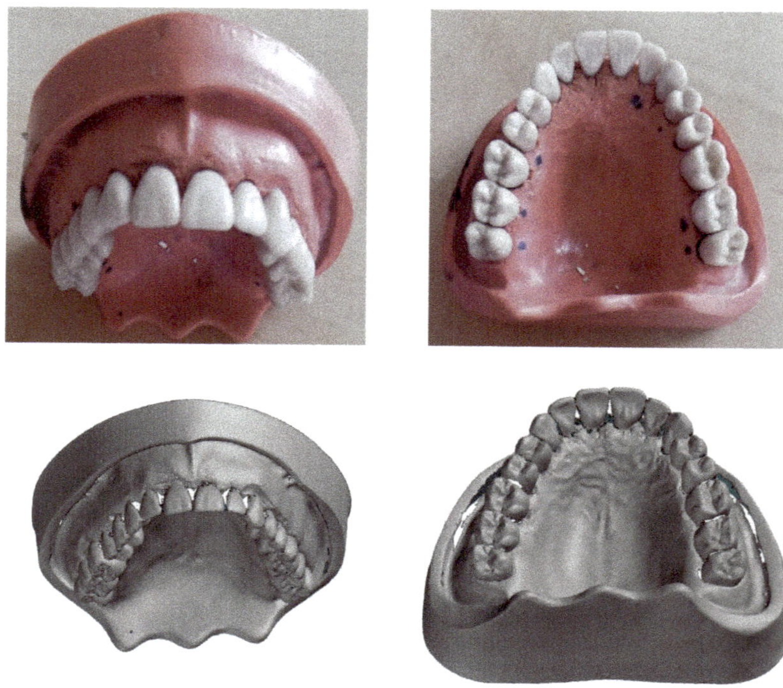

(**a**) (**b**)

**Figure 3.** Dental model of the lower part of human jaw: (**a**) Actual view; (**b**) Digital "model 0".

The next step was to prepare impressions on the human jaw model. The following impression compounds were used in the study: silicone—Express XT Penta Putty (3M Oral Care, St. Paul, MN, USA) and Polyether Impregum Penta (3M Oral Care, St. Paul, MN, USA) (Figure 4). A geometric evaluation of the models obtained using different dental materials was presented by the authors in [31–35]. The present study focuses on a multiscale analysis of the objects considered.

The finished impressions were measured using a photogrammetric measuring system and micro-CT. Plaster models were then cast using Stodent Class II dental plaster (Zhermack S.p.A., Badia Polesine, Italy) (Figure 5). Once the plaster had set, the models were measured using micro-CT before being removed from the impression to identify defects resulting from the separation of the impression compound and the plaster model. The plaster models, after removal from the impressions, were finally measured using an optical scanner and micro-CT.

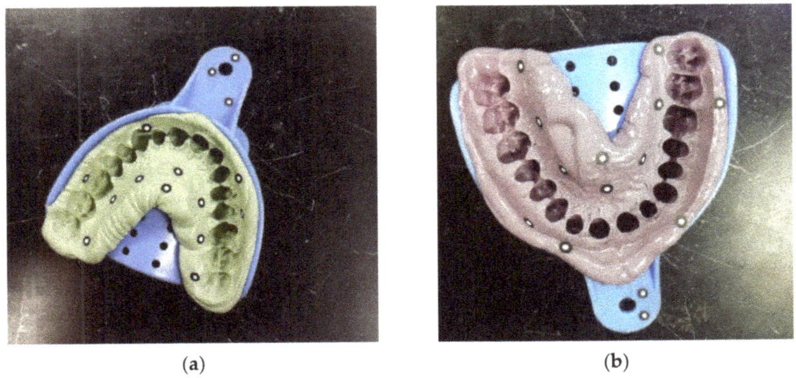

**Figure 4.** Dental impressions from silicone material (**a**) and polyether material (**b**).

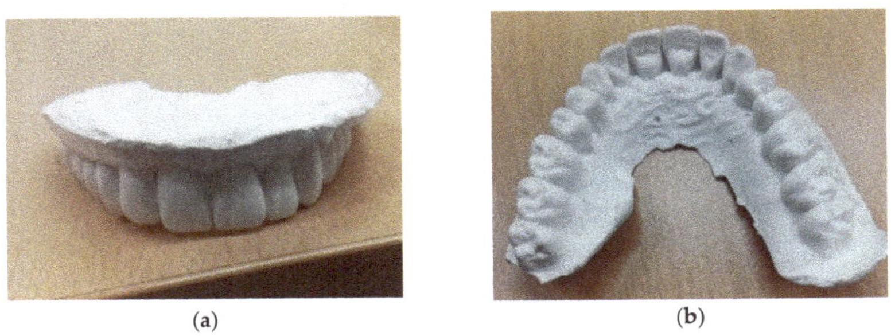

**Figure 5.** Example of a plaster model of a jaw: (**a**) Front view; (**b**) Top view.

As part of the research carried out, we attempted to replace plaster materials with models produced using 3D printing (Figure 6) [40]. The use of rapid prototyping technology allows models to be made based on a jaw's digitized model, which avoids defects associated with the drying process of a model made from dental plaster and from damage caused in the process of separating the plaster model from the impression. The models created during the 3D printing process were made using a ZORTRAX M200 Plus (Zortrax S.A. Olsztyn, Poland) printer.

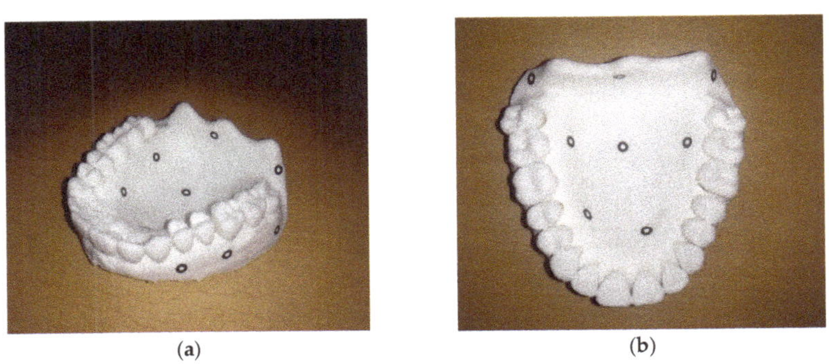

**Figure 6.** Example of a jaw model made using a 3D printer: (**a**) Side view; (**b**) Top view.

As already mentioned, the scanning on the 3D optical scanner resulted in raw data in the form of a point cloud. This model was transformed into a triangular network after polygonization. Some areas of the model were difficult to digitize, such as the interdental spaces and the border between the teeth and the gum. The source of these difficulties lies in the complex geometry of elements, which consists of freeform surfaces arranged in such a way that they become an obstacle for measurements using the optical method. The inability to measure these zones resulted in some gaps in the model. Some of these gaps were closed with special algorithms to estimate the area based on the neighboring rows of triangles around the gap. In other words, in areas where it was not possible to record measured points, the area was calculated mathematically. Not all gaps could be closed, as further modifications to the model would lead to a loss of accuracy. In the case of the model obtained using the CT scanner, a full representation of the jaw model was achieved. Nevertheless, the model from the 3D scanner was adopted as a reference due to its overall higher accuracy. Figure 7 shows a comparison of the two models, with one obtained from the 3D scanner and the other from the micro-CT.

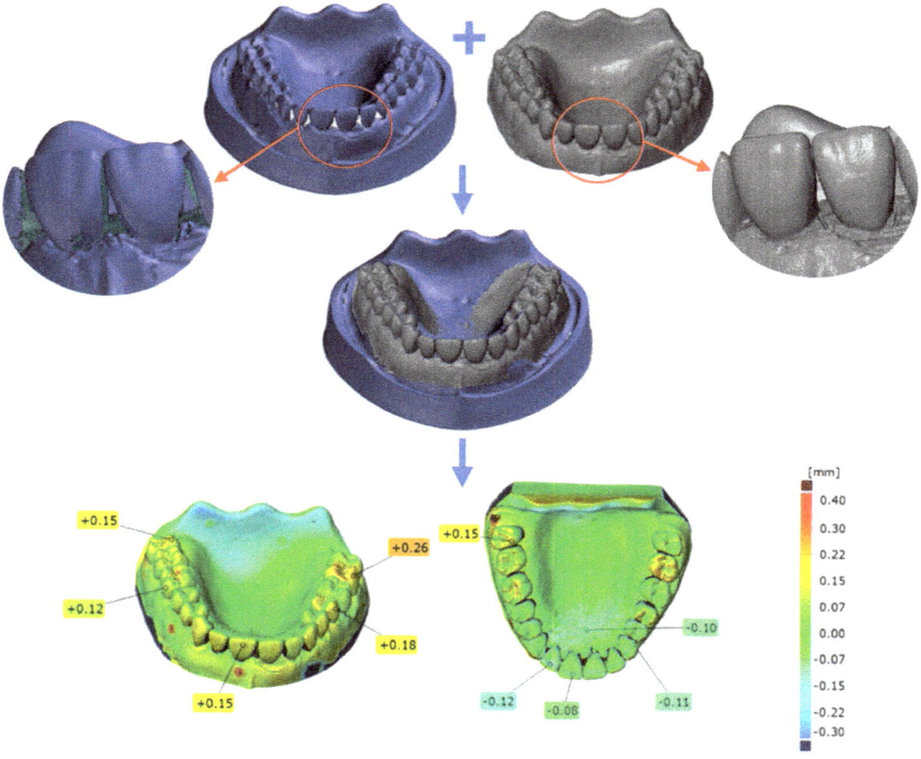


**Figure 7.** Comparison of jaw models digitized on an optical 3D scanner and micro-CT.

Figure 7 shows that the deviations between the 3D scanner and micro-CT ranged from −0.12 mm to 0.26 mm. This result demonstrates the scale of possible misunderstanding related to component deformation at the beginning of the analysis and the importance of accurately defining the reference element.

As previously mentioned, different orthodontic impressions were made based on a real jaw model. Both were digitized using different measurement methods: a 3D scanner and CT scanner. Each digitized piece was compared with the "0 model". A color deviation map is shown in Figure 8 for the silicone material and in Figure 9 for the polyether material.

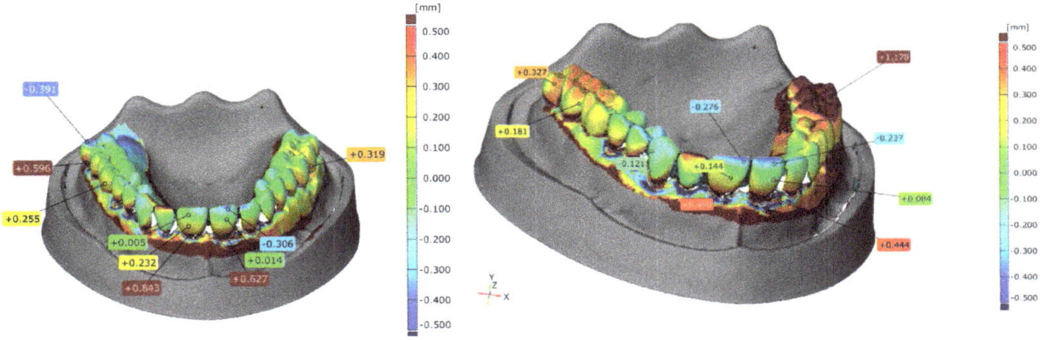


(**a**) (**b**)

**Figure 8.** Comparison of scans of the silicone impression obtained on an optical 3D scanner (**a**) and micro-CT (**b**).

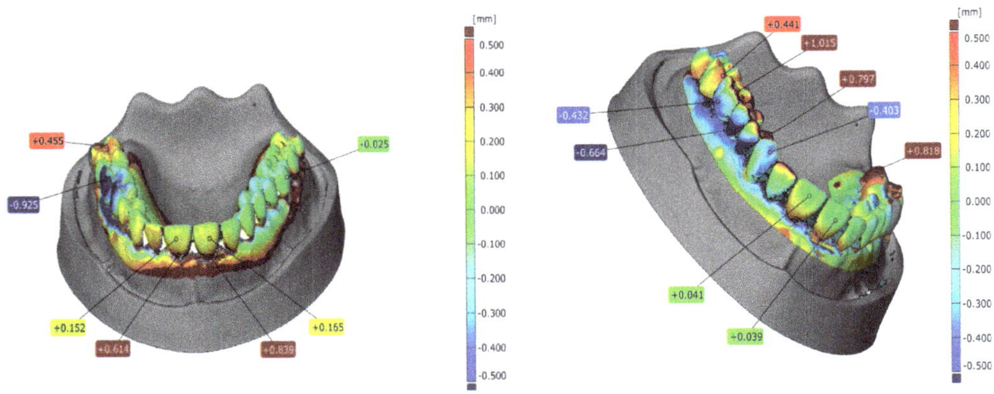


(**a**) (**b**)

**Figure 9.** Comparison of scans of a polyether pulp impression obtained using an optical 3D scanner (**a**) and micro-CT (**b**).

In the presented examples, a significant deviation value of more than 1 mm was observed in the maximum case. When comparing deviations between the dental impression model obtained from the 3D scanner and that obtained from the micro-CT, a similar trend was observed, but the deviation values differed in the examined areas by a few tenths of a millimeter. At this stage of analysis, it should be noted that the orthodontic impression materials were characterized by a certain susceptibility to deformation under external influences, which could be observed by introducing dental plaster materials into the impression.

The next step in the analysis was to measure the plaster model before removal from the impression. The combined elements were digitized using a micro-CT scanner, as shown in Figure 10. The constructed cross-section in the area of the anterior teeth shows how the boundary between the two elements was formed based on the density of the material. The model created from the separation of the digital impression and the plaster did not feature the defects and damage that can occur during separation.

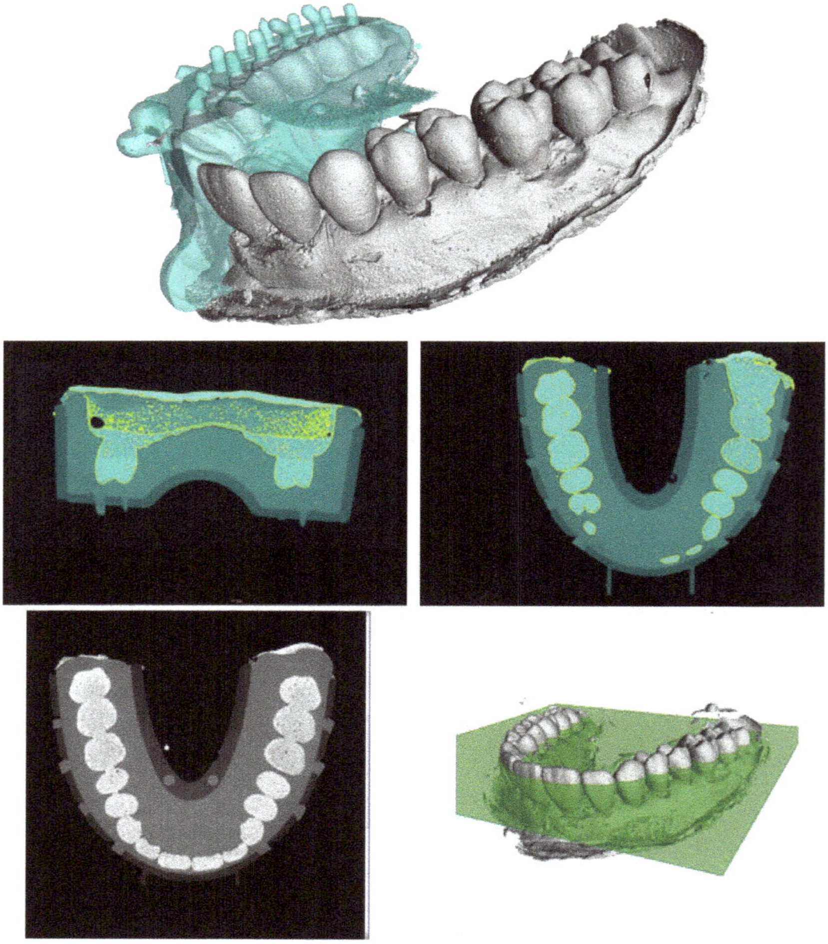

**Figure 10.** Combined orthodontic impression (blue) and dental plaster (grey) digitized using micro-CT.

Once the plaster models were separated from the impression materials, they were digitized using a 3D scanner and micro-CT. The results were analyzed in the same way as the impressions. Color deviation maps to visualize the deformation of the models in relation to the "0 model" are shown in Figures 11 and 12. The results presented show a reasonably uniform match between the plaster model based on the silicone impression matrix and the jaw model on both sides. The third incisal tooth presented a deviation value of −0.17 mm, the highest in the entire dental arch. Here, the poorer fit of the models created via micro-CT is clearly noticeable. Large deviations were noted for the right side of the jaw. Teeth 4, 5, and 6 showed deviations of approximately 0.5 to 1.0 mm at the top. On the other hand, at the base, the deviations ranged from approximately −0.5 mm to 0.8 mm.

Based on a comparison, the geometry of the plaster model cast from the polyether impression with the jaw model did not match very accurately. Here, we can see a worse fit on the right compared to the left, as well as on the chewing surfaces in relation to the buccal surfaces and on the molars. Analyzing the obtained color deviation maps, a better fit was observed for the silicone material than the polyether material. In most combinations, the largest deviations were on the last molars.

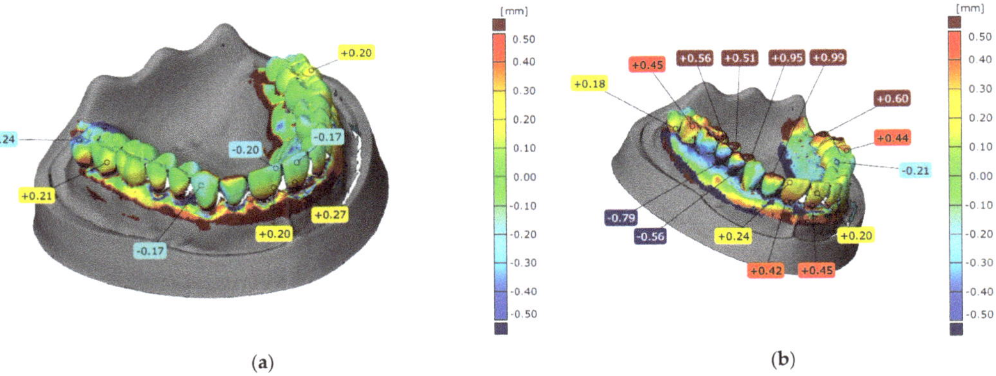


**Figure 11.** Comparison of scans of a plaster model created from a silicone impression obtained on an optical 3D scanner (**a**) and micro-CT (**b**).

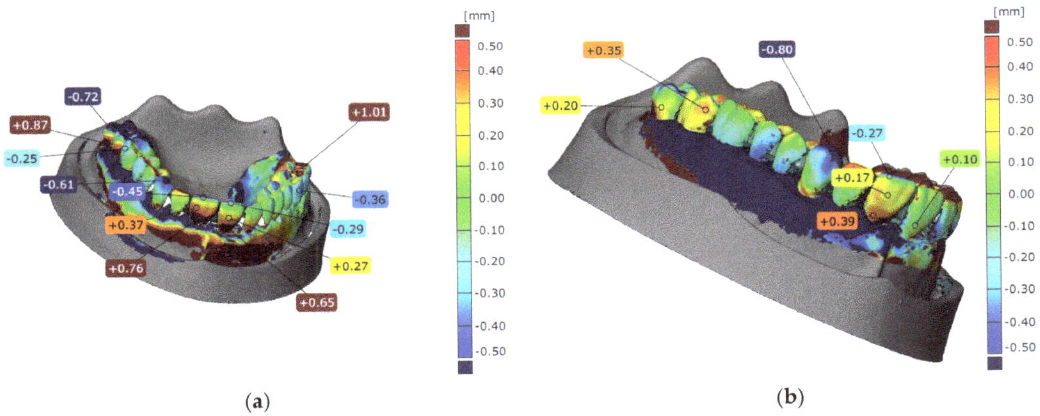


**Figure 12.** Comparison of scans of a plaster model created from a polyether material impression obtained on an optical 3D scanner (**a**) and micro-CT scanner (**b**).

The fit of the gum mapping was not analyzed, as this fit was affected by the irregular filling of the impression with gypsum material. This phenomenon can be clearly seen when analyzing the plaster models created from the polyether impression (Figure 12). Both the 3D scanner and micro-CT scans showed the greatest deviations for the gingival areas.

An important aspect in evaluating the mapping of jaws with impression materials is measurements describing the surface structure on a microscale. Such measurements indicate the quality of the mapped surfaces, which has a significant impact on the fabrication aesthetics of, for example, dental prostheses. The evaluation of the surface structure at the microscale was carried out using an Alicona InfiniteFocus G5 (Alicona Imaging GmbH, Graz, Austria) differential focusing microscope, which is very useful in dental applications [58]. Due to the small measurement range of the device, measurements were limited only to an analysis of molar surfaces, which can be considered representative of the entire impression when analyzed on a microscale. Since the material of the test object is susceptible to damage and scratching, measurements were carried out using a noncontact system.

Analysis of the surface topography was carried out using the MountainsMap (Digital Surf Headquarters, Besançon, France) software. The impression materials and resulting plaster models were analyzed on a microscale. Example results for the silicone material and the corresponding gypsum model are shown in Figure 13, while results for the polyether material are shown in Figure 14. The parameters describing the surface structures of the example considered are shown in Tables 1 and 2.

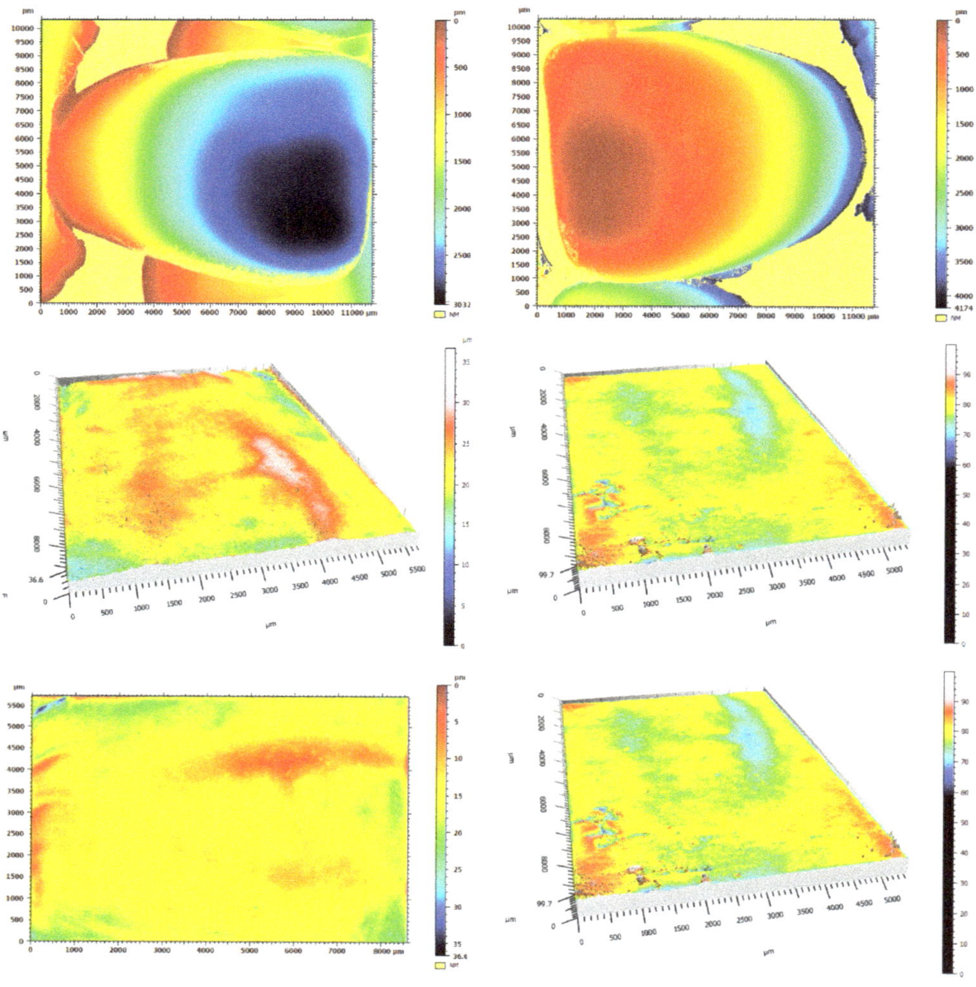

(a) (b)

**Figure 13.** Graphical representation of the surface texture for the silicone impression (**a**) and plaster model (**b**).

Comparing the results for the impression materials and gypsum models, differences in the height parameters describing the surface structure can be clearly observed. These differences are particularly evident for the polyether material and the corresponding gypsum model. The reason for this result may be that air bubbles formed on the surface of the model during the cooling process of the gypsum material.

The final task of this study was an attempt to replace the gypsum materials with models made using 3D printing. In order to determine the accuracy of the reproduction, the obtained model of the jaw was measured using a 3D scanner. Figure 15 shows a comparison between the digitized model made using the incremental method and the model taken as nominal in the form of a color deviation map.

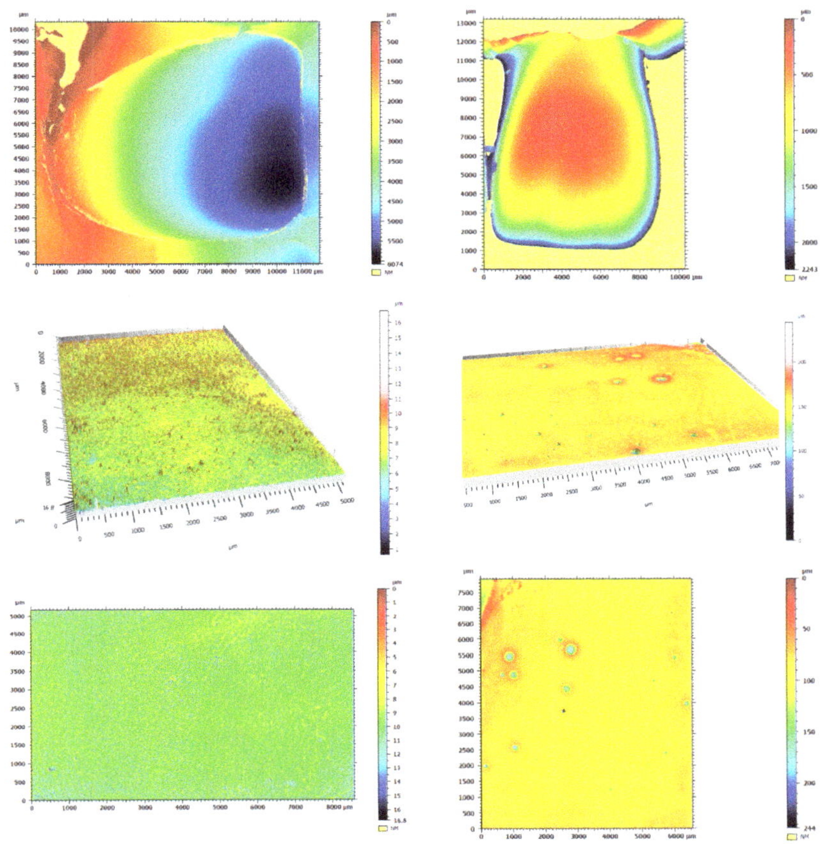

(a) (b)

**Figure 14.** Graphical representation of the surface texture for the polyether material impression (**a**) and plaster model (**b**).

**Table 1.** Summary of the basic surface structure parameters for the silicone impression and plaster model.

| Surface Structure Parameters | Impression | Plaster Model |
|---|---|---|
| Sq (Root Mean Square Height) | 2.97 µm | 2.86 µm |
| Ssk (Skewness) | −1.12 | 0.0587 |
| Sku (Kurtosis) | 60.8 | 32.0 |
| Sp (Maximum peak height) | 50.4 µm | 331 µm |
| Sv (Maximum pit height) | 184 µm | 26 µm |
| Sz (Maximum height) | 234 µm | 357 µm |
| Sa (Arithmetical mean height) | 2.12 µm | 2.13 µm |

**Table 2.** Summary of basic surface structure parameters for the polyether material impression and plaster model.

| Surface Structure Parameters | Impression | Plaster Model |
|---|---|---|
| Sq (Root Mean Square Height) | 1.18 μm | 9.04 μm |
| Ssk (Skewness) | 0.0732 | −3.84 |
| Sku (Kurtosis) | 6.32 | 50.7 |
| Sp (Maximum peak height) | 40.6 μm | 117 μm |
| Sv (Maximum pit height) | 11.1 μm | 165 μm |
| Sz (Maximum height) | 51.7 μm | 282 μm |
| Sa (Arithmetical mean height) | 0.884 μm | 4.23 μm |

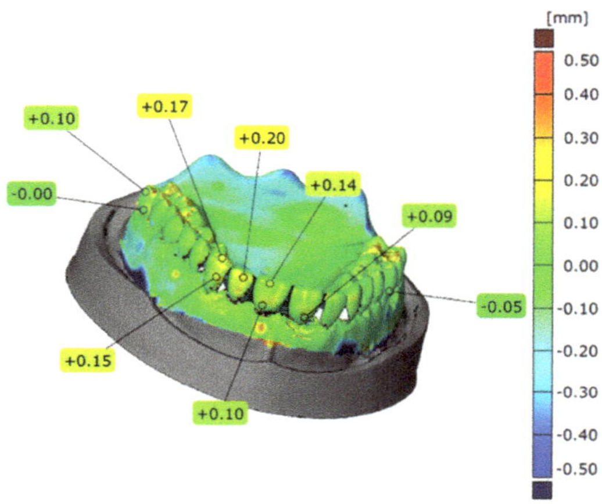


**Figure 15.** Comparison of the digitized jaw model made using the incremental method with the model taken as nominal.

The model resulting from 3D printing clearly offers a very good reproduction compared to the nominal model, with deviations from the nominal model not exceeding 0.2 mm. The results of this model obtained by reverse engineering and rapid prototyping indicate the possibility of using an alternative replacement for plaster models obtained with commonly used dental impressions.

## 4. Conclusions

Due to the wide variety of clinical cases, it is not possible to standardize all activities performed in prosthetics practice. Complicated medical cases with complex geometries and relationships between individual teeth require an unconventional approach to prosthetic design. By using a multiscale assessment, it is possible to better reproduce the patient's jaw geometry to ensure a tight and durable patient–prosthesis connection.

The analysis of the results indicates that a better fit was obtained with the silicone material than with the polyether material. In most comparisons, the largest deviations were observed on the last molar teeth. Several comparisons also demonstrated abnormalities on the left second incisal tooth. For the polyether material, a clear difference in accuracy between the left and right sides could be observed. The largest deviations were observed on the left premolars and first molar. These deviations may be due to the uneven pressing of the material on this side and the inaccurate molding of the teeth. A color-coded deviation map was created by combining the silicone impression, and the plaster model cast showed the best reproduction of geometry. A comparison of the absolute values of deviations for all right and left first incisal teeth in the central part of the labial surface with the absolute values of the deviations of all right and left second premolar teeth on the buccal cusp yielded similar results. It can be observed that at the front of the jaw on the incisors, these deviations were smaller than those at the back on the premolar teeth.

An attempt to use reverse engineering and rapid prototyping technology to obtain a model of the jaws produced satisfactory results. In the future, this method may provide an alternative to commonly used dental materials.

A limitation of this method is the need for specialized equipment, which is not available in prosthetic surgeries. Consequently, qualified personnel are required to digitize and analyze the acquired data. This solution will not be used universally but only for complex and unusual clinical cases. At present, the solution is also dedicated to patients who are prepared to pay a higher cost for a prosthesis, while at the same time being guaranteed a faster prosthesis without the need for longer fitting times through postprocessing, thus representing a higher level of personalization.

In summary, the comprehensive analysis and research carried out using various tools enabled multiscale analysis that directly fits into the ideas of Industry 4.0.

**Author Contributions:** Conceptualization, M.J. and L.M.-P.; methodology, M.J., L.M.-P., B.G. and M.M.; validation, M.J., L.M.-P. and B.G.; formal analysis, M.W.; investigation, M.J., L.M.-P., B.G. and M.M.; resources, M.J. and P.M.; writing—original draft preparation, M.J.; writing—review and editing, M.J., L.M.-P., B.G. and M.W.; visualization, M.J. and L.M.-P.; supervision, M.W.; project administration, M.J.; funding acquisition, M.J. All authors have read and agreed to the published version of the manuscript.

**Funding:** This research was funded by the Ministry of Education and Science in Poland, grant number 02/22/SBAD/1503 and 0614/SBAD/1565.

**Institutional Review Board Statement:** Not applicable.

**Informed Consent Statement:** Not applicable.

**Data Availability Statement:** The data presented in this study are available on request from the corresponding author.

**Acknowledgments:** The authors would also like to acknowledge Martyna Wiczynska and Patrycja Szefer for fabricating the samples.

**Conflicts of Interest:** The funders had no role in the design of the study; in the collection, analyses, or interpretation of data; in the writing of the manuscript; or in the decision to publish the results.

## References

1. Vogel, A.B.; Kilic, F.; Schmidt, F.; Rübel, S.; Lapatki, B.G. Optical 3D scans for orthodontic diagnostics performed on full-arch impressions. Completeness of surface structure representation. *J. Orofac. Orthop.* **2015**, *76*, 493–507. [CrossRef] [PubMed]
2. Ma, T.; Li, J.; Li, Z.; Li, Y. Improvement and Application of Mass Spring Model in Simulation of Gingi-val Soft Tissue Deformation. *J. Comput.-Aided Des. Comput. Graph.* **2020**, *32*, 325–333.
3. Palczewska-Komsa, M.O.; Gapiński, B.; Nowicka, A. The Influence of New Bioactive Materials on Pulp-Dentin Complex Regeneration in the Assessment of Cone Bone Computed Tomography (CBCT) and Computed Micro-Tomography (Micro-CT) from a Present and Future Perspective—A Systematic Review. *J. Clin. Med.* **2022**, *11*, 3091. [CrossRef] [PubMed]
4. Dobrzanski, L.A.; Dobrzanski, L.B. Dentistry 4.0 Concept in the Design and Manufacturing of Prosthetic Dental Restorations. *Processes* **2020**, *8*, 525. [CrossRef]
5. Gonzalez, J. The Evolution of Dental Materials for Hybrid Prosthesis. *Open Dent. J.* **2014**, *8*, 85–94. [CrossRef] [PubMed]
6. Wriedt, S.; Foersch, M.; Muhle, J.D.; Schmidtmann, I.; Wehrbein, H. Multibracket appliance: Impression defaults and their reduction by blocking-out—A three-dimensional study. *Clin. Oral Investig.* **2016**, *20*, 365–372. [CrossRef]
7. Erbe, C.; Ruf, S.; Wöstmann, B.; Balkenhol, M. Dimensional stability of contemporary irreversible hydrocolloids: Humidor versus wet tissue storage. *J. Prosthet. Dent.* **2012**, *108*, 114–122. [CrossRef]
8. Faria, A.C.L.; Rodrigues, R.C.S.; Macedo, A.P.; Mattos, M.G.C.; Ribeiro, R.F. Accuracy of stone casts obtained by different impression materials. *Braz. Oral Res.* **2008**, *22*, 293–298. [CrossRef] [PubMed]
9. Marquezan, M.; Jurach, E.M.; Guimarães, V.D.; Valentim, R.G.A.; Nojima, L.I.; da Cunha Gonçalves Nojima, M. Does the contact time of alginate with plaster cast influence its properties? *Braz. Oral Res.* **2012**, *26*, 197–201. [CrossRef]
10. Nandini, V.V.; Venkatesh, K.V.; Nair, K.C. Alginate impressions: A practical perspective. *J. Conserv. Dent.* **2008**, *11*, 37–41. [CrossRef]
11. Reisbick, M.H.; Johnston, W.M.; Rashid, R.G. Irreversible hydrocolloid and gypsum interactions. *Int. J. Prosthodont.* **1997**, *10*, 7–13.

12. Liczmanski, K.; Stamm, T.; Sauerland, C.; Blanck-Lubarsch, M. Accuracy of intraoral scans in the mixed dentition: A prospective non-randomized comparative clinical trial. *Head Face Med.* **2020**, *16*, 11. [CrossRef] [PubMed]
13. Chalmers, E.V.; McIntyre, G.T.; Wang, W.; Gillgrass, T.; Martin, C.B.; Mossey, P.A. Intraoral 3D scanning or dental impressions for the assessment of dental arch relationships in cleft care: Which is superior? *Cleft Palate–Craniofacial J.* **2016**, *53*, 568–577. [CrossRef]
14. AL-Meraikhi, H.; Yilmaz, B.; McGlumphy, E.; Brantley, W.A.; Johnston, W.M. Distortion of CAD-CAM-fabricated implant-fixed titanium and zirconia complete dental prosthesis frameworks. *J. Prosthet. Dent.* **2018**, *119*, 116–123. [CrossRef]
15. Peng, L.; Chen, L.; Harris, B.T.; Bhandari, B.; Morton, D.; Lin, W.-S. Accuracy and reproducibility of virtual edentulous casts created by laboratory impression scan protocols. *J. Prosthet. Dent.* **2018**, *120*, 389–395. [CrossRef] [PubMed]
16. Nagata, K.; Fuchigami, K.; Okuhama, Y.; Wakamori, K.; Tsuruoka, H.; Nakashizu, T.; Hoshi, N.; Atsumi, M.; Kimoto, K.; Kawana, H. Comparison of digital and silicone impressions for single-tooth implants and two and three-unit implants for a free-end edentulous saddle. *BMC Oral Health* **2021**, *21*, 464. [CrossRef] [PubMed]
17. Glisica, O.; Hoejbjerrea, L.; Sonnesenb, L. A comparison of patient experience, chair-side time, accuracy of dental arch measurements and costs of acquisition of dental models. *Angle Orthod.* **2019**, *89*, 868–875. [CrossRef]
18. Dastoori, M.; Bouserhal, J.P.; Halazonetis, D.J.; Athanasiou, A.E. Anterior teeth root inclination prediction derived from digital models: A comparative study of plaster study casts and CBCT images. *J. Clin. Exp. Dent.* **2018**, *10*, 1069–1074. [CrossRef] [PubMed]
19. Martin, C.B.; Chalmers, E.V.; McIntyre, G.T.; Cochrane, H.; Mossey, P.A. Orthodontic scanners: What is available? *J. Orthod.* **2015**, *42*, 136–143. [CrossRef]
20. Bosio, J.A.; Rozhitsky, F.; Jiang, S.S.; Conte, M.; Mukherjee, P.; Cangialosi, T.J. Comparison of scanning times for different dental cast materials using an intraoral scanner. *J. World Fed. Orthod.* **2017**, *6*, 11–14. [CrossRef]
21. Shah, N.; Bansal, N.; Logani, A. Recent advances in imaging technologies in dentistry. *World J. Radiol.* **2014**, *6*, 794–807. [CrossRef] [PubMed]
22. Elnaghy, R.; Amin, S.; Hasanin, M. Concepts and Clinical Applications of Intraoral 3D Scanning in the Management of Patients with Orofacial Clefts. In *Recent Advances in the Treatment of Orofacial Clefts*; Palone, M., Ed.; IntechOpen: London, UK, 2021.
23. Pereira, M.M.A.; Dini, C.; Souza, J.G.S.; Barão, V.A.R.; de Avila, E.D. Industry support for dental implant research: A metatrend study of industry partnership in the development of new technologies. *J. Prosthet. Dent.* 2022; *in press*. [CrossRef]
24. Burzynski, J.A.; Firestone, A.R.; Beck, F.M.; Fields, H.W., Jr.; Deguchi, T. Comparison of digital intraoral scanners and alginate impressions: Time and patient satisfaction. *Am. J. Orthod. Dentofac. Orthop.* **2018**, *153*, 534–541. [CrossRef] [PubMed]
25. Aly, P.; Mohsen, C. Comparison of the Accuracy of Three-Dimensional Printed Casts, Digital, and Conventional Casts: An In Vitro Study. *Eur. J. Dent.* **2020**, *14*, 189–193. [CrossRef] [PubMed]
26. Ahn, J.S.; Park, A.; Kim, J.W.; Lee, B.H.; Eom, J.B. Development of Three-Dimensional Dental Scanning Apparatus Using Structured Illumination. *Sensors* **2017**, *17*, 1634. [CrossRef] [PubMed]
27. Javaid, M.; Haleem, A.; Kumar, L. Current status and applications of 3D scanning in dentistry. *Clin. Epidemiol. Glob. Health* **2019**, *7*, 228–233. [CrossRef]
28. Faot, F.; Chatterjee, M.; de Camargos, G.V.; Duyck, J.; Vandamme, K. Micro-CT analysis of the rodent jaw bone micro-architecture: A systematic review. *Bone Rep.* **2015**, *2*, 14–24. [CrossRef]
29. Shibli, J.A.; Grassi, S.; de Figueiredo, L.C.; Feres, M.; Marcantonio, E., Jr.; Iezzi, G.; Piattelli, A. Influence of implant surface topography on early osseointegration: A histological study in human jaws. *J. Biomed. Mater. Res.* **2007**, *80*, 377–385. [CrossRef]
30. Uklejewski, R.; Winiecki, M.; Patalas, A.; Rogala, P. Bone Density Micro-CT Assessment during Embedding of the Innovative Multi-Spiked Connecting Scaffold in Periarticular Bone to Elaborate a Validated Numerical Model for Designing Biomimetic Fixation of Resurfacing Endoprostheses. *Materials* **2021**, *14*, 1384. [CrossRef]
31. Emara, A.; Sharma, S.; Halbeisen, F.S.; Msallem, B.; Thieringer, F.M. Comparative evaluation of digitization of diagnostic dental cast (plaster) models using different scanning technologies. *Dent. J.* **2020**, *8*, 79. [CrossRef]
32. Latham, J.; Ludlow, M.; Mennito, A.; Kelly, A.; Evans, Z.; Renne, W. Effect of scan pattern on complete-arch scans with 4 digital scanners. *J. Prosthet. Dent.* **2020**, *123*, 85–95. [CrossRef] [PubMed]
33. Zimmermann, M.; Koller, C.; Rumetsch, M.; Ender, A.; Mehl, A. Precision of guided scanning procedures for full-arch digital impressions in vivo. *J. Orofac. Orthop.* **2017**, *78*, 466–471. [CrossRef] [PubMed]
34. Schenz, N.; Schwarz, V.; Hörmann, R.; Crismani, A.G. Impression material accuracy for palatal orthodontic miniscrews. *J. Orofac. Orthop.* **2020**, *81*, 427–439. [CrossRef]
35. Morris, R.S.; Hoye, L.N.; Elnagar, M.H.; Atsawasuwan, P.; Galang-Boquiren, M.T.; Caplin, J.; Viana, G.C.; Obrez, A.; Kusnoto, B. Accuracy of Dental Monitoring 3D digital dental models using photograph and video mode. *Am. J. Orthod. Dentofac. Orthop.* **2019**, *156*, 420–428. [CrossRef]
36. Lasi, H.; Fettke, P.; Kemper, H.G.; Feld, T.; Hoffmann, M. Industry 4.0. *Bus. Inf. Syst. Eng.* **2014**, *6*, 239–242. [CrossRef]
37. Dietrich, C.A.; Ender, A.; Baumgartner, S.; Mehl, A. A validation study of reconstructed rapid prototyping models produced by two technologies. *Angle Orthod.* **2017**, *87*, 782–787. [CrossRef] [PubMed]
38. Sfondrini, M.F.; Gandini, P.; Malfatto, M.; Di Corato, F.; Trovati, F.; Scribante, A. Computerized Casts for Orthodontic Purpose Using Powder-Free Intraoral Scanners: Accuracy, Execution Time, and Patient Feedback. *BioMed Res. Int.* **2018**, *2018*, 4103232. [CrossRef]

39. Kroma, A.; Mendak, M.; Jakubowicz, M.; Gapiński, B.; Popielarski, P. Non-Contact Multiscale Analysis of a DPP 3D-Printed Injection Die for Investment Casting. *Materials* **2021**, *14*, 6758. [CrossRef]
40. Hassan, W.N.W.; Yusoff, Y.; Mardic, N.A. Comparison of reconstructed rapid prototyping models produced by 3-dimensional printing and conventional stone models with different degrees of crowding. *Am. J. Orthod. Dentofac. Orthop.* **2017**, *151*, 209–218. [CrossRef]
41. Joffe, L. Current Products and Practices OrthoCADTM: Digital models for a digital era. *J. Orthod.* **2004**, *31*, 344–347. [CrossRef] [PubMed]
42. Guzm, J.F.G.; Teramoto Ohara, A. Evaluation of three-dimensional printed virtual setups. *Am. J. Orthod. Dentofac. Orthop.* **2019**, *155*, 288–295.
43. Möhlhenrich, S.C.; Brandt, M.; Kniha, K.; Bock, A.; Prescher, A.; Hölzle, F.; Modabber, A.; Danesh, G. Suitability of virtual plaster models superimposed with the lateral cephalogram for guided paramedian orthodontic mini-implant placement with regard to the bone support. *J. Orofac. Orthop.* **2020**, *81*, 340–349. [CrossRef] [PubMed]
44. Zilberman, O.; Huggare, J.A.V.; Konstantinos, A.P.A. Evaluation of the validity of tooth size and arch width measurements using conventional and three-dimensional virtual orthodontic models. *Angle Orthod.* **2003**, *73*, 301–306. [PubMed]
45. Yuan, T.; Wang, Y.; Hou, Z.; Wang, J. Tooth segmentation and gingival tissue deformation framework for 3D orthodontic treatment planning and evaluating. *Med. Biol. Eng. Comput.* **2020**, *58*, 2271–2290. [CrossRef] [PubMed]
46. Swojak, N.; Wieczorowski, M.; Jakubowicz, M. Assessment of selected metrological properties of laser triangulation sensors. *Measurement* **2021**, *176*, 109190. [CrossRef]
47. Kihara, T.; Yoshimi, Y.; Taji, T.; Murayama, T.; Tanimoto, K.; Nikawa, H. Accuracy of a three-dimensional dentition model digitized from an interocclusal record using a non-contact surface scanner. *Eur. J. Orthod.* **2016**, *38*, 435–439. [CrossRef] [PubMed]
48. Pacheco-Pereira, C.; De Luca Canto, G.; Major, P.W.; Flores-Mird, C. Variation of orthodontic treatment decision-making based on dental model type: A systematic review. *Angle Orthod.* **2015**, *85*, 501–509. [CrossRef]
49. Mullen, S.R.; Martin, C.A.; Ngan, P.; Gladwin, M. Accuracy of space analysis with emodels and plaster models. *Am. J. Orthod. Dentofac. Orthop.* **2007**, *132*, 346–352. [CrossRef]
50. Baan, F.; Bruggink, R.; Nijsink, J.; Maal, T.J.J.; Ongkosuwito, E.M. Fusion of intra-oral scans in cone-beam computed tomography scans. *Clin. Oral Investig.* **2021**, *25*, 77–85. [CrossRef]
51. Gapiński, B.; Janicki, P.; Marciniak-Podsadna, L.; Jakubowicz, M. Application of the computed tomography to control parts made on additive manufacturing process. *Procedia Eng.* **2016**, *149*, 105–121. [CrossRef]
52. Prakoso, A.T.; Basri, H.; Adanta, D.; Yani, I.; Ammarullah, M.I.; Akbar, I.; Ghazali, F.A.; Syahrom, A.; Kamarul, T. The Effect of Tortuosity on Permeability of Porous Scaffold. *Biomedicines* **2023**, *11*, 427. [CrossRef] [PubMed]
53. Park, J.H.; Lee, G.-H.; Moon, D.-N.; Kim, J.-C.; Park, M.; Lee, K.-M. A digital approach to the evaluation of mandibular position by using a virtual articulator. *J. Prosthet. Dent.* **2021**, *125*, 849–853. [CrossRef] [PubMed]
54. Dąbrowski, M.; Rogala, P.; Uklejewski, R.; Patalas, A.; Winiecki, M.; Gapiński, B. Subchondral Bone Relative Area and Density in Human Osteoarthritic Femoral Heads Assessed with Micro-CT before and after Mechanical Embedding of the Innovative Multi-Spiked Connecting Scaffold for Resurfacing THA Endoprostheses: A Pilot Study. *J. Clin. Med.* **2021**, *10*, 2937. [CrossRef] [PubMed]
55. Gapinski, B.; Wieczorowski, M.; Mietliński, P.; Mathia, T.G. Verification of Computed Tomograph for Dimensional Measurements. In *Lecture Notes in Mechanical Engineering*; Springer: Cham, Switzerland, 2022; pp. 142–155. [CrossRef]
56. Wieczorowski, M.; Yago, I.P.; Alejandro, P.D.; Gapiński, B.; Budzik, G.; Diering, M. Comparison of Measurements Realized on Computed Tomograph and Optical Scanners for Elements Manufactured by Wire Arc Additive Manufacturing. In *Lecture Notes in Mechanical Engineering*; Springer: Cham, Switzerland, 2022; pp. 127–141. [CrossRef]
57. Surowska, B.; Ostapiuk, M.; Tarczydło, B. Micro-CT analysis of molar teeth restored by combining conventional and glass fibre reinforced composites. *Eng. Biomater.* **2016**, *19*, 13–19.
58. Schmeidl, K.; Wieczorowski, M.; Grocholewicz, K.; Mendak, M.; Janiszewska Olszowska, J. Frictional properties of the tinbtazro orthodontic wire—A laboratory comparison to popular archwires. *Materials* **2021**, *14*, 6233. [CrossRef]

applied sciences

MDPI

*Article*

# Optical Behavior and Surface Analysis of Dental Resin Matrix Ceramics Related to Thermocycling and Finishing

**Liliana Porojan [1,*], Flavia Roxana Toma [1], Ion-Dragoș Uțu [2] and Roxana Diana Vasiliu [1,*]**

[1] Department of Dental Prostheses Technology (Dental Technology), Center for Advanced Technologies in Dental Prosthodontics, Faculty of Dental Medicine, "Victor Babeș" University of Medicine and Pharmacy Timișoara, Eftimie Murgu Sq. No. 2, 300041 Timișoara, Romania; flavia.toma@umft.ro

[2] Department of Materials and Fabrication Engineering, Politehnica University Timişoara, Bd. Mihai Viteazul nr.1, 300222 Timişoara, Romania; dragos.utu@upt.ro

* Correspondence: sliliana@umft.ro (L.P.); roxana.vasiliu@umft.ro (R.D.V.)

**Abstract:** Color preservation of esthetic dental restorative materials in the oral environment represents, besides longevity, a concern, and there is still limited knowledge related to the effect of aging on the optical behavior of resin matrix ceramics. The study analyzed the finishing and thermocycling of resin matrix ceramic material surfaces, in order to assess their consequences on optical properties. Five resin matrix CAD/CAM ceramics, namely a polymer-infiltrated ceramic and four types of nanoparticle-filled resins, were selected for the study, and finished by polishing and glazing. Thermocycling was chosen as the in vitro aging method. Surface microroughness, optical and hardness evaluations were achieved before and after artificial aging. Statistical analyses were performed with IBM SPSS Statistics software at a significance value of $p < 0.05$. Micro-roughness values increased after thermocycling, but were kept under the clinically accepted values. The optical characteristics of resin matrix ceramics were not significantly modified by thermocycling. Values of the glazed samples became closer to those of the polished ones, after hydrothermal aging, even if the differences were insignificant. Thermocycling significantly decreased the microhardness, mainly for glazed samples. This could be the consequence of glaze removal during thermocycling, which means that glazes provide a surface protection for a limited time.

**Keywords:** resin matrix ceramics; thermocycling; optical properties; surface analysis

**Citation:** Porojan, L.; Toma, F.R.; Uțu, I.-D.; Vasiliu, R.D. Optical Behavior and Surface Analysis of Dental Resin Matrix Ceramics Related to Thermocycling and Finishing. *Appl. Sci.* **2022**, *12*, 4346. https://doi.org/10.3390/app12094346

Academic Editor: Vittorio Checchi

Received: 30 March 2022
Accepted: 23 April 2022
Published: 25 April 2022

**Publisher's Note:** MDPI stays neutral with regard to jurisdictional claims in published maps and institutional affiliations.



## 1. Introduction

Related to the high demand of patients for biomimetic dental restorative materials, ceramics and composites come into question. Longevity is an essential aspect when restoring natural teeth structures and it is important that the physical properties of the restorative materials overlap the tooth structures [1–3]. The rapid development of CAD/CAM technologies provided accurate, repeatable and high-quality dental restorations using a variety of materials. CAD/CAM systems represent an outstanding advancement, offering practitioners the chance to achieve improved dental restorations [4,5].

During the last decade, a new category of dental esthetic materials has been researched, called resin matrix ceramics or hybrid ceramics. These materials consist of an organic matrix with a high content of ceramic particles. These materials are included in the classification of dental ceramics, after the American Dental Association Code on Dental Procedures and Nomenclature (version 2013), which defines the term porcelain/ceramic as "pressed, fired, polished, or milled materials containing predominantly inorganic refractory compounds—including porcelains, glasses, ceramics, and glass-ceramics". The former version of the ADA code did not include materials with resin matrix in the category of ceramic materials [6–9].

The physical properties related to resin matrix ceramics lie very close to those of natural teeth, and between ceramics and composites. The milling time in the CAM unit is shorter compared to other ceramic materials, leading to a longer lifetime of the milling burs. The polymer structure of the material could also prevent crack propagation through the ceramic phase. Well-known resin composites wear out; they lose their surface gloss and color stability overtime more easily compared to ceramic materials [2,10–20].

As surface processing methods of these materials, conventional polishing and glazing for high gloss and gloss stability are designated. Glaze materials are used to seal the surfaces and to obtain smoother and glossy surfaces. This has a great impact in decreasing surface asymmetries, increasing wear resistance, and improving the resistance to staining [21,22]. The surface roughness of a material is important for esthetics and long-term success, but there is a need for more studies related to the effectiveness of glazes on CAD/CAM resin matrix ceramic materials.

Ensuring success in esthetic restorations is a difficult process, because of the optical complexity of tooth structures. To obtain success, basic principles in optical characterization, such as mimicking of the opalescence and translucence of natural teeth, must be taken into consideration [23–25]. Due to the hydrophilic characteristics of resin-based materials, studies demonstrated the relation with their optical properties. Resin-based materials are known for their esthetic appearance, strength, and accessibility, but lack the strength and optical stability of ceramic materials. Thus, resin matrix ceramics were introduced in order to combine the benefits of ceramics and composites. They may limit the absorption of water compared to resin-based materials, and thus preserve optical properties.

Information regarding the properties of resin matrix ceramic materials after a prolonged usage period is limited [18]. The Vickers hardness test is important because it is a predictor of surface wear [26].

Thermocycling is one of the widely used aging methods to investigate restorative materials and there are different in vitro aging protocols. Thermocycling represents the oral environments better than isothermal storage conditions. Temperatures of 5–55 °C are considered the limits for the real situation in the oral cavity. A total of 10,000 cycles were selected for the study, which represent one year of clinical service and are generally used for in vitro studies [27,28].

Dental restorations are exposed to dynamic temperature changes in the oral cavity. The different thermal expansion coefficients of the filler particles and resin matrix induce internal stresses in the material during continual temperature changes. Resulting cracks and gaps damage the mechanical properties over time, accelerating aging. Additionally, in materials with nano-zirconia filler, zirconia may undergo a low-temperature degradation with a phase transition from tetragonal to monoclinic phase at oral temperature, overlapping the abovementioned degradation [29–31]. It was demonstrated that a definite water content of enamel and dentine structures is mandatory for their physical characteristics and biomechanical behavior, providing stability and robustness. Water absorption induces a greater risk of decomposition of the molecular structure on the microscale, and is considered to change the physical properties and the lifetime of dental restorative materials. Accordingly, the impact of water content on dental materials represents a challenge, as well as their susceptibility to degradation in water and aging [32–34]. Polymer networks can be strongly altered by the wet oral environment [35]. There is still limited information regarding the effect of aging on the optical stability of these materials [36–42] Color preservation of esthetic dental restorative materials in the oral environment represents besides longevity a concern in the use of esthetic dental restorative materials. Restorations should reproduce the optical properties of natural teeth and maintain this natural appearance over time. These are directly related to optical harmony with natural teeth and to the color stability of the material. Spectrophotometers are currently used to evaluate the color change ($\Delta E^*$) of dental materials by quantifying the color coordinates in the CIELAB color space: $L^*$, $a^*$ and $b^*$. The $L^*$ coordinate is an indicator of brightness, the $a^*$ coordinate indicates the red–green component (negative $a^*$ represents greenness and positive $a^*$ indicates redness), and the $b^*$ coordinate corresponds to yellowness or blueness (negative $b^*$ indicates blueness and positive $b^*$ represents yellowness). $L^*$ coordinates are the most important parameters in the optical appearance of restorations, because the lightness has the greatest effect on esthetics [43–45].

The study aimed to conduct a surface analysis of resin matrix ceramic materials related to finishing and thermocycling, and to assess their consequences on optical properties. The study included hybrid materials that were tested after hydrothermal aging for changes in the optical properties such as translucency and opalescence, and as well for surface and mechanical properties.

The null hypothesis is that the optical and surface properties of the hybrid ceramic included in this study are influenced by the hydrothermal aging.

## 2. Materials and Methods

### 2.1. Specimen Preparation

Five resin matrix CAD/CAM ceramic materials were selected for the study: a polymer infiltrated network ceramic (Vita Enamic VITA Zahnfabrik, Bad Säckingen, Germany) (E) and four types of ceramic nanoparticle-filled resins (Lava Ultimate, 3M ESPE, St. Paul, MN, USA (L), Cerasmart, GC Corporation, Tokyo, Japan (C), Shofu HC, Shofu, Kyoto, Japan (S), and Hyramic Upcera, Liaoning, China (H)) were selected for the study (Table 1), with shades A2 or 2M2 and translucency HT. The CAD/CAM blocks were sliced into rectangular-shaped plates ($n$ = 16) per material using a machine (Orthoflex PI Dental, Budapest, Hungary) that provides millimeter accuracy. The samples were polished using silicon carbide papers (600–2000 grit) and the final thickness (1 mm) of each plate was checked with a digital caliper.

**Table 1.** Composition and manufacturer specifications of tested materials [20,45,46].

| Material | Type | Manufacturer | Filler | Monomer | Shade/Translucency |
|---|---|---|---|---|---|
| Vita Enamic (E) | Hybrid ceramic | VITA Zahnfabrik, Bad Säckingen, Germany | Feldspar ceramic enriched with aluminum oxide 86% | UDMA, TEGDMA | A2/MT |
| Lava Ultimate (L) | CAD/CAM composite resin | 3M ESPE, Seefeld, Germany | $SiO_2$, $ZrO_2$, aggregated $ZrO_2/SiO_2$ cluster 80% | UDMA, Bis-GMA, Bis-EMA, TEGDMA | A2/MT |
| Cerasmart (C) | CAD/CAM composite resin | GC Corporation, Tokyo, Japan | Silica, barium glass 71% | UDMA, Bis-MEPP, DMA | A2/MT |
| Shofu HC (S) | CAD/CAM composite resin | Shofu, Kyoto, Japan | Silica, silicate, zirconium silicate 61% | UDMA, TEGDMA | A2/MT |
| Hyramic (H) | CAD/CAM composite resin | Upcera, Liaoning, China | Inorganic Filler 55–85% | Resin Polymers | |

The surfaces were finally polished with a low-speed handpiece using a diamond polishing paste, Renfert polish all-in-one (Renfert, Hilzingen, Germany). Half of the specimens from each material were kept polished ($p$) and half were glazed (g). Resin Glaze Primer (Shofu, Kyoto, Japan) was applied to the surfaces for 60 s and allowed to dry. After that, two thin layers of the glaze Resin Glaze Liquid (Shofu, Kyoto, Japan) were applied with a soft brush in the same direction in order to eliminate air bubbles and were light cured for 180 s in the device SibariSr 620 (Sirio Dental, Meldola, Italy). After the surface finishing protocols, all plates were ultrasonically cleaned for 10 min and degreased in alcohol.

### 2.2. Hydrothermal Aging Protocol

Prior to baseline measurements, all samples were immersed in distilled water at 37 °C for 24 h to allow full hydration. Further specimens were submitted to 5000 cycles in baths filled with distilled water at 55 °C and 5 °C. Each cycle lasted 80 s; 30 s was the dwelling time in the5 °C bath, 10 s were needed for transfer to the other bath, 30 s was the time in the 55 °C bath, and 10 s were needed to transfer of the samples back to the 5 °C bath (t1). The other 5000 cycles were followed using the same protocol (t2).

The hydrothermal aging protocol has an indication for this type of dental materials. This method is used to simulate the in vivo aging of the dental restorative materials by subjecting them to repeated cold and warm water baths [47]. These water baths simulate the changes that occur in the oral cavity of the patients.

### 2.3. Surface Microroughness Evaluation

Surface microroughness was measured with a 2 μm contact stylus profilometerSurftest SJ-201 (Mitutoyo, Kawasaki, Japan) before (w) and after each step of aging (t1 and t2). Arithmetic average roughness (Ra) [48,49] evaluations were performed in five different directions, all data were recorded and mean values of the five measurements were calculated for each surface. The used sampling length was 0.3 mm, and a force of 0.7 mN was applied.

### 2.4. Optical and Color Changes Measurements

Translucency (TP) and opalescence (OP) values were calculated for all samples, on both types of surfaces (polished and glazed), before (w) and after each step of aging (t1 and t2). Optical parameters were registered under a D65 illuminant, using a Vita Easyshade IV spectrophotometer (Vita Zahnfabrick, Bad Säckingen, Germany). It was calibrated before each measurement.

To assess the measurements, two different backgrounds, black (b) and white (w), were selected, using the grey card WhiBal G7 (White Balance Pocket Card). L* represents the lightness–darkness of the material (L* = 0 for a perfect black and L* = 100 for a perfect white). a* represents the measure of greenness (negative value) or redness (positive value), and b* measures the blueness (negative value) or the yellowness (positive value) [50–53].

TP values were calculated using Equation (1).

$$TP = [(L_b - L_w)^2 + (a_b - a_w)^2 + (b_b - b_w)^2]^{1/2} \quad (1)$$

OP values were calculated using Equation (2).

$$OP = [(a_b - a_w)^2 + (b_b - b_w)^2]^{1/2} \quad (2)$$

The CR (contrast ratio) value was achieved by Equation (3).

$$CR = Y_b/Y_w \ Y = [(L^* + 16)/116]^3 \times 100 \quad (3)$$

w and b correspond to the white and black backgrounds, respectively. CR = 0 is equivalent to transparent, and CR = 1 to totally opaque [54].

The color changes (ΔE*), which represent the color difference between two stages, were calculated based on the CIE L*a*b*color system, for a black background, according to Equation (4).

$$\Delta E^* = [(\Delta L^*)^2 + (\Delta a^*)^2 + (\Delta b^*)^2]^{1/2} \quad (4)$$

The National Bureau of Standards (NBS) system quantifies the levels of color change, relating to a clinical standard. ΔE* values were thus converted into NBS units: NBS unit = ΔE* × 0.92 [52,55–59].

### 2.5. Microhardness Evaluation

Samples were evaluated for the Vickers microhardness before (w) and after aging (t2). Measurements were made on selected points using the digital camera of the tester, with the micro-hardness tester DM 8/DM 2 (Yang Yi Technology Co., Ltd., Tainan City 70960, Taiwan) using a diamond pyramidal indenter with 300 g load, for 10 s. After lifting the indenter, the indentation dimensions were microscopically recorded (40× magnifications). Five measurements were done on each surface, and mean values were calculated. The formula used for the Vickers microhardness calculation is the following (5):

$$HV = 1.8544\ F/d^2 \quad (5)$$

where HV is the Vickers hardness value, F is the applied load value and d is the diagonal length of the indentation [60].

### 2.6. Statistical Analysis

IBM SPSS Statistics software (IBM, New York, NY, USA) was selected to achieve statistical analysis. For all studied materials as well as for all surface processing procedures, mean values for color parameters, roughness, surface hardness, SDs and 95% confidence intervals were subsequently calculated related to hydrothermal aging stages. Statistical evaluation for material type and surface processing was performed. Comparison of different aging stages was conducted using a paired samples *t* test. Differences were considered significant if the corresponding $p$ value was <0.05. A statistical correlation (Spearman) was used to establish relationships between optical parameters. It measures the strength of correlations between variables and the direction of the relationship. The significance was calculated as follows: 0–0.19 "very weak", 0.20–0.39 "weak", 0.40–0.59 "moderate", 0.60–0.79 "strong", and 0.80–1.0 "very strong".

## 3. Results

Before thermocycling (w), average roughness values (Ra) showed significant differences between polished and glazed samples for L ($p = 0.035$) and H ($p = 0.033$). Glazing increased roughness values in L, C, and S samples and decrease them in E and H. The roughness values increased as follows: Sp < Ep < Lp < Hp < Cp, Hg < Eg < Sg < Cg < Lg. Differences were significant between Cp and Sp ($p = 0.003$), Ep ($p = 0.014$), and Lp ($p = 0.029$), respective Lg and Hg ($p = 0.036$).

Related to different surface finishing methods, after hydrothermal aging polished surfaces had significantly lower roughness than glazed ones for C ($p = 0.007$) and H ($p = 0.001$). The values increased as follows: Hp < Sp < Cp < Ep < Lp, Lg < Sg < Eg < Cg < Hg. Related to thermocycling, Ra values increased significant for Ep, Lp, and Sp, respective Eg, Sg, and Hg (Figure 1).

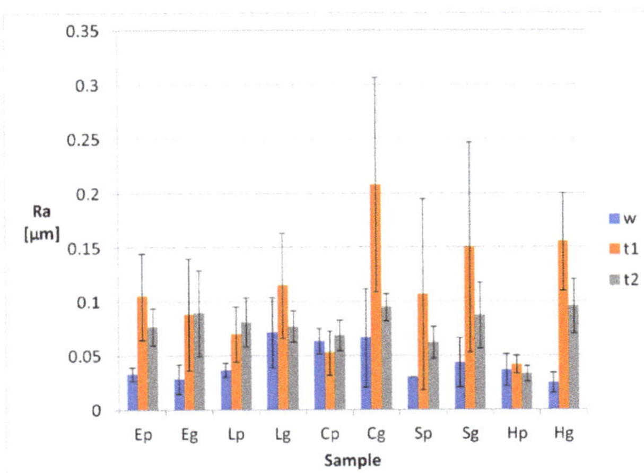


**Figure 1.** Mean Ra roughness values and SD values of the samples, before and after thermal aging.

Related to surface processing, TP and OP values increased and CR decreased for glazed samples, with results being significant before thermocycling and insignificant after.

Mean calculated optical parameters ranged between 17.01 and 24.79 for TP, 4.40 and 8.05 for OP, and 0.46 and 0.60 for CR (Figures 2–4, Tables 2–4). TP, OP and CR values were insignificantly changed by thermocycling.

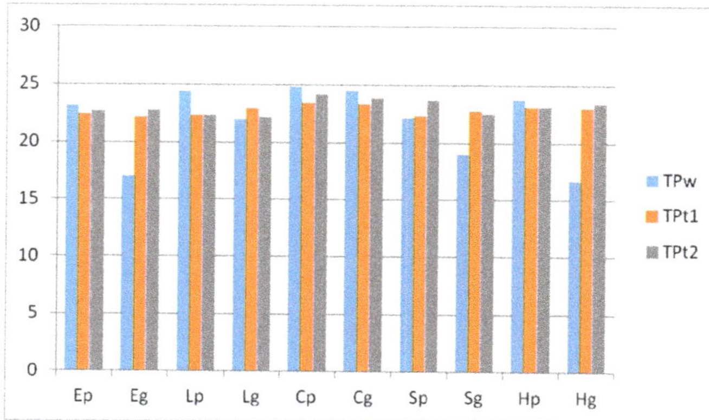


**Figure 2.** Mean values of the TP parameter, before and after thermal aging.

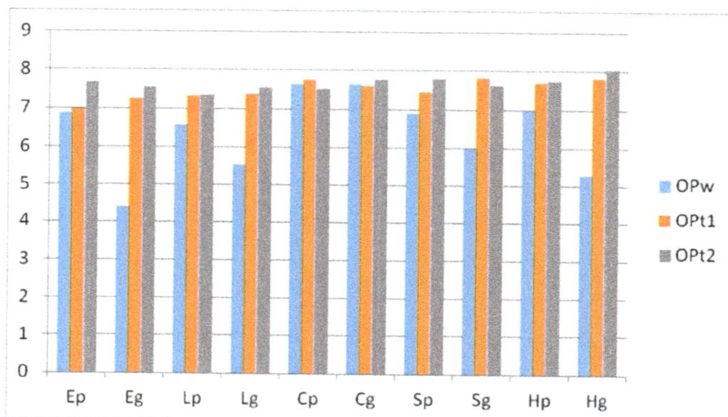


**Figure 3.** Mean values of the OP parameter, before and after thermal aging.

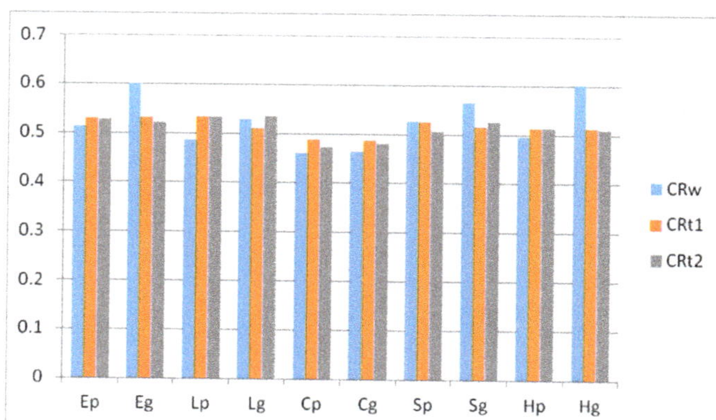


**Figure 4.** Mean values of the CR parameter, before and after thermal aging.

TP and OP values were very strongly positively correlated before thermocycling (0.891), strongly correlated after the first step (0.648), and moderately correlated after the second (0.455). TP and CR values were very strongly negatively correlated before thermocycling (−1), after the first step (−0.927), and after the second (−0.988). OP and CR values are very strongly negatively correlated before thermocycling (−0.891), and moderately correlated after the first (−0.552), and after the second thermocycling step (−0.442).

**Table 2.** Mean TP values of samples after water immersion, before thermocycling (w), after thermocycling for 5000 cycles (t1) and after thermocycling for 10,000 cycles (t2). *,a,b significant changes after hydrothermal aging.

| Sample | Ep | Eg | Lp | Lg | Cp | Cg | Sp | Sg | Hp | Hg |
|---|---|---|---|---|---|---|---|---|---|---|
| TPw | 23.14 * | 17.01 * | 24.45 a | 21.97 a | 24.79 | 24.52 | 22.21 | 19.00 | 23.71 b | 16.74 b |
| TPt1 | 22.42 | 22.19 | 22.32 | 22.95 | 23.41 | 23.33 | 22.38 | 22.74 | 23.13 | 23.03 |
| TPt2 | 22.66 | 22.75 | 22.35 | 22.21 | 24.15 | 23.82 | 23.64 | 22.50 | 23.11 | 23.41 |

**Table 3.** Mean OP values of samples after water immersion, before thermocycling (w), after thermocycling for 5000 cycles (t1) and after thermocycling for 10,000 cycles (t2). *,a significant changes after hydrothermal aging.

| Sample | Ep | Eg | Lp | Lg | Cp | Cg | Sp | Sg | Hp | Hg |
|---|---|---|---|---|---|---|---|---|---|---|
| OPw | 6.89 * | 4.40 * | 6.58 a | 5.54 a | 7.66 | 7.64 | 6.90 | 5.99 | 6.98 | 5.28 |
| OPt1 | 6.98 | 7.24 | 7.33 | 7.37 | 7.74 | 7.60 | 7.44 | 7.82 | 7.71 | 7.83 |
| OPt2 | 7.67 | 7.56 | 7.34 | 7.55 | 7.53 | 7.78 | 7.80 | 7.62 | 7.76 | 8.05 |

**Table 4.** Mean CR values of samples after water immersion, before thermocycling (w), after thermocycling for 5000 cycles (t1) and after thermocycling for 10,000 cycles (t2).

| Sample | Ep | Eg | Lp | Lg | Cp | Cg | Sp | Sg | Hp | Hg |
|---|---|---|---|---|---|---|---|---|---|---|
| CRw | 0.51 | 0.60 | 0.48 | 0.52 | 0.46 | 0.46 | 0.52 | 0.56 | 0.49 | 0.60 |
| CRt1 | 0.52 | 0.53 | 0.53 | 0.51 | 0.48 | 0.48 | 0.52 | 0.51 | 0.51 | 0.51 |
| CRt2 | 0.52 | 0.52 | 0.53 | 0.53 | 0.47 | 0.48 | 0.50 | 0.52 | 0.51 | 0.51 |

The calculated NBS levels of color change registered marked changes (NBS units > 3) only for Lp samples, after thermocycling (t1 and t2).

Microhardness values were significantly lower for *p* than g samples before thermocycling, for all resin nanoceramic materials ($p < 0.05$). For E the values were similar ($p = 0.094$). After thermocycling the differences between *p* and g remained significant for L and H. Related to thermocycling, the microhardness values decreased significantly for all samples, excepting Sp (Figure 5).

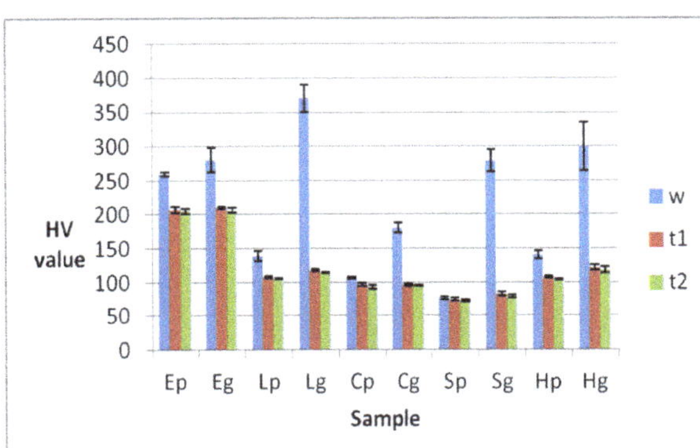


**Figure 5.** Mean microhardness values and SD of the samples, before and after thermocycling.

Related to materials, for *p* samples before thermocycling, the values decreased significantly as follows: Ep > Hp > Lp > Cp > Sp, except from Hp to Lp. For g samples they decreased as follows: Lg > Hg > Eg > Sg > Cg, being significant only between Sg and Cg.

After thermocycling, values decreased as follows: Ep > Lp > Hp > Cp > Sp, being insignificant between Lp and Hp, and Cp and Sp. For glazed samples they decreased as follows: Eg > Hg> Lg > Cg > Sg, being insignificant between Hg and Lg.

## 4. Discussion

Based on the results of this in vitro study the null hypothesis was confirmed, namely that all of the materials included in this study were influenced by the hydrothermal aging.

Based on the results, thermocycling significantly decreased the Vickers hardness. Thermocycling may cause water absorption in the resin material structure. A consequence is an expansion of the network and decreasing of the frictional forces between polymer chains. Studies made suppositions that the assimilated water would lead to hydrolysis of the silane coupling agent, altering the chemical bond between the fillers and the resin matrix [19,61,62]. Other studies speculated that differences in the thermal expansion coefficients of the two phases could induce stress at the network interfaces. Experiments demonstrated that an equilibrium should be reached after 30 days and further storage in water did not alter more the mechanical properties [63].

The hardness of polished samples decreased with the decrease of the inorganic filler content, both before and after thermocycling, and for glazed samples after thermocycling, because the glaze was not kept on the surface. Glaze temporary increased the microhardness, but was removed by thermocycling. This means that aging due to thermocycling affecting the materials differently in relation to surface processing and glazing should be avoided. Other studies showed that different materials behave differently under thermocycling [63]. Related to the studied materials, PICN ceramic (E) was obtained through infiltration of presintered ceramic with resin, inducing a higher density. This could be another reason that supports the higher microhardness of this material. On the other hand, resin nanoceramic materials contain hydrophobic elements such asurethane dimethacrylate (UDMA), or hydrophilic elements such as triethylene glycol dimethacrylate (TEGDMA), and bisphenol A-glycidyl methacrylate (Bis-GMA), which can explain the decreased microhardness caused by an increase of the susceptibility to water sorption [13,63,64]. Ethoxylatedbisphenol A diglycidyl methacrylate (Bis-EMA) is a type of ethoxylatedBis-GMA that is highly hydrophilic and has no reactive hydroxyl group in its main polymer chains. It should therefore exhibit insignificant water sorption. Studies investigated composites with different filler particles and showed that those with larger fillers are more susceptible to color changes related to water sorption than those with smaller filler particles, which is due to the hydrolysis at the filler–matrix interface [19,27,65,66]. All of these previous studies support the results of this study, because hydrophobic elements are included in the matrix of resin nanoceramics and the filler particles size is also small.

Related to microroughness, all Ra values increased after thermocycling, but they were kept under the clinically accepted value, just below 0.1 μm after the second step of thermocycling. Ra values below 0.2 μm are generally clinical accepted [3,67].

Translucency allows passing of light, and it is known as the state between opacity and transparency. Opalescence is related to the light scattering of short wave-lengths from the visible spectrum in translucent materials. This characteristic gives a material a bluish-white aspect in reflected light and an orange–brown aspect in transmitted light. Restorative materials should have similar opalescent properties to natural tooth structures. Among all of the optical properties, translucency is known as a key factor for the natural outcome of esthetic restorations [68–73].

Previous studies registered mean TP values for 1 mm thick human enamel as 18.7 and for human dentine as 16.4 [74–76] The TP values for the studied resin matrix ceramic samples lie between 17.01 and 24.79. The OP value of the enamel–dentin complex was reported to be 4.8, and that of enamel, 7.4 [77–79]. The values for the studied resin matrix ceramic samples lay between 4.40 and 8.05. The CR and TP values of esthetic dental materials were compared in different studies. CR was negatively correlated to TP ($r = -0.93$). The calculated correlation was also very strong during all of the tested periods [70,79]. All of the color parameters were insignificantly changed by thermocycling. The values of the glazed samples became closer to those of the polished ones, even if the differences were insignificant between *p* and g samples. This could be a consequence of the glaze being removed after thermocycling. A marked color change was registered only for Lp.

One of the limitations of the investigations is related to the applied aging method, which is limited related to the complex clinical conditions. Another limitation of this study could be the selection of one shade (A2 or 2M2) and translucency (HT) for the tested materials. Considering that besides water absorption and the thermal changes many other factors age dental restorative materials, further studies are needed that evaluate the restorative materials using various and complex aging procedures, in order to simulate as close as possible the real oral environment [18,80,81].

However, in vitro tests can exhibit useful indications for newly developed materials as long as the testing protocol is accurate, the investigations are well-conducted and the results are carefully interpreted, taking into account the limitations [82–84].

## 5. Conclusions

Within the mentioned limitations of this in vitro study, the following conclusions can be drawn:

1. The optical properties of resin matrix ceramic materials are not significantly modified by thermocycling.
2. Roughness values, even if they increase after aging, are kept under the clinically accepted values.
3. Thermocycling significantly decreases the Vickers hardness.
4. Glaze provides surface protection for a short time, because it is removed during thermocycling.
5. This research stands as a starting point for future research because of the various hybrid materials included in this text and of the significant results. Taking everything into consideration, we can only encourage further investigations so that the results of different studies can be compared and analyzed properly.

**Author Contributions:** Conceptualization, L.P. methodology, L.P.; software, L.P.; investigation, I.-D.U., R.D.V., and F.R.T.; data curation, L.P.; writing—original draft preparation, L.P.; writing—review and editing, L.P. and R.D.V.; supervision, L.P. All authors have read and agreed to the published version of the manuscript.

**Funding:** This research received no external founds.

**Conflicts of Interest:** The authors declare no conflict of interest.

## References

1. Niem, T.; Youssef, N. Influence of accelerated ageing on the physical properties of CAD/CAM restorative materials. *Clin. Oral. Investig.* **2020**, *24*, 2415–2425. [CrossRef] [PubMed]
2. Seyidaliyeva, A.; Rues, S. Color stability of polymer-infiltrated-ceramics compared with lithium disilicatece-ramics and composite. *J. Esthet. Restor. Dent.* **2020**, *32*, 43–50. [CrossRef] [PubMed]
3. Valizadeh, S.; Asiaie, Z. Color stability of self-adhering composite resins in different solutions. *Dent. Med. Probl.* **2020**, *57*, 31–38. [CrossRef] [PubMed]
4. Hampe, R.; Lümkemann, N.; Sener, B.; Stawarczyk, B. The effect of artificial aging on Martens hardness and indentation modulus of different dental CAD/CAM restorative materials. *J. Mech. Behav. Biomed. Mater.* **2018**, *86*, 191–198. [CrossRef]
5. Miyazaki, T.; Hotta, Y. A reviewof dental CAD/CAM: Current status and future perspectives from years of experience. *Dent. Mater. J.* **2009**, *28*, 44–56. [CrossRef]
6. Bajraktarova-Valjakova, E.; Korunoska-Stevkovska, V. Contemporary Dental Ceramic Materials, A Review: Chemical Composition, Physical and Mechanical Properties, Indications for Use. *Open Access Maced. J. Med. Sci.* **2018**, *6*, 1742–1755. [CrossRef]

7. Silva, L.H.; Lima, E. Dental ceramics: A review of new materials and processing methods. *Braz Oral. Res.* **2017**, *31* (Suppl. e58), 133–146. [CrossRef]
8. Gracis, S.; Thompson, V.P. A new classification system for all-ceramic and ceramic-like restorative materials. *Int. J. Prosthodont.* **2015**, *28*, 227–235. [CrossRef]
9. Fasbinder, D.J. Chairside CAD/CAM: An overview of restorative material options. *Compend. Contin. Educ. Dent.* **2012**, *33*, 50, 52–58. [PubMed]
10. American Dental Association. CDT: Code on Dental Procedures and Nomenclature. Available online: http://www.ada.org/en/publications/cdt/ (accessed on 9 July 2019).
11. He, L.H.; Swain, M. A novel polymer infiltrated ceramic dental material. *Dent. Mater.* **2011**, *27*, 527–534. [CrossRef]
12. Yin, R.; Kim, Y.K. Comparative evaluation of the mechanical properties of CAD/CAM dental blocks. *Odontology* **2019**, *107*, 360–367. [CrossRef] [PubMed]
13. Choi, J.W.; Song, E.J.; Shin, J.H.; Jeong, T.S.; Huh, J.B. In vitro investigation of wear of CAD/CAM polymeric materials against primary teeth. *Materials* **2017**, *10*, 1410–1422. [CrossRef] [PubMed]
14. Xu, Z.; Yu, P.; Arola, D.D.; Min, J.; Gao, S. A comparative study on the wear behavior of a polymer infiltrated ceramic network (PICN) material and tooth enamel. *Dent. Mater.* **2017**, *33*, 1351–1361. [CrossRef] [PubMed]
15. Zhi, L.; Bortolotto, T.; Krejci, I. Comparative in vitro wear resistance of CAD/CAM composite resin and ceramic materials. *J. Prosthet. Dent.* **2016**, *115*, 199–202. [CrossRef]
16. Ruse, N.D.; Sadoun, M.J. Resin-composite blocks for dental CAD/CAM applications. *J. Dent. Res.* **2014**, *93*, 1232–1234. [CrossRef]
17. Conrad, H.J.; Seong, W.J. Current ceramic materials and systems with clinical recommendations: A systematic review. *J. Prosthet. Dent.* **2007**, *98*, 389–404. [CrossRef]
18. Lauvahutanon, S.; Takahashi, H. Mechanical properties of composite resin blocks for CAD/CAM. *Dent. Mater. J.* **2014**, *33*, 705–710. [CrossRef]
19. Sonmez, N.; Gultekin, P. Evaluation of five CAD/CAM materials by microstructural characterization and me-chanical tests: A comparative in vitro study. *BMC Oral. Health* **2018**, *18*, 5. [CrossRef]
20. Al Amri, M.D.; Labban, N. In Vitro Evaluation of Translucency and Color Stability of CAD/CAM Polymer-Infiltrated Ceramic Materials after Accelerated Aging. *J. Prosthodont.* **2021**, *30*, 318–328. [CrossRef]
21. Arnetzl, G.; Arnetzl, G.V. Hybrid materials offer new perspectives. *Int. J. Comput. Dent.* **2015**, *18*, 177–186.
22. Kaizera, M.R.; Oliveira-Ogliaria, A. Do nanofill or submicron composites show improved smoothness and gloss? A systematic review of in vitro studies. *Dent. Mater.* **2014**, *30*, 41–78. [CrossRef]
23. Tekçe, N.; Pala, K.; Tuncer, S.; Demirci, M. The effect of surface sealant application and accelerated aging on posterior restorative surfaces: An SEM and AFM study. *Dent. Mater. J.* **2017**, *36*, 182–189. [CrossRef] [PubMed]
24. Nogueira, A.D.; Della Bona, A. The effect of a coupling medium on color and translucency of CAD-CAM ceramics. *J. Dent.* **2013**, *41*, e18–e23. [CrossRef] [PubMed]
25. Vichi, A.; Louca, C.; Corciolani, G.; Ferrari, M. Color related to ceramic and zirconia restorations: A review. *Dent. Mater.* **2011**, *27*, 97–108. [CrossRef] [PubMed]
26. Lee, Y.-K. Opalescence of human teeth and dental esthetic restorative materials. *Dent. Mater. J.* **2016**, *35*, 845–854. [CrossRef]
27. Ardu, S.; Feilzer, A.J.; Devigus, A.; Krejci, I. Quantitative clinical evaluation of esthetic properties of incisors. *Dent. Mater.* **2008**, *24*, 333–340. [CrossRef]
28. Sulaiman, T.A.; Suliman, A.A. Optical properties of bisacryl-, composite-, ceramic-resin restorative materials: An aging simulation study. *J. Esthet. Restor. Dent.* **2021**, *33*, 913–918. [CrossRef]
29. Fontes, S.T.; Fernández, M.R.; De Moura, C.M.; Meireles, S.S. Color stability of a nanofillcomposite: Effect of different immersion media. *J. Appl. Oral Sci.* **2009**, *17*, 388–391. [CrossRef]
30. Bagheri, R.; Burrow, M.; Tyas, M. Influence of food-simulating solutions and surface finish on susceptibility to staining of aesthetic restorative materials. *J. Dent.* **2005**, *33*, 389–398. [CrossRef]
31. Murakami, M. Surface properties of an indirect composite polymerized with five laboratory light polymerization systems. *J. Oral. Sci.* **2009**, *51*, 215–221. [CrossRef]
32. Kahler, B.; Swain, M.V. Fracture-toughening mechanisms responsible for differences in work to fracture of hydrated and dehydrated dentine. *J. Biomech.* **2003**, *36*, 229–237. [CrossRef]
33. Lohbauer, U.; Frankenberger, R.; Krämer, N.; Petschelt, A. Time-dependent strength and fatigue resistance of dental direct restorative materials. *J. Mater. Sci. Mater. Electron.* **2003**, *14*, 1047–1053. [CrossRef] [PubMed]
34. Lohbauer, U.; Belli, R.; Ferracane, J. Factors Involved in Mechanical Fatigue Degradation of Dental Resin Composites. *J. Dent. Res.* **2013**, *92*, 584–591. [CrossRef] [PubMed]
35. Ferracane, J.L. Hygroscopic and hydrolytic effects in dental polymer networks. *Dent. Mater.* **2006**, *22*, 211–222. [CrossRef]
36. Münchow, E.A.; Ferreira, A.C.A.; Machado, R.; Ramos, T.S.; Rodrigues-Junior, S.A.; Zanchi, C.H. Effect of Acidic Solutions on the Surface Degradation of a Micro-Hybrid Composite Resin. *Braz. Dent. J.* **2014**, *25*, 321–326. [CrossRef]
37. Della Bona, A.; Corazza, P.H. Characterization of a polymer infiltrated ceramic network material. *Dent. Mater.* **2014**, *30*, 564–569. [CrossRef]
38. Zarslan, M.M.; Büyükkaplan, U.S. Effects of different surface finishing procedures on the change in surface roughness and color of a polymer infiltrated ceramic network material. *J. Adv. Prosthodont.* **2016**, *8*, 16–20. [CrossRef]

39. Buyukkaplan, S.U.; Özarslan, M.M.; Barutcigil, Ç.; Arslan, M.; Barutcigil, K.; Yoldan, E.E. Effects of staining liquids and finishing methods on translucency of a hybrid ceramic material having two different translucency levels. *J. Adv. Prosthodont.* **2017**, *9*, 387–393. [CrossRef]
40. Yan, Y.; Chen, C.; Chen, B.; Shen, J.; Zhang, H.; Xie, H. Effects of hydrothermal aging, thermal cycling, and water storage on the mechanical properties of a machinable resin-based composite containing nano-zirconia fillers. *J. Mech. Behav. Biomed. Mater.* **2019**, *102*, 103522. [CrossRef]
41. Chevalier, J.; Gremillard, L.; Virkar, A.V.; Clarke, D.R. The Tetragonal-Monoclinic Transformation in Zirconia: Lessons Learned and Future Trends. *J. Am. Ceram. Soc.* **2009**, *92*, 1901–1920. [CrossRef]
42. Weir, M.D.; Moreau, J.L. Nanocomposite containing $CaF_2$ nanoparticles: Thermal cycling, wear and long-term water-aging. *Dent. Mater.* **2012**, *28*, 642–652. [CrossRef]
43. Badra, V.V.; Faraoni, J.J.; Ramos, R.P.; Palma-Dibb, R.G. Influence of different beverages on the microhardness and surface roughness of resin composites. *Oper. Dent.* **2015**, *30*, 213–219.
44. Zanetti, F.; Zhao, X.; Pan, J.; Peitsch, M.C.; Hoeng, J.; Ren, Y.-F. Effects of cigarette smoke and tobacco heating aerosol on color stability of dental enamel, dentin, and composite resin restorations. *Quintessence Int.* **2018**, *50*, 156–166.
45. Bagis, B.; Turgut, S. Optical properties of current ceramics systems for laminate veneers. *J. Dent.* **2013**, *41*, e24–e30. [CrossRef] [PubMed]
46. Minami, H.; Hori, S.; Kurashige, H.; Murahara, S.; Muraguchi, K.; Minesaki, Y.; Tanaka, T. Effects of Thermal Cycling on Surface Texture of Restorative Composite Materials. *Dent. Mater. J.* **2007**, *26*, 316–322. [CrossRef] [PubMed]
47. Jones, C.S.; Billington, R.W.; Pearson, G.J. The in vivo perception of roughness of restorations. *Br. Dent. J.* **2004**, *196*, 42–45. [CrossRef]
48. Porojan, L.; Vasiliu, R.D.; Bîrdeanu, M.I.; Porojan, S.D. Surface Characterisation of Dental Resin Composites Related to Conditioning and Finishing. *Polymers* **2021**, *13*, 4236. [CrossRef]
49. Nguyen, J.-F.; Migonney, V.; Ruse, N.D.; Sadoun, M. Resin composite blocks via high-pressure high-temperature polymerization. *Dent. Mater.* **2012**, *28*, 529–534. [CrossRef]
50. Porojan, L.; Vasiliu, R.-D.; Bîrdeanu, M.-I.; Porojan, S.-D. Surface Characterization and Optical Properties of Reinforced Dental Glass-Ceramics Related to Artificial Aging. *Molecules* **2020**, *25*, 3407. [CrossRef] [PubMed]
51. Kurt, M.; Güngör, M.B.; Nemli, S.K.; Bal, B.T. Effects of glazing methods on the optical and surface properties of silicate ceramics. *J. Prosthodont. Res.* **2019**, *64*, 202–209. [CrossRef]
52. Hallmann, L.; Ulmer, P.; Lehmann, F.; Wille, S.; Polonskyi, O.; Johannes, M.; Köbel, S.; Trottenberg, T.; Bornholdt, S.; Haase, F.; et al. Effect of surface modifications on the bond strength of zirconia ceramic with resin cement resin. *Dent. Mater.* **2016**, *32*, 631–639. [CrossRef] [PubMed]
53. Paravina, R.; Powers, J. *Esthetic Color Training in Dentistry*; Elsevier Mosby: St. Louis, MO, USA, 2004; pp. 51–78.
54. Porojan, L.; Toma, F.R.; Vasiliu, R.D.; Topală, F.-I.; Porojan, S.D.; Matichescu, A. Optical Properties and Color Stability of Dental PEEK Related to Artificial Ageing and Staining. *Polymers* **2021**, *13*, 4102. [CrossRef] [PubMed]
55. Shirani, M.; Savabi, O.; Mosharraf, R.; Akhavankhaleghi, M.; Hebibkhodaei, M.; Isler, S. Comparison of translucency and opalescence among different dental monolithic ceramics. *J. Prosthet. Dent.* **2021**, *126*, 446.e1–446.e6. [CrossRef]
56. Fang, D.; Zhang, N.; Chen, H.; Bai, Y. Dynamic stress relaxation of orthodontic thermoplastic materials in a simulated oral environment. *Dent. Mater. J.* **2013**, *32*, 946–951. [CrossRef]
57. Agarwal, M.; Wible, E.; Ramir, T.; Altun, S.; Viana, G.; Evans, C.; Lukic, H.; Megremis, S.; Atsawasuwan, P. Long-term effects of seven cleaning methods on light transmittance, surface roughness, and flexural modulus of polyurethane retainer material. *Angle Orthod.* **2018**, *88*, 355–362. [CrossRef]
58. Nguyen-Tri, P.; Prud'Homme, R.E. Nanoscale analysis of the photodegradation of polyester fibers by AFM-IR. *J. Photochem. Photobiol. A Chem.* **2018**, *371*, 196–204. [CrossRef]
59. Biron, M. *Thermoplastics and Thermoplastic Composites*, 3rd ed.; Detailed Accounts of Thermoplastic Resins; William Andrew: Oxford, UK, 2018; pp. 203–766.
60. Porojan, L.; Vasiliu, R.-D.; Porojan, S.-D.; Bîrdeanu, M.-I. Surface Quality Evaluation of Removable Thermoplastic Dental Appliances Related to Staining Beverages and Cleaning Agents. *Polymers* **2020**, *12*, 1736. [CrossRef]
61. Vasiliu, R.D.; Uţu, I.D.; Porojan, L. The effect of thermocycling on microhardness and surface roughness of two zirconia reinforced lithium silicate glass-ceramics. *Mater. Today Proc.* **2021**, *45*, 4247–4249. [CrossRef]
62. He, L.H.; Purton, D. A novel polymer infiltrated ceramic for dental stimulation. *J. Mater. Sci. Mater. Med.* **2011**, *22*, 1639–1643. [CrossRef]
63. Druck, C.C.; Pozzobon, J.L.; Callegari, G.L.; Dorneles, L.S.; Valandro, L.F. Adhesion to Y-TZP ceramic: Study of silica nanofilm coating on the surface of Y-TZP. *J. Biomed. Mater. Res. Part B Appl. Biomater.* **2014**, *103*, 143–150. [CrossRef]
64. Arif, R.; Yilmaz, B.; Johnston, W.M. In vitro color stainability and relative translucency of CAD-CAM restorative materials used for laminate veneers and complete crowns. *J. Prosthet. Dent.* **2019**, *122*, 160–166. [CrossRef]
65. Coldea, A.; Swain, M.; Thiel, N. Mechanical properties of polymer-infiltrated-ceramic-network materials. *Dent. Mater.* **2013**, *29*, 419–426. [CrossRef] [PubMed]
66. Yap, A.U.J.; Wee, K.E.C. Effects of cyclic temperature changes on water sorption and solubility of composite restoratives. *Oper. Dent.* **2002**, *27*, 147–153. [PubMed]

67. Nasoohi, N.; Hoorizad, M. Effect of tea and coffee on color change of two types composite resins: Nanofilled and micro hybrid. *J. Res. Dent. Sci.* **2011**, *7*, 18–22.
68. Beltrami, R.; Ceci, M.; De Pani, G.; Vialba, L.; Federico, R.; Poggio, C.; Colombo, M. Effect of different surface finishing/polishing procedures on color stability of esthetic restorative materials: A spectrophotometric evaluation. *Eur. J. Dent.* **2018**, *12*, 49–56. [CrossRef] [PubMed]
69. Köroğlu, A.; Sahin, O.; Dede, D.; Yilmaz, B. Effect of different surface treatment methods on the surface roughness and color stability of interim prosthodontic materials. *J. Prosthet. Dent.* **2015**, *115*, 447–455. [CrossRef] [PubMed]
70. Ahin, O.; Koroglu, A. Effect of surface sealant agents on the surface roughness and color stability of denture base materials. *J. Prosthet. Dent.* **2016**, *116*, 610–616.
71. Kelly, J.R.; Benetti, P. Ceramic materials in dentistry: Historical evolution and current practice. *Aust. Dent. J.* **2011**, *56* (Suppl. 1), 84–96. [CrossRef] [PubMed]
72. PanzeriPires-de-Souza, F.d.C.; Casemiro, L.A. Color stability of dental ceramics submitted to artificial accelerated aging after repeated firings. *J. Prosthet. Dent.* **2009**, *101*, 13–18. [CrossRef]
73. Yu, B.; Ahn, J.-S.; Lee, Y.-K. Measurement of translucency of tooth enamel and dentin. *Acta Odontol. Scand.* **2009**, *67*, 57–64. [CrossRef]
74. Yu, B.; Lee, Y.-K. Difference in opalescence of restorative materials by the illuminant. *Dent. Mater.* **2009**, *25*, 1014–1021. [CrossRef]
75. Cho, M.-S.; Yu, B.; Lee, Y.-K. Opalescence of all-ceramic core and veneer materials. *Dent. Mater.* **2009**, *25*, 695–702. [CrossRef] [PubMed]
76. Gunal, B.; Ulusoy, M.M. Optical properties of contemporary monolithic CAD-CAM restorative materials at different thicknesses. *J. Esthet. Restor. Dent.* **2018**, *30*, 434–441. [CrossRef] [PubMed]
77. Lee, Y.-K. Translucency of human teeth and dental restorative materials and its clinical relevance. *J. Biomed. Opt.* **2015**, *20*, 45002. [CrossRef] [PubMed]
78. Akar, G.C.; Pekkan, G.; Çal, E.; Eskitaşçıoğlu, G.; Özcan, M. Effects of surface-finishing protocols on the roughness, color change, and translucency of different ceramic systems. *J. Prosthet. Dent.* **2014**, *112*, 314–321. [CrossRef]
79. Monaco, C.; Arena, A.; Ozcan, M. Effect of Prophylactic Polishing Pastes on Roughness and Translucency of Lithium Disilicate Ceramic. *Int. J. Periodontics Restor. Dent.* **2014**, *34*, e26–e29. [CrossRef] [PubMed]
80. Lee, S.-H.; Lee, Y.-K.; Lim, B.-S. Influence of thermocycling on the optical properties of laboratory resin composites and an all-ceramic material. *J. Mater. Sci. Mater. Electron.* **2004**, *15*, 1221–1226. [CrossRef]
81. Alp, G.; Subasi, M.G. Effect of surface treatments and coffee thermal cycling on the color and translucency of CAD-CAM monolithic glassceramic. *J. Prosthet Dent.* **2018**, *120*, 263–268. [CrossRef]
82. Morresi, A.L.; D'Amario, M.; Capogreco, M.; Gatto, R.; Marzo, G.; D'Arcangelo, C.; Monaco, A. Thermal cycling for restorative materials: Does a standardized protocol exist in laboratory testing? A literature review. *J. Mech. Behav. Biomed. Mater.* **2014**, *29*, 295–308. [CrossRef]
83. Egilmez, F.; Ergun, G.; Cekic-Nagas, I.; Vallittu, P.K.; Lassila, L.V. Does artificial aging affect mechanical properties of CAD/CAM composite materials. *J. Prosthodont. Res.* **2018**, *62*, 65–74. [CrossRef]
84. El-Araby, A.M.; Talic, Y.F. The effect of thermocycling on the adhesion of self-etching adhesives on dental enamel and dentin. *J. Contemp. Dent. Pract.* **2007**, *8*, 17–24. [CrossRef]

*applied sciences*

MDPI

*Article*

# Amorphous Calcium Magnesium Fluoride Phosphate—Novel Material for Mineralization in Preventive Dentistry

**Erik Unosson [1], Daniel Feldt [2], Wei Xia [2] and Håkan Engqvist [2,*]**

[1] Psilox AB, Vallvägen 4A, 756 51 Uppsala, Sweden; unosson.erik@gmail.com
[2] Department of Materials Science and Engineering, Division of Applied Materials Science, Uppsala University, 751 21 Uppsala, Sweden
* Correspondence: hakan.engqvist@angstrom.uu.se

**Featured Application: The article presents a novel fluoride particle technology for rapid remineralization, applicable for caries prevention and treatment of dentin hypersensitivity.**

**Abstract:** This paper describes novel and innovative amorphous calcium magnesium fluoride phosphate (ACMFP) core-shell microparticles that may be applied in preventive dentistry for the prevention of caries and the treatment of dentin hypersensitivity. The particles can be synthesized with varied fluoride content, up to approximately 6 wt%, without any observable differences in morphology or crystallinity. Fluoride release from the particles is correlated to the fluoride content, and the particles are readily converted to fluoride-substituted hydroxyapatite or fluorapatite in a simulated saliva solution. The remineralization and dentin tubule occlusion potential of the particles was evaluated in vitro on acid-etched dentin specimens, and treatment with the ACMFP particles resulted in complete tubule occlusion and the formation of a dense mineralization layer. The acid resistance of the mineralization layer was improved compared to treatment with analogous particles without fluoride inclusion. A cross-sectional evaluation of dentin specimens after treatment revealed the formation of high aspect ratio fluorapatite crystals and poorly crystalline hydroxyapatite, respectively. The particles of the current study provide a single source vehicle of readily available calcium, phosphate, and fluoride ions for the potential remineralization of carious lesions as well as exposed dentin tubules for the reduction of hypersensitivity.

**Keywords:** caries; dentin hypersensitivity; preventive dentistry; amorphous calcium phosphate; fluoride; remineralization

**Citation:** Unosson, E.; Feldt, D.; Xia, W.; Engqvist, H. Amorphous Calcium Magnesium Fluoride Phosphate—Novel Material for Mineralization in Preventive Dentistry. *Appl. Sci.* **2023**, *13*, 6298. https://doi.org/10.3390/app13106298

Academic Editor: Vittorio Checchi

Received: 4 May 2023
Revised: 19 May 2023
Accepted: 20 May 2023
Published: 22 May 2023



## 1. Introduction

Caries (tooth decay or dental cavities) is a major global healthcare issue, and according to the 2019 Global Burden of Disease Study, it is estimated that 2.03 billion people have caries in their permanent teeth and that 520 million children have caries in their primary teeth, making it the most prevalent non-communicable disease in the world [1,2]. Caries is a result of plaque formation on the tooth surface, where bacteria excrete acids while metabolizing fermentable carbohydrates. This causes demineralization of the enamel and dentin and, if allowed to progress, will cause the formation of cavities. In order to prevent caries, it is important to reduce the daily intake of dietary sugars and to exercise regular dental hygiene care, such as tooth brushing and flossing. Tooth brushing should be performed with a fluoridated toothpaste, which can prevent and arrest the progression of caries by forming fluorapatite, i.e., inhibiting demineralization [3,4]. Demineralization of dentin and enamel may be countered by remineralization, in which calcium and phosphate ions present in the saliva can deposit to form new mineral. This requires a local supersaturation of ions to form hydroxyapatite. If fluoride is present, the newly formed mineral may be fluorapatite rather than hydroxyapatite, making it less soluble and more resistant to acid erosion [5,6].

Repeated acid attacks or poor salivary flow may, however, tip the scale towards continued demineralization, leading to a net mineral loss. This has prompted the need for additional calcium phosphate sources and the development of specialized oral care products [7]. Different calcium phosphate technologies and particles have thus been introduced in the past 20 years to promote the remineralization of enamel as well as the occlusion of dentin tubules for the reduction of dentin hypersensitivity [8,9]. Dentin hypersensitivity is generally triggered by thermal, mechanical, or evaporative stimuli of the tooth and is highly prevalent among adults, reported at 34% in a recent study [10]. It is a clinical condition that can cause significant oral discomfort and pain, and the underlying cause is that the dentin tubules have become exposed due to gingival recession or loss of enamel, which is in turn caused by, e.g., abrasion or acid erosion, excessive tooth brushing or flossing, pocket reduction surgery, or as a secondary reaction to periodontal disease [10,11]. According to the generally accepted hydrodynamic theory, occluding the dentin tubules will hinder fluid movement within the tubules, which otherwise excites nerve endings in the pulp, causing the sensation of pain [12]. For a long-lasting and minimally invasive treatment of dentin hypersensitivity, the tubules should therefore ideally be deeply occluded with an acid-resistant mineralization layer resistant to both abrasion and erosion, and it should preferably be easy to apply at home or as a topical desensitizer product at the dental office. Successful treatment and prevention of both caries and dentin hypersensitivity thus rely on effective remineralization, requiring adequate access to calcium, phosphate, and fluoride ions.

There are a number of products and technologies on the market today that deliver various forms of calcium phosphate to the tooth surface, the most prevalent being hydroxyapatite (as nano- or microparticles, available in many kinds of toothpaste), different bioglasses (e.g., NovaMin®), and casein phosphopeptide–amorphous calcium phosphate (CPP–ACP, marketed as RECALDENT™). All of these technologies have successful clinical track records and have been demonstrated to be effective as remineralization agents in multiple studies [9,13,14]. They are regularly combined with fluoride in oral care products for daily caries protection. Each of these technologies has drawbacks or limitations, however, ranging from poor solubility (hydroxyapatite) to coarse particles (bioglass) [15] and milk protein allergy (CPP–ACP). A recent comparative study showcased the efficacy in dentin mineralization and tubule occlusion of an alternative technology based on stabilized microparticles of amorphous calcium magnesium phosphate (ACMP, marketed as CAPOSAL®) [16]. In the study, CAPOSAL® was the only technology resulting in complete occlusion and deep mineralization of the dentin tubules. The mineralization layer was also able to withstand an acid challenge, increasing the chances for long-term sensitivity relief. The mode of action of these particles, as well as the characteristics of intra-tubular mineralization layers, have been demonstrated in separate studies [17,18]. Combined, these studies demonstrate that the application of ACMP particles is one of the most effective approaches for promoting dentin remineralization and tubule occlusion, caused by the high aqueous solubility that supplies a high local concentration of calcium and phosphate ions. The metastable nature of ACMP particles also means that they are easily transformed into more stable calcium phosphate phases in situ, such as hydroxyapatite. In fact, amorphous calcium phosphate has long been considered a precursor to natural apatite in teeth and bone and therefore plays an important role in endogenous mineralization [19,20], and its unique properties have rendered it a highly interesting material for dental and other biomedical applications [21,22]. With the innovative CAPOSAL® technology, the previously elusive nature of amorphous calcium phosphate particles as a functional ingredient in oral care products has been made commercially available. Until now, however, the ACMP particles have relied on separate application and external supply of fluoride ions to form the more acid- and caries-resistant fluorapatite mineralization layer [18]. In the current study, we present a development of the ACMP particles to also contain a fluoride inclusion, making the particles essentially self-sustaining in the process of remineralizing dentin for the proposed reduction of dentin hypersensitivity and the prevention of caries.

## 2. Materials and Methods

### 2.1. Particle Synthesis

The amorphous calcium magnesium fluoride phosphate (ACMFP) particles described in this study were produced based on the development of a previously described method for the synthesis of ion-substituted calcium phosphate particles [17,23–25]. The amorphous nature of the particles is obtained by substituting $Mg^{2+}$ for $Ca^{2+}$, which inhibits the nucleation and growth of hydroxyapatite during synthesis. The particles may be synthesized by heating a phosphate buffer containing calcium and substitution ions or by a continuous flow mixing process of pre-heated calcium/magnesium and phosphate/fluoride salt solutions. Both methods result in the precipitation of core-shell particles with a hollow interior, with the latter method generating finer particles and being better suited for large-scale production as it allows for higher throughput. The fluoride content in the current particles was adjusted by changing the relative fluoride concentration in the appropriate starting solution. The formed particles were collected by filtration and washed with deionized water to remove any salt residues. To obtain long-term stability, the resulting particle slurry was mixed with glycerol, and residual water was evaporated by drying the mixture in a forced convection oven. The dried product was then homogenized to obtain a viscous paste consisting of stabilized and well-dispersed ACMFP particles in glycerol, suitable for use in the formulation of oral care products.

### 2.2. Characterization

The appearance and elemental composition of the synthesized particles were evaluated using the in-lens secondary electron detector of a field emission scanning electron microscope (SEM, Zeiss LEO 1530) equipped with an energy-dispersive X-ray spectroscopy system (EDS, Oxford AZtec). In preparation for analysis, the particles were dispersed in alcohol by ultrasound, pipetted onto sample stubs, and sputter coated with a thin Au/Pd conductive layer. Imaging was conducted using an acceleration voltage of 2 keV and a working distance of approximately 3 mm, whereas EDS data was collected using an acceleration voltage of 6 keV and a working distance of 8 mm. Crystallinity of the particles was evaluated on powder samples by X-ray diffraction (XRD, Bruker D8 ADVANCE), using CuK$\alpha$-radiation and scanning $2\theta$ from 10 to 60° with a step size of 0.0125°. Particle size distribution was evaluated using dynamic light scattering (DLS, Malvern Zetasizer Nano) after dispersing a fine amount of particles by ultrasound in ethanol. The Brunauer–Emmett–Teller (BET) particle-specific surface area was measured using $N_2$ adsorption (Micromeritics TriStar II). In addition to the EDS measurements, the content of Ca, Mg, and P in the particles was quantified using inductively coupled plasma optical emission spectroscopy (ICP-OES, Perkin Elmer Avio 200) after dissolution in 5% $HNO_3$. The instrument was calibrated with stock standard solutions (Perkin Elmer) and corresponding blanks. Fluoride concentration was additionally determined using a calibrated fluoride ion selective electrode coupled to a benchtop meter (Hanna Instruments HI 4110, HI 5522-02), measuring in total ionic strength adjustment buffer (TISAB II) after dissolving the particles in diluted HCl. Fluoride release from the particles was analyzed by adding 50 mg of particles to 100 mL of TISAB II under stirring and measuring the fluoride concentration in solution after 1, 5, 10, and 30 min.

### 2.3. In Vitro Mineralization and Dentin Tubule Occlusion

Bioactivity of the ACMFP particles, in terms of their propensity to transform/crystallize into hydroxyapatite or fluorapatite in biological conditions, was evaluated by submerging the particles in a simulated saliva solution composed as described in Table 1 (pH 7). Particles were left static in the solution for 18 h at 37 °C, then filtered, dried, and characterized in SEM and by XRD. Phase composition analysis of the crystallized material was performed using Rietveld refinement (Profex v4.3.5 software, an open source software, available from www.profex-xrd.org, accessed on 3 May 2023), quantifying hydroxyapatite and fluorapatite.

**Table 1.** Composition of the simulated saliva solution.

| Salt | Conc. (mM) |
|---|---|
| NaCl | 30 |
| KCl | 3 |
| $CaCl_2 \cdot 2H_2O$ | 1.5 |
| $MgCl_2 \cdot 6H_2O$ | 0.5 |
| $Na_2HPO_4 \cdot 2H_2O$ | 2.9 |
| $KH_2PO_4$ | 2.1 |

In vitro mineralization and dentin tubule occlusion testing were performed based on a previously described protocol [16]. Dentin specimens were sectioned from extracted human molars without any caries or anatomical defects using a water-cooled low-speed saw (Buehler IsoMet 2000). The sectioning was performed in the buccolingual plane, yielding specimens with approximate dimensions of 1 × 8 × 8 mm. Utilization of human molars in the study was performed in compliance with guidelines from the Swedish Ethical Review Authority (2016/039). After sectioning, the dentin specimens were etched in 30% phosphoric acid for 15 s to remove the smear layer and expose the tubules, followed by a thorough rinsing in deionized water. The dentin specimens were then subjected to a mineralization treatment with formulas containing glycerol and either 5% ACMFP particles or 5% ACMP particles (without fluoride) for comparison. A blank treatment formula without any mineralizing particles was also included for reference. Each treatment formula was applied to two dentin specimens twice daily for seven days, using a soft-bristled toothbrush and manual brushing with light hand pressure for approximately 30 s at each application. In between applications, the dentin specimens were stored in a simulated saliva solution (Table 1) at 37 °C, which was exchanged daily. Upon completion of the treatment, one specimen of each treatment formula was subjected to an acid challenge by swirling in a 2% citric acid solution (pH 2) for 30 s. The specimens were then rinsed, vacuum dried, mounted on sample stubs, and sputter coated with a thin conductive Au/Pd layer to allow SEM evaluation. One dentin specimen for each treatment cycle was evaluated, for a total of six specimens. Cross-sectional images of the dentin tubules were taken after manually breaking the specimens.

## 3. Results

The EDS elemental composition of ACMFP particles synthesized with various fluoride contents is listed in Table 2. The fluoride concentration ranged from essentially 0 wt% in ACMP particles synthesized without fluoride to nearly 6 wt% in the particles denoted ACMFP-4. Results from ICP-OES analysis were in general agreement with EDS data for Ca, P, and Mg content, whereas fluoride ion selective electrode measurements indicated a lower F content than those quantified with EDS (Table 3).

**Table 2.** Elemental composition of particles according to EDS analysis.

| Sample | O (wt%) | Ca (wt%) | P (wt%) | Mg (wt%) | F (wt%) |
|---|---|---|---|---|---|
| ACMP | 54.3 ± 0.8 | 23.2 ± 1.0 | 14.6 ± 0.1 | 7.9 ± 1.8 | 0.1 ± 0.1 |
| ACMFP-1 | 48.4 ± 2.0 | 25.6 ± 0.6 | 19.0 ± 1.0 | 5.9 ± 0.1 | 1.2 ± 0.2 |
| ACMFP-2 | 50.2 ± 1.5 | 23.0 ± 1.5 | 17.9 ± 2.3 | 6.4 ± 0.4 | 2.6 ± 0.3 |
| ACMFP-3 | 50.3 ± 3.3 | 24.7 ± 0.8 | 15.5 ± 3.3 | 6.3 ± 0.0 | 3.2 ± 0.7 |
| ACMFP-4 | 48.6 ± 1.8 | 25.7 ± 1.5 | 12.8 ± 0.6 | 7.1 ± 0.8 | 5.8 ± 0.2 |

Morphology of synthesized particles is shown in Figure 1, demonstrating a generally spherical shape and a mixture of singular and fused particles with diameters ranging from 100 to 300 nm. The DLS z-average particle size of approximately 360 nm (Table 3) reflects the aggregation of particles. There were no apparent differences in the appearance between

ACMP particles (Figure 1A) and ACMFP particles (Figure 1B,C), demonstrating that the fluoride inclusion did not affect the particle morphology.

**Table 3.** Characteristics of ACMFP-2 particles. Elemental composition according to ICP-OES (Ca, P, and Mg) and fluoride ion selective electrode (F). Z-average particle size according to DLS and specific surface area according to $N_2$ BET analysis.

| Sample | Ca (wt%) | P (wt%) | Mg (wt%) | F (wt%) | Z-Avg. Particle Size (nm) | BET Surface Area (g/m$^2$) |
|---|---|---|---|---|---|---|
| ACMFP-2 | 21.5 ± 0.3 | 20.0 ± 0.5 | 6.9 ± 0.1 | 1.51 ± 0.05 | 362 ± 38 | 24.5 ± 1.1 |

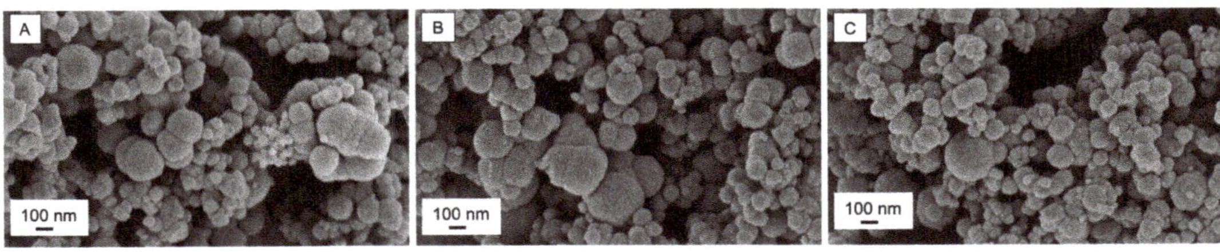


**Figure 1.** SEM images of particles: (**A**) ACMP synthesized without fluoride; (**B**) ACMFP-2 particles; (**C**) ACMFP-4 particles.

XRD analysis of the same particles demonstrated that they were amorphous, with identical spectra regardless of fluoride inclusion (Figure 2A). Fluoride release, however, as shown in Figure 2B, demonstrates a significant difference between particles synthesized with and without fluoride. The relative fluoride release from particles was reflective of the concentrations listed in Table 2. The particles can be stabilized after synthesis by suspension in glycerol, with no observed changes in particle morphology or crystallinity after six months of storage at 40 °C.

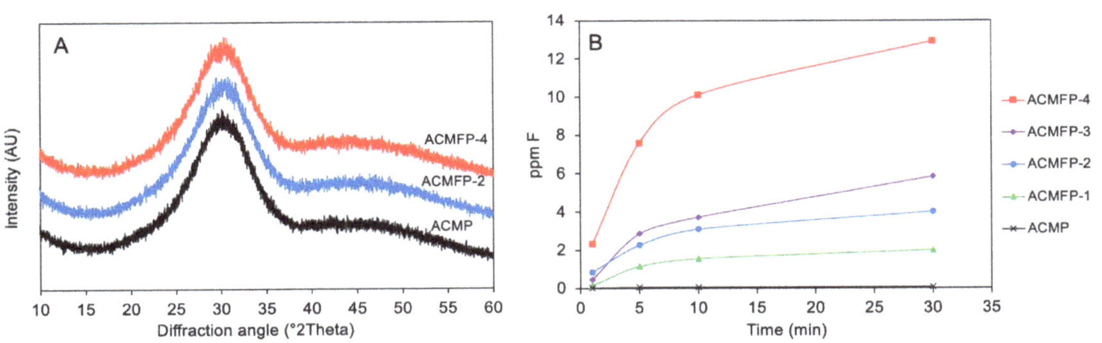


**Figure 2.** (**A**) XRD spectra of ACMP, ACMFP-2, and ACMFP-4 particles; (**B**) Fluoride release curves from ACMP and ACMFP particles with varied fluoride content.

The gradual transformation of ACMFP particles from amorphous core-shell particles to crystalline bundles of fluoride-substituted hydroxyapatite in simulated saliva solution is shown in Figure 3A–C. In Figure 3A, protrusions of high aspect ratio crystals are observed stemming directly from the ACMFP particle surfaces, with the image capturing an early phase of the transformation process. In Figure 3B, some features of the origin of ACMFP particles are still visible, but sharp crystals dominate the appearance. In Figure 3C, the particles are completely crystallized, demonstrating the final phase of transformation. All three SEM images in Figure 3 were captured from the same sample after static incubation for 18 h, and the global crystallinity of the sample is demonstrated in the XRD spectrum in Figure 3D. Phase identification of the crystalline part using Rietveld refinement yielded a share of approximately 58% fluorapatite and 42% hydroxyapatite.

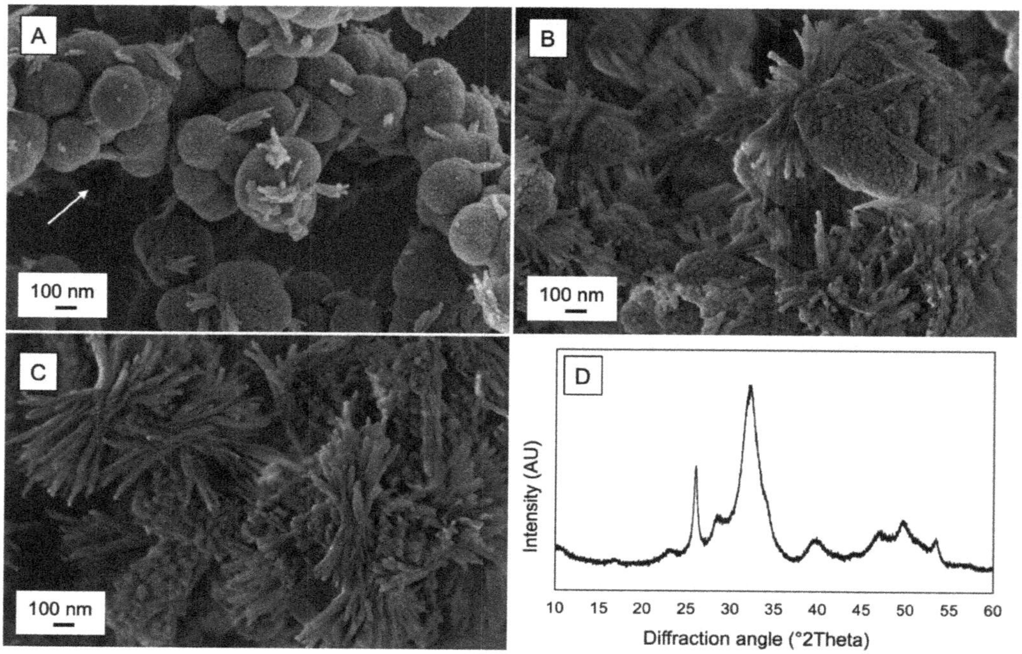


**Figure 3.** (**A–C**) SEM images of ACMFP particles at different stages of crystallization in simulated saliva. Arrow in (**A**) displays a hollow particle core; (**D**) XRD spectrum of crystallized particles.

The results of the in vitro mineralization and dentin tubule occlusion tests are shown in Figure 4. The top panel (Figure 4A–C) displays a reference dentin surface and a tubule in cross-section after treatment with a blank formula without any mineralizing particles. The tubules were fully exposed both before and after the acid challenge, demonstrating that the simulated saliva solution used for storage was not sufficiently mineralizing to have any notable effect. The middle panel (Figure 4D–F) shows the dentin surface and the mineralization product within a tubule after treatment with ACMP particles, i.e., without any fluoride inclusion. The tubules were completely occluded with a mineralized layer before the acid challenge (Figure 4D), but the orifices became partly visible again after the acid challenge (Figure 4E). The mineralized material both on the surface and within the tubules was characteristic of poorly crystalline nano-hydroxyapatite, as observed in previous studies [17,18]. Treatment with the ACMFP particles also resulted in complete tubule occlusion (Figure 4G) but with the added feature of resisting dissolution during the acid challenge (Figure 4H). The mineralization product within the tubules was dense and characterized by high aspect ratio crystals extending from the peritubular wall (Figure 4I), similar in appearance to the crystallized particles shown in Figure 3C as well as to fluoride-substituted hydroxyapatite structures reported in previous studies [16,18]. The deep (>10 μm) mineralization within the dentin tubules was unaffected by the acid challenge.

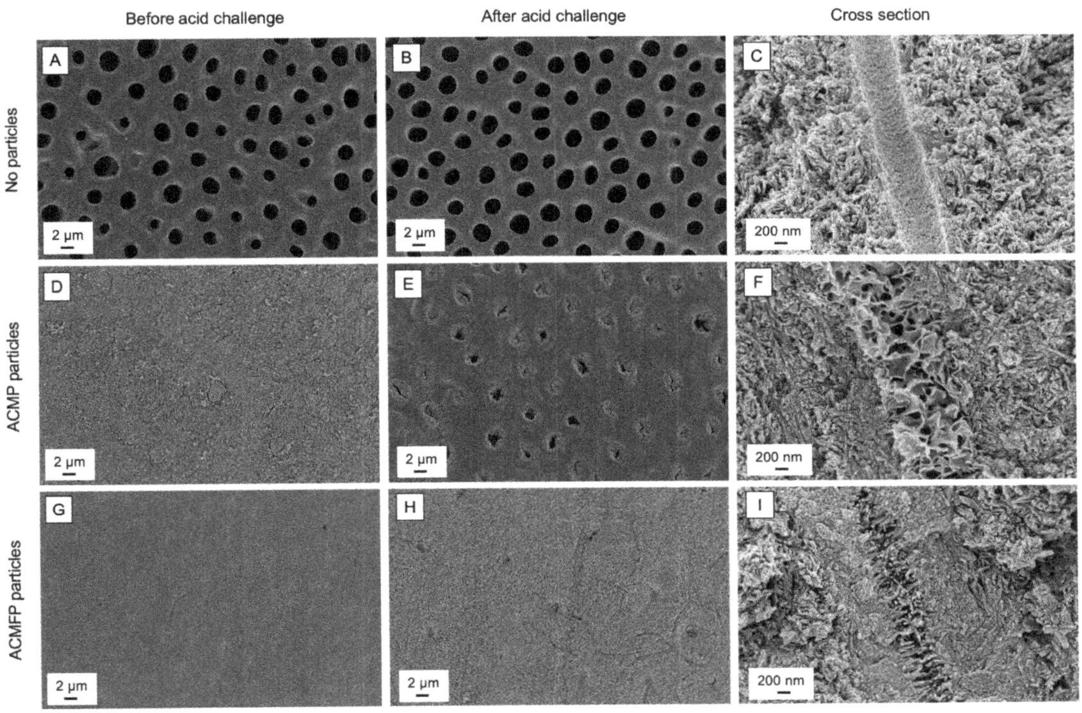


**Figure 4.** SEM images of dentin surfaces and dentin tubules in cross-section: Top panel (**A–C**) shows appearance after treatment with blank formula (no particles); Middle panel (**D–F**) shows appearance after treatment with the ACMP formula; Bottom panel (**G–I**) shows appearance after treatment with the ACMFP formula. The left-hand panel (**A**,**D**,**G**) shows surfaces before the acid challenge, and the center panel (**B**,**E**,**H**) after the acid challenge. Cross-section images of dentin tubules beneath the treated surface are shown in the right-hand panel (**C**,**F**,**I**).

## 4. Discussion

Fluoride treatment is the gold standard when it comes to caries prevention, and brushing with fluoridated toothpaste is at the core of a sound oral care routine. Much of the effectiveness of fluoride in preventing caries and helping maintain good oral health depends on its capacity to enhance the remineralization of dentin and enamel and subsequently inhibit demineralization due to increased acid resistance [5]. For remineralization to be effective, there should be a net mineral gain in the tooth structure, i.e., the degree of apatite deposition should outweigh the dissolution caused by plaque bacteria. Facilitating the right conditions to remineralize or repair early enamel defects such as sub-surface lesions ("white spots") may be complex, as it generally depends on ion diffusion through a more intact surface layer. A key aspect of reversing sub-surface demineralization is thus to clear the acid-producing plaque and allow saliva to contact the surface, which can neutralize the area and provide calcium and phosphate ions. If the saliva is supersaturated with calcium and phosphate, ions may then diffuse back into the lesion and remineralize partially demineralized crystals in a process that is accelerated in the presence of fluoride [26,27]. To create conditions that favor remineralization, especially in areas subjected to repeated acid challenges or in cases of poor salivary flow, supplementing the saliva and the lesion surface with readily available calcium, phosphate, and fluoride ions is therefore crucial. Application of a successful remineralization therapy may often be sufficient to stop caries progression and repair early lesions, reducing the need for costly and irreversible restorations [26]. As such, there is evidently a need for the development of calcium phosphate technologies that can contribute to the remineralization process in an effective way.

The ACMFP particles of the current study present an opportunity to deliver a single source vehicle of readily available calcium, phosphate, and fluoride ions for remineralization of carious lesions as well as exposed dentin tubules for the reduction of hypersensitivity. The particles may also be produced in a simple and cost-effective way. The unique spherical shape and sub-micron size of the particles make them especially suitable for dentin tubule occlusion, as they enable deep penetration and mineralization that can resist both abrasion and acid erosion. The prospect of having all key remineralization ions from a single source that is readily converted into fluoride-substituted hydroxyapatite could make products for preventive dentistry more effective and potentially safer, as excessive use of fluoride during tooth development may lead to fluorosis. The potential risk of fluorosis should not deter from the proper use of fluoride, however, as the benefits clearly outweigh the risks [3–5]. Nevertheless, the current findings demonstrate that the degree of fluoride inclusion in the particles and subsequent fluoride release can be adjusted without altering their characteristic features in terms of morphology and crystallinity (Figures 1 and 2), which effectively allows tailoring of the particles to suit a wide range of applications. The fluoride inclusion may be high to maximize the fluoride release and remineralization potential of the particles, or it can be optimized at a lower level to reduce overall fluoride exposure. As the direct crystallization and remineralization triggered by the particles are independent of long-range fluoride ion diffusion from other sources, the ACMFP particles can offer local remineralization with a lower overall fluoride concentration.

The rapid in vitro conversion from amorphous core-shell particles into crystalline fluorapatite-like mineral depicted in Figure 3 illustrates the bioactive and remineralizing properties of the ACMFP particles. Several mechanisms of the conversion process from ACP to apatite in aqueous media have been proposed in the literature, including dissolution–reprecipitation, reorganization of Posner's clusters, and surface-mediated transformation triggered by phosphate hydrolysis, leading to apatite nucleation and growth supported by surface ion migration [22]. It is plausible that all these processes occur to a varying degree at different stages of conversion of the particles, i.e., once apatite is nucleated at the particle surface, the rate of dissolution–reprecipitation increases. It is further established that this conversion process is accelerated in the presence of fluoride [22,27]. The corresponding conversion was demonstrated in an in vitro mineralization and tubule occlusion test, showing that the ACMFP particles generated a more acid-resistant mineralization layer than the fluoride-free ACMP particles (Figure 4). It should be noted that similar mineralization and tubule occlusion results have been observed in previous studies [16,18], but only when the ACMP particles have been applied in combination with an external fluoride source, e.g., successive application of a toothpaste containing sodium fluoride. Although the current findings are based on in vitro data from a limited set of dentin specimens, the results indicate that a similarly effective remineralization and dentin tubule occlusion effect can be obtained by the sole use of the ACMFP particles, eliminating the need for external or additional fluoride sources.

## 5. Conclusions

This study briefly describes the development, characteristic features, and potential application of ACMFP core-shell particles for use as a remineralization agent in preventive dentistry. It is demonstrated that the particles may be synthesized with a varied fluoride content and thereby allow fine-tuning and optimization for various needs and indications related to caries prevention. The amorphous particles are rapidly converted into fluorapatite structures in simulated saliva, and in vitro analysis demonstrates the formation of an acid-resistant mineralization layer both on the dentin surface and deep within dentin tubules. Based on the hydrodynamic theory, the complete tubule occlusion observed after the application of the ACMFP particles makes them a viable option for the effective treatment of dentin hypersensitivity.

**Author Contributions:** Conceptualization, E.U., W.X. and H.E.; methodology, E.U., D.F. and W.X.; investigation, E.U. and D.F.; resources, E.U. and H.E.; writing—original draft preparation, E.U.; writing—review and editing, E.U., D.F., W.X. and H.E.; visualization, E.U.; supervision, E.U. and W.X. All authors have read and agreed to the published version of the manuscript.

**Funding:** This research received no external funding.

**Institutional Review Board Statement:** The use of extracted human molars was approved according to the guidelines from the Regional Ethics Review Board in Uppsala (Sweden) (2016/039).

**Informed Consent Statement:** The study did not involve any interventions or handling of personal data that are covered in the Swedish Ethics Review Act (2006:615). The use of would-be discarded extracted molars for scientific purposes was therefore waived on the condition of anonymity, and provisions regarding personal consent did not apply to the use of human samples in the study.

**Data Availability Statement:** Data presented in the study are available upon request from the authors.

**Conflicts of Interest:** E.U., W.X. and H.E. are connected to Psilox AB, which has developed the material family (CAPOSAL®) evaluated in the study. E.U. is employed by the company, and W.X. and H.E. are shareholders. D.F. has no conflict of interest.

## References

1. Qin, X.; Zi, H.; Zeng, X. Changes in the global burden of untreated dental caries from 1990 to 2019: A systematic analysis for the Global Burden of Disease study. *Heliyon* **2022**, *8*, e10714. [CrossRef]
2. Pitts, N.B.; Twetman, S.; Fisher, J.; Marsh, P.D. Understanding dental caries as a non-communicable disease. *Brit. Dent. J.* **2021**, *231*, 749–753. [CrossRef]
3. Tenuta, L.M.A.; Cury, J.A. Fluoride: Its role in dentistry. *Braz. Oral Res.* **2010**, *24*, 9–17. [CrossRef]
4. Cate, J.M.T. Contemporary perspective on the use of fluoride products in caries prevention. *Brit. Dent. J.* **2013**, *214*, 161–167. [CrossRef]
5. Featherstone, J.D.B. Prevention and reversal of dental caries: Role of low level fluoride. *Community Dent. Oral* **1999**, *27*, 31–40. [CrossRef]
6. Pajor, K.; Pajchel, L.; Kolmas, J. Hydroxyapatite and Fluorapatite in Conservative Dentistry and Oral Implantology—A Review. *Materials* **2019**, *12*, 2683. [CrossRef]
7. Neel, E.A.A.; Aljabo, A.; Strange, A.; Ibrahim, S.; Coathup, M.; Young, A.M.; Bozec, L.; Mudera, V. Demineralization–remineralization dynamics in teeth and bone. *Int. J. Nanomed.* **2016**, *11*, 4743–4763. [CrossRef]
8. Philip, N. State of the Art Enamel Remineralization Systems: The Next Frontier in Caries Management. *Caries Res.* **2019**, *53*, 284–295. [CrossRef]
9. Meyer, F.; Amaechi, B.T.; Fabritius, H.-O.; Enax, J. Overview of Calcium Phosphates used in Biomimetic Oral Care. *Open. Dent. J.* **2018**, *12*, 406–423. [CrossRef]
10. Alcântara, P.M.; Barroso, N.F.F.; Botelho, A.M.; Douglas-de-Oliveira, D.W.; Gonçalves, P.F.; Flecha, O.D. Associated factors to cervical dentin hypersensitivity in adults: A transversal study. *BMC Oral. Health* **2018**, *18*, 155. [CrossRef]
11. Davari, A.; Ataei, E.; Assarzadeh, H. Dentin hypersensitivity: Etiology; diagnosis; treatment; a literature review. *J. Dent. Shiraz Iran.* **2013**, *14*, 136–145.
12. Bartold, P. Dentinal hypersensitivity: A review. *Aust. Dent. J.* **2006**, *51*, 212–218. [CrossRef]
13. Chen, L.; Al-Bayatee, S.; Khurshid, Z.; Shavandi, A.; Brunton, P.; Ratnayake, J. Hydroxyapatite in Oral Care Products—A Review. *Materials* **2021**, *14*, 4865. [CrossRef]
14. Li, J.; Xie, X.; Wang, Y.; Yin, W.; Antoun, J.S.; Farella, M.; Mei, L. Long-term remineralizing effect of casein phosphopeptide-amorphous calcium phosphate (CPP-ACP) on early caries lesions in vivo: A systematic review. *J. Dent.* **2014**, *42*, 769–777. [CrossRef]
15. LaTorre, G.; Greenspan, D.C. The role of ionic release from NovaMin (calcium sodium phosphosilicate) in tubule occlusion: An exploratory in vitro study using radio-labeled isotopes. *J. Clin. Dent.* **2010**, *21*, 72–76.
16. Berg, C.; Unosson, E.; Engqvist, H.; Xia, W. Comparative Study of Technologies for Tubule Occlusion and Treatment of Dentin Hypersensitivity. *J. Funct. Biomater.* **2021**, *12*, 27. [CrossRef]
17. Berg, C.; Unosson, E.; Engqvist, H.; Xia, W. Amorphous Calcium Magnesium Phosphate Particles for Treatment of Dentin Hypersensitivity: A Mode of Action Study. *Acs Biomater. Sci. Eng.* **2020**, *6*, 3599–3607. [CrossRef]
18. Berg, C.; Unosson, E.; Riekehr, L.; Xia, W.; Engqvist, H. Electron microscopy evaluation of mineralization on peritubular dentin with amorphous calcium magnesium phosphate microspheres. *Ceram. Int.* **2020**, *46*, 19469–19475. [CrossRef]
19. Posner, A.S.; Betts, F. Synthetic amorphous calcium phosphate and its relation to bone mineral structure. *Acc. Chem. Res.* **1975**, *8*, 273–281. [CrossRef]
20. Boskey, A.L. Amorphous Calcium Phosphate: The Contention of Bone. *J. Dent. Res.* **1997**, *76*, 1433–1436. [CrossRef]

21. Zhao, J.; Liu, Y.; Sun, W.; Zhang, H. Amorphous calcium phosphate and its application in dentistry. *Chem. Cent. J.* **2011**, *5*, 40. [CrossRef]
22. Combes, C.; Rey, C. Amorphous calcium phosphates: Synthesis, properties and uses in biomaterials. *Acta Biomater.* **2010**, *6*, 3362–3378. [CrossRef] [PubMed]
23. Xia, W.; Grandfield, K.; Schwenke, A.; Engqvist, H. Synthesis and release of trace elements from hollow and porous hydroxyapatite spheres. *Nanotechnology* **2011**, *22*, 305610. [CrossRef] [PubMed]
24. Xia, W.; Qin, T.; Suska, F.; Engqvist, H. Bioactive Spheres: The Way of Treating Dentin Hypersensitivity. *ACS Biomater. Sci. Eng.* **2016**, *2*, 734–740. [CrossRef] [PubMed]
25. Mellgren, T.; Qin, T.; Öhman-Mägi, C.; Zhang, Y.; Wu, B.; Xia, W.; Engqvist, H. Calcium Phosphate Microspheres as a Delivery Vehicle for Tooth-Bleaching Agents. *J. Dent. Res.* **2018**, *97*, 283–288. [CrossRef]
26. Featherstone, J. Dental caries: A dynamic disease process. *Aust. Dent. J.* **2008**, *53*, 286–291. [CrossRef]
27. Cate, J.M.T.; Featherstone, J.D.B. Mechanistic Aspects of the Interactions between Fluoride and Dental Enamel. *Crit. Rev. Oral Biol. Med.* **1991**, *2*, 283–296. [CrossRef]

applied sciences

MDPI

*Systematic Review*

# Effect of Plasma Treatment on Root Canal Sealers' Adhesion to Intraradicular Dentin—A Systematic Review

**Inês Ferreira [1,2], Cláudia Lopes [3,4], Armando Ferreira [3,4], Filipe Vaz [3,4], Irene Pina-Vaz [5,*] and Benjamín Martín-Biedma [6]**

1 School of Medicine and Dentistry, University of Santiago de Compostela, 15705 Santiago de Compostela, Spain; iferreira@fmd.up.pt
2 CINTESIS, Faculty of Dental Medicine, University of Porto, 4200-393 Porto, Portugal
3 Physics Centre of Minho and Porto Universities (CF-UM-UP), University of Minho, 4710-057 Braga, Portugal; fvaz@fisica.uminho.pt (F.V.)
4 LaPMET—Laboratory of Physics for Materials and Emergent Technologies, University of Minho, 4710-057 Braga, Portugal
5 CINTESIS@RISE, Faculty of Dental Medicine, University of Porto, 4200-393 Porto, Portugal
6 Oral Sciences Research Group, Endodontics and Restorative Dentistry Unit, School of Medicine and Dentistry, Health Research Institute of Santiago (IDIS), University of Santiago de Compostela, 15705 Santiago de Compostela, Spain; benjamin.martin@usc.es
* Correspondence: igvaz@fmd.up.pt

**Abstract:** This investigation aimed to assess, through a systematic review, the effect of non-thermal plasma treatments on root canal sealers' adhesion to dentin. This study followed the 2020 Preferred Reporting Items for Systematic Reviews and Meta-Analyses (PRISMA) guidelines. A literature search was undertaken without limits on time or language, until May 2023, in PubMed–MEDLINE, Scopus, Web of Science, OpenGrey, and three endodontic journals. The included studies underwent quality assessment and data extraction. Out of an initial 188 articles, 4 studies were included. Three of these studies based the adhesion ability on the push-out test in human extracted teeth, while the other used bovine dentin samples to measure the contact angle with the sealer (wettability). While there was no consensus about the effect of non-thermal plasma (NTP) on the AH Plus sealer's adhesion to radicular dentin, NTP seemed to positively influence the adhesion ability of BioRoot RCS and Endosequence BC. The findings of the present review should be interpreted cautiously due to the scarcity of studies on the topic. The NTP parameters should be optimized to obtain a stronger evidence base in endodontics on its role as an adjuvant tool to increase sealers' adhesion to dentin.

**Keywords:** adhesion; gutta-percha; plasma treatments; root canal filling; root canal obturation; root canal therapy; root canal sealers

**Citation:** Ferreira, I.; Lopes, C.; Ferreira, A.; Vaz, F.; Pina-Vaz, I.; Martín-Biedma, B. Effect of Plasma Treatment on Root Canal Sealers' Adhesion to Intraradicular Dentin—A Systematic Review. *Appl. Sci.* **2023**, *13*, 8655. https://doi.org/10.3390/app13158655

Academic Editor: Vittorio Checchi

Received: 3 June 2023
Revised: 14 July 2023
Accepted: 24 July 2023
Published: 27 July 2023



## 1. Introduction

Endodontic therapy, generally focused on root canal treatment, has a major goal directed to the cure or prevention of periradicular periodontitis. Orthograde endodontic treatment includes cleaning and shaping of the root canal system, preparing it for the subsequent filling, with the aim of maintaining disinfection and preventing reinfection. The latter is achieved by a core—most often gutta-percha—and an endodontic sealer, under well-defined criteria of length and density. The treatment is completed by an adequate coronal restoration [1].

A dentin sealer's adhesion is its ability to adhere to the root canal's walls and promote the union of the filling materials to dentin. Different sealers and filling techniques (e.g., single cone, lateral compaction, or thermoplastic obturation) have been reported to produce an impact in the penetration of the sealer into dentinal tubules, thereby influencing dentin sealers' adhesion [2]. Optimal adhesion of the root filling to the intraradicular dentin leads to fewer gap-containing regions, which would allow fluid infiltration within either sealer–dentin or sealer–core–filling material interfaces [3]. Consequently, it also avoids sealer dislodgment during operative procedures, increasing endodontic treatment success rates [3]. It is widely accepted that sealing ability is of utmost importance to successful outcomes of root canal treatments [3].

A great variety of endodontic sealers are available commercially. They are divided into different groups according to their chemical composition, properties, or therapeutic additives, which influence their performance [4]. Studies have also shown that the sealers' bond strength to dentin may be affected by the pretreatment of canal walls and the type of sealer used [5].

The physicochemical properties of sealers interfere with their ability to adhere to dentin [6]. The epoxy-resin-based sealer AH Plus (Dentsply DeTrey GmbH, Konstanz, Germany) is the gold-standard sealer due to its extensively studied physical properties, such as its high bond strength to dentin [6]. This advantage has been justified by epoxy-resin-based sealers' chemical bonding to exposed collagen and their great capacity to form smooth and compact tags inside dentinal tubules [6,7]. MTA Fillapex is composed of a salicylate–resin matrix filled with MTA, natural resin, bismuth oxide, and silica [8]. This sealer's composition is primarily resin, which raises doubts concerning its classification as a true calcium-silicate-based sealer or MTA-based sealer [4]. Nevertheless, it is reported that the set sealer releases calcium and hydroxyl ions. When the material comes into contact with phosphate-containing fluids, these ions cause the formation of apatite, which may deposit within collagen fibrils, promoting controlled mineral nucleation on dentin, seen as the formation of an interfacial layer with tag-like structures [7,8]. MTA Fillapex's low bond strength could be due to the low adhesion capacity of these tag-like structures [9].

Calcium-silicate-based sealers, such as BioRoot RCS and Endosequence BC, have become popular in endodontics, mainly due to their biocompatibility and bioactivity [10]. These sealers have the potential to adhere chemically to dentin through the production of hydroxyapatite during setting [6]. Although they have undergone great development to improve their performance, there is still a lack of consensus regarding their bond strength to intraradicular dentin [6,11].

Plasma, considered to be the fourth state of matter, is an electrically conductive medium that responds to electric and magnetic fields and is also a source of large quantities of highly reactive species such as electrons, ions, electronically excited neutrons, and free radicals [12]. Plasmas are generally classified as thermal and non-thermal (or cold plasma), based on the relative temperatures and energy of the different plasma species (electrons, ions, and neutrons) [12]. In thermal plasmas, electrons and heavy particles are in thermal equilibrium, while in non-thermal plasma (NTP), electrons are hotter than ions and neutrons are at room temperature [12]. NTP can be used under vacuum or atmospheric conditions, using inert gases like argon (Ar) or helium (He), reactive gases such as oxygen ($O_2$) or nitrogen ($N_2$), or a mixture of two or more gases [13,14]. Plasma treatments provide an effective and clean technology for surface activation without changing the materials' original structure and functional properties [15]. Previous studies have shown that NTP is efficient for cleaning/decontaminating and sterilizing instruments [16] and tooth whitening [17], and it seems to be a promising tool in combating dental biofilms [18]. Moreover, this technology has been shown to increase the wettability and hydrophilicity of different surfaces, such as dentin, enamel, and composites, improving their adhesive features or etching dentinal tubules, ensuring higher mechanical retention of root canal sealers [19].

To the best of our knowledge, to date, no systematic review has evaluated the influence of NTP on the adhesion between endodontic sealers and intraradicular dentin. Thus, this work aimed to assess, through a systematic review, the effect of NTP treatments on root canal sealers' adhesion to dentin.

## 2. Materials and Methods

This systematic review followed the recommendations of the 2020 Preferred Reporting Items for Systematic Reviews and Meta-Analyses (PRISMA) guidelines [20].

### 2.1. Eligibility Criteria

This study was conducted to answer the PICO question "Does the NTP treatment affect sealers' adhesion to dentin compared to no treatment?", with the following parameters: extracted teeth as the participants, plasma treatment as the intervention, no treatment as the comparison, and evaluating root canal sealers' adhesion to dentin as the outcome.

Only in vitro studies that treated dentin with plasma technology and assessed the effects of NTP treatments on root canal sealers' adhesion to dentin were included. Studies that did not use a control group (without plasma treatment) were excluded.

### 2.2. Search Strategy

The search was carried out in May 2023 on PubMed (Medline), Scopus, and Web of Science. The electronic search combined Medical Subject Heading (MeSH) terms, text words (tw), and truncation terms. The Boolean operators "AND" and "OR" were used to create the search strategy (Table 1). No language or publication date restrictions were applied. Additionally, gray literature was investigated through OpenGrey, and a manual search of the *Journal of Endodontics*, *International Endodontic Journal*, and *Australian Endodontic Journal* was performed to find any additional papers. Moreover, an additional search was conducted using the reference lists of all included papers. References from different databases were imported into the EndNote X9 software (Thomson Reuters, New York, NY, USA), which automatically removed duplicate records.

**Table 1.** Search strategy in different databases.

| Database | Search Strategy | Findings |
|---|---|---|
| PubMed | #1 ((non-thermal plasma[Title/Abstract]) or (nonthermal plasma[Title/Abstract]) or (Plasma Gases[Title/Abstract]) or (plasma treatment[Title/Abstract]) or plasma[Title/Abstract] or (Plasma Gases[MeSH Terms]) or plasma[MeSH Terms]) | |
| | #2 ((dental cements[MeSH Terms]) or (root canal sealants[MeSH Terms]) or (dental cement *[Title/Abstract]) or (root canal seal *[Title/Abstract]) or (endodontic seal *[Title/Abstract]) or (root canal fill *[Title/Abstract]) or (seal*[Title/Abstract])) | |
| | #3 ((endodontic *[Title/Abstract]) or (root canal[Title/Abstract]) or (endodontic treatment[Title/Abstract]) or (root canal treatment[Title/Abstract]) or (Root Canal Therapy[Title/Abstract]) or (Root Canal Therapy[MeSH Terms]) or (Endodontics[MeSH Terms]) | |
| | #1 and #2 and #3 | 96 |
| Scopus | #1 TITLE-ABS-KEY("non-thermal plasma" or "nonthermal plasma" or "Plasma Gases" or "plasma treatment" or plasma) | |
| | #2 TITLE-ABS-KEY("dental cements" or "root canal sealants" or "dental cement *" or "root canal seal *" or "endodontic seal *" or "root canal fill *" or "seal *") | |
| | #3 TITLE-ABS-KEY("endodontic *" or "root canal" or "endodontic treatment" or "root canal treatment" or "Root Canal Therapy") | |
| | #1 and #2 and #3 | 140 |
| Web of Science | #1 TS = ("non-thermal plasma" or "nonthermal plasma" or "Plasma Gases" or "plasma treatment" or plasma) | |
| | #2 TS = ("dental cements" or "root canal sealants" or "dental cement *" or "root canal seal*" or "endodontic seal *" OR "root canal fill *" or "seal *") | |
| | #3 TS = ("endodontic *" or "root canal" or "endodontic treatment" or "root canal treatment" or "Root Canal Therapy") | |
| | #1 and #2 and #3 | 83 |

## 2.3. Selection of the Studies

Two reviewers independently assessed the searched titles and abstracts and discarded the non-eligible papers. When the title and abstract were insufficient to confirm or exclude a particular study, they read the full text. In case of divergence, a third author decided whether the paper should be included.

## 2.4. Data Extraction

The following information was extracted and recorded from each included study: tooth type, non-thermal treatment (i.e., gas/application time, plasma mode, device used, distance, pressure, and power applied), methodology for testing adhesion ability (push-out testing parameters (i.e., filling materials used, storage, canal segments analyzed, slice thickness, plunger diameter, and plunger loading direction) and contact angle analysis), and main results.

## 2.5. Risk-of-Bias Assessment

Two authors independently evaluated the risk of bias in each selected study. The risk of bias assessment method was adapted from a previously published systematic review [21]. The following parameters were considered: (1) randomization, (2) blinding, (3) standardization of specimen selection, (4) standardized preparation (single operator), and (5) reporting of data. If the above parameters were mentioned, the risk of bias was recorded as low; if the parameters were not mentioned, it was recorded as high; if their mention was not clear, it was recorded as unclear. Disagreements among authors were resolved through discussion with a third author.

# 3. Results

Figure 1 shows the flow diagram of the search strategy. After duplicates were removed, the search generated 188 studies. After the analysis of titles and abstracts, five were selected. After comprehensive reading of these studies, one was excluded due to not treating dentin with plasma technology [22]. Therefore, four studies fulfilled the eligibility criteria and were included in this systematic review.

Table 2 shows the results of the included papers' risk of bias. All studies had a high risk of bias with respect to blinding, randomization process, and standardized sample preparation (single operator), because these parameters were not mentioned. All of the studies reported all results and performed sample standardization, so they were considered to have a low risk of bias in these parameters. None of the included studies had a low risk of bias in all parameters evaluated, so the overall risk of bias of the selected studies was high. Table 3 summarizes the included studies.

**Table 2.** Quality assessment of the included studies [13,23–25].

| Author (Year) | Randomization | Blinding | Standardization of Sample Selection | Standardization Preparation (Single Operator) | Reporting of Data |
|---|---|---|---|---|---|
| Prado et al., 2016 | High | High | Low | High | Low |
| Menezes et al., 2017 | High | High | Low | High | Low |
| Yeter et al., 2020 | High | High | Low | High | Low |
| Garlapati et al., 2021 | High | High | Low | High | Low |

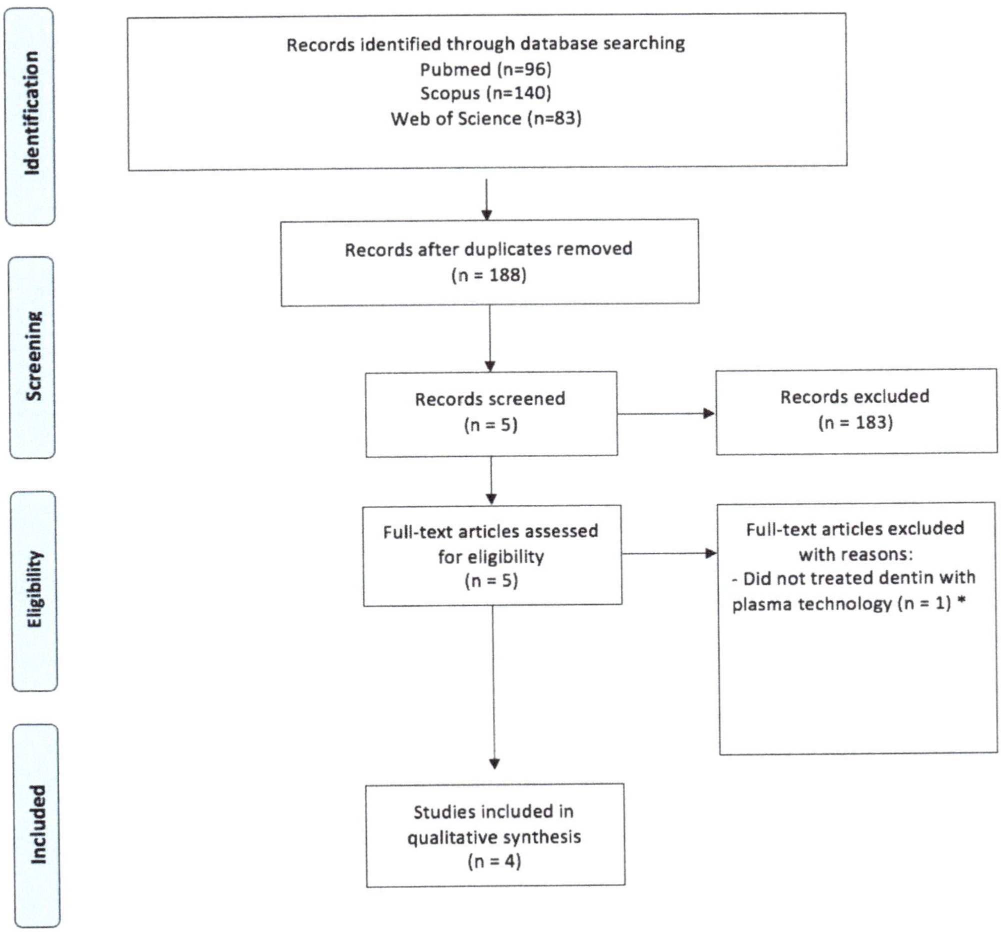


**Figure 1.** Flow diagram of the search strategy. * Record excluded [22].

### 3.1. NTP Treatment Methodology

Three studies used human single-rooted extracted teeth [23–25]. Only one used bovine teeth [13]. Prado, et al. [13] and Garlapati, et al. [25] applied NTP treatments under vacuum conditions using a glass reactor, while Yeter, et al. [23] and Menezes, et al. [24] used an atmospheric-pressure plasma jet. Under vacuum conditions, a power of 60 W was applied to generate the plasma, with a working pressure of 10 Pa and a base pressure of 2 Pa. For plasma application through a plasma jet mode, the gas pressure was kept at 6 bar and 2.5 bar; the distance between the tip of the plasma jet and the dentin was approximately 5 mm. Two studies used argon plasma [13,23], while the other two applied a mixture of gases [24,25]. The application time was 30 s, except in the study of Menezes, et al. [24], where it was 1 min.

**Table 3.** Characteristics of the included studies (GP: gutta-percha; Ar: argon; $O_2$: oxygen; He: helium; P: pressure; SFE: surface free energy, SE: sealer wettability) [13,23–25].

| Author | Tooth Type | Non-Thermal Treatment | | | | | Methodology for Testing Dentin-Sealer Adhesion Capacity | | | | | | | | | Main Results |
|---|---|---|---|---|---|---|---|---|---|---|---|---|---|---|---|---|
| | | | | | | | Bond Strength Analysis—Push-Out Test | | | | | | | | Contact Angle Analysis | |
| | | Gas | Plasma Mode | Application Time | Distance | Power | Pressure | Filling Material | Storage and Duration | Canal Segments | Slice Thickness | Plunger Diameter | Crosshead Speed | Plunger Loading Direction | | |
| Prado et al., 2016 | Bovine incisors | Argon | Vacuum | 30 s | - | 60 W | $P_{base}$ = 2 Pa $P_{work}$ = 10 Pa | AH Plus | - | - | - | - | - | - | Wettability—contact angle between the dentin and the AH Plus sealer | Argon plasma increased the wettability of AH Plus, favoring its bonding to dentin |
| Menezes et al., 2017 | Human single-rooted premolars | Mixture of 98% He and 2% $O_2$ | Jet | 1 min | 5 mm | - | 6 bars | GP + AH Plus GP + MTA Fillapex | 100% humidity for 2 days | Coronal; middle; apical | 1 mm | 0.76 mm coronal; 0.60 mm middle; 0.40 mm apical | 0.5 mm/min | Unclear | - | Regarding AH Plus, bond strength was similar in the plasma and control groups. For MTA Fillapex, the bond strength decreased with plasma treatment |
| Yeter et al., 2020 | Human single-rooted mandibular premolars | Argon | Jet | 30 s | 5 mm | - | 2.5 bars | GP + AH Plus GP + Endosequence BC | 100% humidity for 7 days | Coronal; middle | Unclear | Unclear | 0.5 mm/min | Apical–coronal | - | Argon plasma did not influence the bond strength of AH Plus to dentin. The Endosequence BC showed a better bond strength than the AH Plus after argon plasma treatment |
| Garlapati et al., 2021 | Human single-rooted mandibular premolar | Mixture of He and Ar | Vacuum | 30 s | - | 60 W | $P_{base}$ = 2 Pa $P_{work}$ = 10 Pa | GP + AH Plus GP + BioRoot RCS | Not mentioned | Middle | 2 mm | 1 mm | 1 mm/min | Unclear | - | Plasma treatment enhanced the bond strength of BioRoot RCS and AH Plus |

### 3.2. Dentin Sealers' Adhesion Assessment

- Push-out test [23–25]
    (a) Filling material and sample storage: Three studies filled the canal with gutta-percha and sealer [23–25]. The storage time ranged from 2 to 7 days, and the specimens were kept in an incubator at 37 °C and 100% humidity. Garlapati, et al. [25] did not mention the storage conditions and time.
    (b) Slice thickness and canal segments: The thickness of the slices varied between 1 and 2 mm. Yeter, et al. [23] did not clearly describe the slice thickness. Menezes, et al. [24] used apical, middle, and coronal thirds, Garlapati, et al. [25] used only the middle third, and Yeter, et al. [23] used the coronal and middle thirds.
    (c) Plunger diameter, speed, and direction: Menezes, et al. [24] used three plunger sizes to equal the diameter of each root third, Garlapati, et al. [25] used a plunger of 1 mm, and Yeter, et al. [23] did not mention the plunger diameter used. The plunger's loading direction was unclear in two studies. Yeter, et al. [23] applied an apical–coronal direction. The crosshead speed varied between 0.5 mm/min and 1 mm/min.
- Contact angle analysis [13].

In one of the studies, adhesion was assessed based on the wettability of the resin-based sealer AH Plus. It was calculated through the contact angle between the dentin surfaces and the sealer [13].

### 3.3. Influence of NTP on Dentin Sealers' Adhesion

The epoxy-resin-based sealer AH Plus was tested in all of the included studies. The other sealers tested were MTA Fillapex [24], BioRoot RCS [25], and Endosequence BC [23]. In two studies, plasma treatment did not influence the bond strength of AH Plus to dentin [23,24]. On the other hand, Garlapati, et al. [25] and Prado, et al. [13] concluded that plasma treatment improved the AH Plus–dentin adhesion. The bond strength of BioRoot RCS and Endosequence BC was positively influenced by plasma treatment. For MTA Fillapex, the bond strength decreased with plasma treatment.

## 4. Discussion

Root canal filling materials' adhesion to dentin has been widely tested using the push-out bond strength (POBS) test, also called dislodgement resistance [26]. Well-controlled experiments are challenging when using biological samples, due to the substantial effects of the inherent biological, physical, and chemical variances imposed by natural samples. A recent study investigated the reliability of using bovine teeth as an alternative to human teeth for testing the POBS of sealers to dentin and concluded that the dentin substrate did not influence the sealers' bond strength [27]. Only one of the studies included in our review used bovine teeth [13]. The variations in push-out methodology are a concern because they prevent the comparison of results from different researchers [26]. Generally, studies have followed two philosophies: the root canals are either filled with the sealer alone or combined with gutta-percha with the filling techniques of cold lateral compaction, single-cone filling, or specific obturation systems such as Resilon/Epiphany [28,29]. Three studies included in this review filled the samples with gutta-percha and sealer [23–25]. According to some authors, filling the canals only with sealer ensures that there are no confounding factors and that the adhesion strength tested is that of the sealer [28].

The adhesion processes are mostly influenced by the relative surface free energy, which determines the predisposition of the material's surface for establishing new interactions/bonds with the surrounding medium. In the same way, wettability is influenced by the interfacial tensions and, in turn, by the surface free energy [30]. Thus, contact angle evaluation has been widely used to measure the surface wettability of different materials [22]. The contact angle has an inverse relationship with the surface free energy (wettability), i.e., the lower the contact angle, the greater the surface free energy and, hence, likely greater adhesion [13]. Prado, et al. [13] observed increased surface free energy, correlated with the higher wettability of bovine dentin with AH Plus after 30 s of argon NTP, compared to the control (i.e., without NTP). They also reported a chemical change based on FTIR results. Argon plasma treatment reduced the organic compounds of dentin (amide I and II bands) and increased the inorganic component (the carbonade band), due to its ability to etch dentin surfaces; no associated topographical changes occurred. Based on these findings, the authors concluded that argon treatment favored the bonding of the sealer to dentin surfaces [13]. However, only the resinous AH Plus sealer was evaluated.

There is no consensus or sufficient data about NTP's effect on radicular dentin in terms of endodontic sealers' adhesion. In the present investigation, a systematic review was conducted to answer the following PICO question: Does the NTP treatment affect sealers' adhesion to dentin compared to no treatment? A few ex-vivo studies met the selection criteria, even though some disparity in the materials and methodologies was registered, which prevented a meta-analysis from being performed. Our findings indicate that NTP on dentin root walls might positively impact sealers' adhesion, considering the increased POBS or surface energy and wettability values reported in the selected literature.

The bioceramic sealer (BioRoot RCS) showed the highest POBS values, followed by the epoxy-resin-based sealer (AH Plus), after mixing helium and argon atmospheres on dentin surfaces [25]. Moreover, the NTP dentin groups showed an increase in bond strength more than two times higher than the non-plasma-treated dentin (control groups), independent of the sealer [25]. The better bond strength of the bioceramic sealer after NTP, compared to the resinous AH Plus [25], was also corroborated by other authors who stressed its good performance, particularly in the middle region of the root canal [23]. Albeit with different plasma applications, both studies included two recently developed calcium-silicate-based sealers: BioRoot RCS [25] and Endosequence [23], reported to have adhesive characteristics and bioactivity. A recent review of current sealers points out that tricalcium silicate sealers are associated with the lowest relative microleakage compared to the standard AH Plus [4]. The higher POBS values obtained can derive from the chemical nature of bioceramic sealers, affecting properties such as fluidity, their easy spread over the dentin walls due to their low contact angle, or an increase in dentin wettability after NTP [15,23,31]. It was reported that the dentin surface modification after NTP, such as enhanced wettability and chemical interaction, could favor dentinal tubule penetration and the bioceramic sealer's bond strength [23]. Although the authors did not explain the minor influence of NTP on the POBS evaluation of AH Plus [23], other factors, such as the chemical and structural alterations that different irrigating solutions can produce in dentin surfaces, might have affected the results [32].

There are other endodontic procedures aimed to open plasma treatments that can be created under low pressure or atmospheric pressure and increase wettability, such as the standard chelating agent EDTA [33]. However, the additional NTP generally increased these properties, acting as an adjuvant procedure, as shown by the higher POBS values or wettability observed after EDTA exposure [13,25]. Conversely, in the study of Yeter, et al. [23], the final flush was performed with NaOCl. NaOCl may have caused a deproteinization, causing a hydrophilic surface that did not favor the resinous sealer's hydrophilicity [32]. With a similar irrigating solution sequence (EDTA followed by NaOCl), Menezes, et al. [24] found similar bonding values to the control for the NTP groups with either AH Plus or MTA Fillapex. The type of sealer might also have influenced the results.

NTP has been reported to reach deep into the dentinal tubules, similar to or further than bacteria, creating reactive oxygen species and damaging the remaining microorganisms, in addition to cleaning/etching [19]. Thus, it seems to ensure higher mechanical retention and adhesion. This rationale was corroborated by Menezes, et al. [24], Prado, et al. [13], and Garlapati, et al. [25], who reported improved adhesion of NTP surfaces.

Plasma treatments can be carried out at low pressure or atmospheric pressure. The main difference lies in the pressure at which they operate, which affects the plasma density, confinement, and particle behavior [34]. Low-pressure plasmas are generated and sustained in a vacuum or low-pressure environment using vacuum chambers. The benefit of low-pressure plasmas is that the mean free path of the particles (i.e., atoms, ions, and electrons) is relatively long, meaning that they can travel greater distances between collisions. The conditions are much more controllable and reproducible compared to atmospheric-pressure conditions (typically close to 1 atmosphere, where the particles' mean free path is much shorter than in low-pressure plasmas due to the higher gas density), which could compensate (at least partially) for the practical drawbacks of using low-pressure plasma—especially the need for expensive vacuum equipment [35,36]. On the other hand, atmospheric-pressure plasmas have become very attractive because they are generated in an open environment and can be easily implemented [37]. Nevertheless, if particular precautions are not taken, they tend to become thermal, i.e., hot plasmas that can damage heat-sensitive materials or burn living tissues [38]. In the included studies, Prado, et al. [13] and Garlapati, et al. [25] applied NTP treatments under vacuum conditions using a glass reactor, while Yeter, et al. [23] and Menezes, et al. [24] used an atmospheric-pressure plasma jet.

Using low-pressure plasma in dental applications offers several advantages, such as enhanced control over the plasma parameters (e.g., gas composition, pressure, and power), deeper penetration into complex dental structures, access to confined spaces, and uniform treatments due to the better diffusion of the reactive species [22,39–41]. Furthermore, the reduced heat and controlled plasma conditions make low-pressure plasma treatments suitable for treating delicate dental components, such as resin-based composites, polymer-based materials, or dental implants [22,39–41]. However, the potential drawbacks of plasma treatments must be carefully considered. Excessive exposure or high-energy plasma can damage the dentin structure, limiting the treatment's effectiveness and durability. Moreover, implementing plasma treatments requires specialized equipment and expertise, which can increase the cost and complexity of dental procedures. Despite these considerations, plasma treatments offer advantages such as enhanced bonding, improved biocompatibility, effective sterilization, and reduced dentin hypersensitivity [34]. Dental professionals should understand the potential benefits and challenges so as to make informed decisions about incorporating plasma treatments into their practice.

Plasma treatments offer a promising avenue for enhancing dentin surfaces, and the choice of gas composition (e.g., low-pressure processes) plays a crucial role in determining the treatment outcomes [42]. Gas mixing can lead to synergistic effects, creating chemical reactions or interactions that are more effective than using each gas individually [43]. Also, mixing gases expands the range of possible low-pressure plasma treatments and allows for selective treatments [43]. One common gas mixture used in low-pressure plasma treatments is argon (Ar) and oxygen ($O_2$), which provides several benefits [43]. Ar, like helium (He), is an inert gas with low thermal conductivity, which helps minimize the thermal effects on dentin during plasma treatment. It also acts as a carrier gas, facilitating the transport and interaction of reactive species within the plasma [42]. Oxygen, on the other hand, introduces additional reactive species, enabling more effective cleaning, surface modification, or chemical reactions with the dentin surface [42]. The Ar + $O_2$ or He + $O_2$ combination is also an effective sterilization method [18]. The reactive species generated in plasma, such as oxygen radicals, have antimicrobial properties, enabling them to eliminate bacteria, viruses, and other pathogens [18]. This sterilization capability is particularly valuable in infection control during dental procedures, reducing the risk of post-treatment infections [18]. If gases are carefully selected and mixed, the plasma parameters can be controlled, allowing for fine-tuning of the treatment process. Thus, dental professionals can optimize the treatment conditions, ensuring efficient and effective results while minimizing potential risks and adverse effects.

Compared to untreated dentin, i.e., not subjected to plasma treatment, the studies included in this systematic review suggest—albeit with low-certainty evidence—that plasma treatment may be a promising tool for improving the adhesion of endodontic sealers to dentin. Some of the parameters used, such as the time of NTP application, were based on investigations of dental composites' adhesion, because there are insufficient data on root canal dentin–sealer adhesion [14,23]. The type of plasma atmosphere, exposure time, and assessment tools might need to be unified to optimize NTP. However, its high cost has been highlighted.

The findings of the present review should be interpreted cautiously, due to the scarcity of studies on the topic. Moreover, a quantitative analysis was not feasible due to the heterogeneity of the study designs in terms of the plasma treatment (i.e., type of devices used; plasma parameters like power, frequency, gas type, and application time), adhesion methodology, and type of sealers used. Although a total of 188 studies were obtained from the electronic search, only 4 were included after applying the eligibility criteria. Nonetheless, the overall risk of bias of the included studies was high. However, the strict selection of the studies enabled an overview of this contemporary topic, highlighting its potential.

## 5. Conclusions

The studies included in this systematic review suggest that plasma treatment may be a promising tool for improving endodontic sealers' adhesion to dentin. There is a need to optimize NTP's parameters to develop a stronger evidence base in endodontics on its role as an adjuvant tool to increase sealers' adhesion to dentin. This optimization could help improve the outcomes of root canal treatments.

**Author Contributions:** Conceptualization, I.F., I.P.-V. and B.M.-B.; methodology, I.F., C.L. and A.F.; data curation, I.F., C.L. and A.F.; writing—original draft preparation, I.F., C.L. and A.F.; writing—review and editing, F.V., I.PV. and B.M.-B.; supervision, I.PV. and B.M.-B.; funding acquisition, I.P.-V. All authors have read and agreed to the published version of the manuscript.

**Funding:** This article was supported by National Funds through the FCT—Fundação para a Ciência e a Tecnologia, I.P., within CINTESIS, R&D Unit (reference UIDP/4255/2020).

**Institutional Review Board Statement:** Not applicable.

**Informed Consent Statement:** Not applicable.

**Data Availability Statement:** The data presented in this study are available from the corresponding author upon reasonable request.

**Conflicts of Interest:** The authors declare no conflict of interest.

## References

1. European Society of Endodontology. Quality guidelines for endodontic treatment: Consensus report of the European Society of Endodontology. *Int. Endod. J.* **2006**, *39*, 921–930. [CrossRef]
2. Abdellatif, D.; Amato, A.; Calapaj, M.; Pisano, M.; Iandolo, A. A novel modified obturation technique using biosealers: An ex vivo study. *J. Conserv. Dent.* **2021**, *24*, 369–373. [CrossRef]
3. Schwartz, R.S. Adhesive dentistry and endodontics. Part 2: Bonding in the root canal system-the promise and the problems: A review. *J. Endod.* **2006**, *32*, 1125–1134. [CrossRef]
4. Komabayashi, T.; Colmenar, D.; Cvach, N.; Bhat, A.; Primus, C.; Imai, Y. Comprehensive review of current endodontic sealers. *Dent. Mater. J.* **2020**, *39*, 703–720. [CrossRef]
5. Fernandes Zancan, R.; Hadis, M.; Burgess, D.; Zhang, Z.J.; Di Maio, A.; Tomson, P.; Hungaro Duarte, M.A.; Camilleri, J. A matched irrigation and obturation strategy for root canal therapy. *Sci. Rep.* **2021**, *11*, 4666. [CrossRef] [PubMed]
6. Silva, E.; Canabarro, A.; Andrade, M.; Cavalcante, D.M.; Von Stetten, O.; Fidalgo, T.; De-Deus, G. Dislodgment Resistance of Bioceramic and Epoxy Sealers: A Systematic Review and Meta-analysis. *J. Evid.-Based Dent. Pract.* **2019**, *19*, 221–235. [CrossRef]
7. BaechtoldI, M.S.; MazaroI, A.F.; CrozetaI, B.M.; LeonardiI, D.P.; TomazinhoI, F.S.F.; Baratto-FilhoI, F.; HaragushikuI, G.A. Adhesion and formation of tags from MTA Fillapex compared with AH Plus® cement. *RSBO* **2014**, *11*, 71–76.
8. Silva, E.J.; Rosa, T.P.; Herrera, D.R.; Jacinto, R.C.; Gomes, B.P.; Zaia, A.A. Evaluation of cytotoxicity and physicochemical properties of calcium silicate-based endodontic sealer MTA Fillapex. *J. Endod.* **2013**, *39*, 274–277. [CrossRef]
9. Sagsen, B.; Ustün, Y.; Demirbuga, S.; Pala, K. Push-out bond strength of two new calcium silicate-based endodontic sealers to root canal dentine. *Int. Endod. J.* **2011**, *44*, 1088–1091. [CrossRef] [PubMed]
10. Al-Haddad, A.; Che Ab Aziz, Z.A. Bioceramic-Based Root Canal Sealers: A Review. *Int. J. Biomater.* **2016**, *2016*, 9753210. [CrossRef] [PubMed]

11. Silva Almeida, L.H.; Moraes, R.R.; Morgental, R.D.; Pappen, F.G. Are Premixed Calcium Silicate-based Endodontic Sealers Comparable to Conventional Materials? A Systematic Review of In Vitro Studies. *J. Endod.* **2017**, *43*, 527–535. [CrossRef]
12. Lata, S.; Chakravorty, S.; Mitra, T.; Pradhan, P.K.; Mohanty, S.; Patel, P.; Jha, E.; Panda, P.K.; Verma, S.K.; Suar, M. Aurora Borealis in dentistry: The applications of cold plasma in biomedicine. *Mater. Today Bio* **2022**, *13*, 100200. [CrossRef] [PubMed]
13. Prado, M.D.; Roizenblit, R.N.; Pacheco, L.V.; Barbosa, C.A.d.M.; Lima, C.O.d.; Simão, R.A. Effect of Argon Plasma on Root Dentin after Use of 6% NaOCl. *Braz. Dent. J.* **2016**, *27*, 41–45. [CrossRef]
14. Ritts, A.C.; Li, H.; Yu, Q.; Xu, C.; Yao, X.; Hong, L.; Wang, Y. Dentin surface treatment using a non-thermal argon plasma brush for interfacial bonding improvement in composite restoration. *Eur. J. Oral Sci.* **2010**, *118*, 510–516. [CrossRef]
15. Chen, M.; Zhang, Y.; Sky Driver, M.; Caruso, A.N.; Yu, Q.; Wang, Y. Surface modification of several dental substrates by non-thermal, atmospheric plasma brush. *Dent. Mater.* **2013**, *29*, 871–880. [CrossRef] [PubMed]
16. Whittaker, A.G.; Graham, E.M.; Baxter, R.L.; Jones, A.C.; Richardson, P.R.; Meek, G.; Campbell, G.A.; Aitken, A.; Baxter, H.C. Plasma cleaning of dental instruments. *J. Hosp. Infect.* **2004**, *56*, 37–41. [CrossRef] [PubMed]
17. Nam, S.H.; Lee, H.W.; Cho, S.H.; Lee, J.K.; Jeon, Y.C.; Kim, G.C. High-efficiency tooth bleaching using non-thermal atmospheric pressure plasma with low concentration of hydrogen peroxide. *J. Appl. Oral Sci. Rev. FOB* **2013**, *21*, 265–270. [CrossRef]
18. Jungbauer, G.; Moser, D.; Müller, S.; Pfister, W.; Sculean, A.; Eick, S. The Antimicrobial Effect of Cold Atmospheric Plasma against Dental Pathogens-A Systematic Review of In-Vitro Studies. *Antibiotics* **2021**, *10*, 211. [CrossRef]
19. Lehmann, A.; Rueppell, A.; Schindler, A.; Zylla, I.-M.; Seifert, H.J.; Nothdurft, F.; Hannig, M.; Rupf, S. Modification of Enamel and Dentin Surfaces by Non-Thermal Atmospheric Plasma. *Plasma Process. Polym.* **2013**, *10*, 262–270. [CrossRef]
20. Moher, D.; Liberati, A.; Tetzlaff, J.; Altman, D.G. Preferred reporting items for systematic reviews and meta-analyses: The PRISMA statement. *J. Clin. Epidemiol.* **2009**, *62*, 1006–1012. [CrossRef]
21. Augusto, C.M.; Cunha Neto, M.A.; Pinto, K.P.; Barbosa, A.F.A.; Silva, E.; Dos Santos, A.P.P.; Sassone, L.M. Influence of the use of chelating agents as final irrigant on the push-out bond strength of epoxy resin-based root canal sealers: A systematic review. *Aust. Endod. J.* **2022**, *48*, 347–363. [CrossRef] [PubMed]
22. Prado, M.; Menezes, M.S.O.; Gomes, B.; Barbosa, C.A.M.; Athias, L.; Simão, R.A. Surface modification of gutta-percha cones by non-thermal plasma. *Mater. Sci. Eng. C Mater. Biol. Appl.* **2016**, *68*, 343–349. [CrossRef] [PubMed]
23. Yeter, K.Y.; Gunes, B.; Terlemez, A.; Seker, E. The effect of nonthermal plasma on the push-out bond strength of two different root canal sealers. *Niger. J. Clin. Pract.* **2020**, *23*, 811–816. [CrossRef]
24. Menezes, M.; Prado, M.; Gomes, B.; Gusman, H.; Simão, R. Effect of photodynamic therapy and non-thermal plasma on root canal filling: Analysis of adhesion and sealer penetration. *J. Appl. Oral Sci. Rev. FOB* **2017**, *25*, 396–403. [CrossRef]
25. Garlapati, R.; Chandra, K.M.; Gali, P.K.; Nagesh, B.; Vemuri, S.; Gomathi, N. Effect of nonthermal atmospheric plasma on the push-out bond strength of epoxy resin-based and bioceramic root canal sealers: An in vitro study. *J. Conserv. Dent. JCD* **2021**, *24*, 41–45. [CrossRef]
26. Brichko, J.; Burrow, M.F.; Parashos, P. Design Variability of the Push-out Bond Test in Endodontic Research: A Systematic Review. *J. Endod.* **2018**, *44*, 1237–1245. [CrossRef]
27. Silva, E.; Carvalho, N.K.; Prado, M.C.; Senna, P.M.; Souza, E.M.; De-Deus, G. Bovine teeth can reliably substitute human dentine in an intra-tooth push-out bond strength model? *Int. Endod. J.* **2019**, *52*, 1063–1069. [CrossRef]
28. Neelakantan, P.; Subbarao, C.; Subbarao, C.V.; De-Deus, G.; Zehnder, M. The impact of root dentine conditioning on sealing ability and push-out bond strength of an epoxy resin root canal sealer. *Int. Endod. J.* **2011**, *44*, 491–498. [CrossRef]
29. Ferreira, I.; Braga, A.C.; Pina-Vaz, I. Effect of Gutta-percha Solvents on the Bond Strength of Sealers to Intraradicular Dentin: A Systematic Review. *Iran. Endod. J.* **2021**, *16*, 17–25. [PubMed]
30. Prado, M.; de Assis, D.F.; Gomes, B.P.; Simão, R.A. Effect of disinfectant solutions on the surface free energy and wettability of filling material. *J. Endod.* **2011**, *37*, 980–982. [CrossRef] [PubMed]
31. Gade, V.J.; Belsare, L.D.; Patil, S.; Bhede, R.; Gade, J.R. Evaluation of push-out bond strength of endosequence BC sealer with lateral condensation and thermoplasticized technique: An in vitro study. *J. Conserv. Dent.* **2015**, *18*, 124–127. [CrossRef]
32. de Assis, D.F.; Prado, M.; Simão, R.A. Evaluation of the interaction between endodontic sealers and dentin treated with different irrigant solutions. *J. Endod.* **2011**, *37*, 1550–1552. [CrossRef]
33. Qian, W.; Shen, Y.; Haapasalo, M. Quantitative analysis of the effect of irrigant solution sequences on dentin erosion. *J. Endod.* **2011**, *37*, 1437–1441. [CrossRef]
34. Cha, S.; Park, Y.S. Plasma in dentistry. *Clin. Plasma Med.* **2014**, *2*, 4–10. [CrossRef]
35. Šimončicová, J.; Kryštofová, S.; Medvecká, V.; Ďurišová, K.; Kaliňáková, B. Technical applications of plasma treatments: Current state and perspectives. *Appl. Microbiol. Biotechnol.* **2019**, *103*, 5117–5129. [CrossRef] [PubMed]
36. Samanta, K.; Jassal, M.; Agrawal, A.K. Atmospheric pressure glow discharge plasma and its applications in textile. *Indian J. Fibre Text. Res.* **2006**, *31*, 83–98.
37. Kim, J.-H.; Lee, M.-A.; Han, G.-J.; Cho, B.-H. Plasma in dentistry: A review of basic concepts and applications in dentistry. *Acta Odontol. Scand.* **2014**, *72*, 1–12. [CrossRef] [PubMed]
38. Borges, A.C.; Kostov, K.G.; Pessoa, R.S.; de Abreu, G.M.A.; Lima, G.d.M.G.; Figueira, L.W.; Koga-Ito, C.Y. Applications of Cold Atmospheric Pressure Plasma in Dentistry. *Appl. Sci.* **2021**, *11*, 1975. [CrossRef]

39. Fu, Q.; Gabriel, M.; Schmidt, F.; Müller, W.D.; Schwitalla, A.D. The impact of different low-pressure plasma types on the physical, chemical and biological surface properties of PEEK. *Dent. Mater. Off. Publ. Acad. Dent. Mater.* **2021**, *37*, e15–e22. [CrossRef] [PubMed]
40. Abreu, J.L.B.d.; Prado, M.; Simão, R.A.; Silva, E.M.d.; Dias, K.R.H.C. Effect of non-thermal argon plasma on bond strength of a self-etch adhesive system to NaOCl-Treated Dentin. *Braz. Dent. J.* **2016**, *27*, 446–451. [CrossRef]
41. Sevilla, P.; Lopez-Suarez, C.; Pelaez, J.; Tobar, C.; Rodriguez-Alonso, V.; Suarez, M.J. Influence of low-pressure plasma on the surface properties of CAD-CAM leucite-reinforced feldspar and resin matrix ceramics. *Appl. Sci.* **2020**, *10*, 8856. [CrossRef]
42. Strazzi-Sahyon, H.B.; Suzuki, T.Y.U.; Lima, G.Q.; Delben, J.A.; Cadorin, B.M.; Nascimento, V.D.; Duarte, S.; Santos, P.H.D. In vitro study on how cold plasma affects dentin surface characteristics. *J. Mech. Behav. Biomed. Mater.* **2021**, *123*, 104762. [CrossRef] [PubMed]
43. Izdebska-Podsiadły, J. Study of Argon and Oxygen Mixtures in Low Temperature Plasma for Improving PLA Film Wettability. *Coatings* **2023**, *13*, 279. [CrossRef]

MDPI
St. Alban-Anlage 66
4052 Basel
Switzerland
www.mdpi.com

*Applied Sciences* Editorial Office
E-mail: applsci@mdpi.com
www.mdpi.com/journal/applsci

www.ingramcontent.com/pod-product-compliance
Lightning Source LLC
Chambersburg PA
CBHW061440210926
51850CB00008B/1564
*9783036597768*